Venous Catheters
A Practical Manual

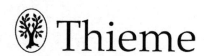

To

*Johannes H. P. Pieters and Ruth Ellen Pieters, who, through their love,
have made everything possible for me*

*Andrea Abbott Pieters, who, through her love,
has given me a wonderful life*

*Kelsea, Chloe, and Jackson Pieters, who, through their love,
make everything worthwhile and every day a pleasure*

—P. C. P.

*Samantha, Melissa, and Jamie for their continued
love, support, and encouragement,*

and Clarice for the same

—J. T.

my wife Pat, for her love and understanding,

and my children Lauren and David, for being two great kids

—M.A.M.

Venous Catheters
A Practical Manual

Edited by

Philip C. Pieters, M.D.

Radiology Associates of Richmond
Director
Interventional Radiology
Henrico Doctors Hospitals

Clinical Assistant Professor
Medical College of Virginia
Virginia Commonwealth University
Richmond, Virginia

Jaime Tisnado, M.D., F.A.C.R., F.A.C.C., F.S.I.R.

Professor
Departments of Radiology, Cardiovascular and
Interventional Radiology, and Surgery
Medical College of Virginia
Virginia Commonwealth University

Consultant Cardiovascular
and Interventional Radiologist
McGuire Veterans Administration
Medical Center
Richmond, Virginia

and

Matthew A. Mauro, M.D., F.A.C.R., F.S.I.R.

Professor
Departments of Radiology and Surgery
Vice-Chairman
Department of Radiology
University of North Carolina
School of Medicine
Chapel Hill, North Carolina

Thieme
New York • Stuttgart

Thieme Medical Publishers, Inc.
333 Seventh Ave.
New York, NY 10001

Editor: Felicity Edge
Editorial Assistant: Diane Sardini
Director, Production and Manufacturing: Anne Vinnicombe
Production Editor: Anita Kaufman
Marketing Director: Phyllis Gold
Sales Manager: Ross Lumpkin
Chief Financial Officer: Peter van Woerden
President: Brian D. Scanlan
Compositor: Alden Bookset
Printer: Edwards Brothers

Library of Congress Cataloging-in-Publication Data

Venous catheters : a practical manual / edited by Philip C. Pieters, Jaime Tisnado, and
Matthew A. Mauro.
　　　p. cm
　　　Includes bibliographical references and index.
　　　ISBN 0-86577-921-X (US : TNY : hardcover) – ISBN 3-13-124821-1 (Germany : GTV : hardcover)
　　　　　1. Intravenous catheterization–Handbooks, manuals, etc. 2.
Blood-vessels–Cutdown–Handbooks, manuals, etc. 3. Arteriovenous shunts,
Surgical–Handbooks, manuals, etc. I. Pieters, Philip C., 1958- II. Tisnado, Jaime., 1937- III.
Mauro, Matthew A., 1951-

　　　RD598.5. V465 2002
　　　607.4'14059–dc21

2002035976

Important note: Medical knowledge is ever-changing. As new research and clinical experience broaden our knowledge, changes in treatment and drug therapy may be required. The authors and editors of the material herein have consulted sources believed to be reliable in their efforts to provide information that is complete and in accord with the standards accepted at the time of publication. However, in view of the possibility of human error by the authors, editors, or publisher of the work herein, or changes in medical knowledge, neither the authors, editors, or publisher, nor any other party who has been involved in the preparation of this work, warrants that the information contained herein is in every respect accurate or complete, and they are not responsible for any errors or omissions or for the results obtained from use of such information. Readers are encouraged to confirm the information contained herein with other sources. For example, readers are advised to check the product information sheet included in the package of each drug they plan to administer to be certain that the information contained in this publication is accurate and that changes have not been made in the recommended dose or in the contraindications for administration. This recommendation is of particular importance in connection with new or infrequently used drugs.

　　Some of the product names, patents, and registered designs referred to in this book are in fact registered trademarks or proprietary names even though specific reference to this fact is not always made in the text. Therefore, the appearance of a name without designation as proprietary is not to be construed as a representation by the publisher that it is in the public domain.

Printed in the United States of America
54321

TNY ISBN 0-86577-921-X
GTV ISBN 3-13-124821-1

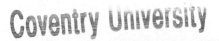

Contents

Preface

The number of patients requiring central venous access continues to grow by leaps and bounds. As the management of oncology, dialysis, trauma, and other patients improves, their life expectancy is prolonged. The result is a larger population of patients who are in critical need of reliable venous access. These catheters are often a virtual "life-line" for patients in a wide array of circumstances. It follows that the number of individuals with limited venous access is also increasing.

The ability of the vascular and interventional radiologists to obtain venous access and place catheters, often under circumstances where other specialists have been unable to achieve success, has allowed the radiologists to become important contributors to the management and care of patients. Furthermore, the ability to place catheters in the angiography suite, in a cost-effective and timely manner, has made radiologic placement of catheters even more desirable to both referring physicians and patients. Because of imaging expertise and because of the well-documented advantages of the radiologic placement of catheters, many diagnostic radiologists are now being requested to place venous catheters to meet the needs of patients. Therefore, this book is intended to be helpful not only to the vascular and interventional radiologists, but also diagnostic radiologists, radiology residents, and medical students, as well as other members of the vascular-access team. Other physicians and medical personnel who place venous catheters, or who have patients with venous catheters, can also benefit from this material.

This book emphasizes the complete care of patients and their catheters, not only catheter placement. Although critically important, catheter placement is only one step in the process of providing reliable venous access for patients. The venous access service _**must**_ provide consultation and expertise on all of the following:

- Familiarity with all catheter options available, including the advantages and disadvantages of the various devices
- Choosing the best catheter for each patient, considering the circumstances of each patient and the requirements of the catheter
- Evaluating venous patency and choosing the ideal site for venous access
- Proper preparation of the patients for the procedures
- Assuring sterility during catheter placement and maintenance
- Obtaining venous access and successfully placing the device
- Diagnosing and treating early and late complications associated with venous access devices
- Assuring proper care after placement
- Providing regular follow-up and consultation after placement
- Diagnosing and treating malfunctioning catheters
- Removal of catheters

Certainly, there is a lot to know! Although there is an abundance of literature available, the information is scattered, with no practical single source to learn from the "experts." As a result, many radiologists have learned this subject by trial and error.

This book will, hopefully, provide most of the information needed for the reader to become an "expert." **Helpful Hints** have been inserted by the editors and authors as "pearls" of wisdom from the experts.

The objectives of the book are to provide a comprehensive review of venous access and each of the steps mentioned above, so the readers may become experts; to furnish state-of-the-art care to patients; and supply a critical service to the medical community. The authors have worked diligently and happily to complete the material, which, we hope, is simple, succinct, practical, and useful to the readers.

Philip C. Pieters, M.D.
Jaime Tisnado, M.D.
Matthew A. Mauro, M.D.

Acknowledgments

Writing a book is not an easy task. Writing a good book is even more difficult. It takes a long time and considerable effort from inception until actual publication. The process may take years to be completed, and numerous individuals from different disciplines and occupations may be involved.

It is a great feeling for the authors when their work is completed and sent to the publisher. The authors usually have the privilege and satisfaction of acknowledging the work and cooperation of others. This would seem to be an easy task but in reality it is not. It would be too easy for the authors to say: "Thank you, to everyone who helped to make this book possible." But in doing so, people who should be recognized are not, and some people who should not be recognized may be.

Therefore, we must acknowledge and thank the people who truly made this book possible. To decide in what order people should be acknowledged is a particularly difficult task. Every author has some mixed feelings about this. Among the most important members of the "writing team" are the secretaries. Without them, we could not function properly or do the job right. They support us in all actions and purposes. We are very fortunate to have outstanding ladies such as Joanne Braat (secretary for PCP), Margie Smith (secretary for JT), and Wilma Melville (secretary for MAM). To these ladies we extend our heartfelt thanks for the thousands of hours spent in front of the keyboard typing and re-typing the manuscripts, looking at the references, obtaining information, contacting hundreds of individuals, and so on.

The authors would like to recognize the tireless labor of Laurie Persson for his outstanding diagrams and artwork. Carlos Chazo must be commended for his excellent photographic work.

We extend our gratitude to our teachers, for their enthusiasm in making sure we learned from the "masters," and to our residents and trainees who keep us "on our toes" with their questions and curiosity.

The work of an interventional radiologist is based on a team approach. This team includes IR technologists, IR nurses, angiographic equipment, and interventional radiologists. We would like to acknowledge the support of these people in the different institutions where we work.

We are grateful for the constant support and assistance of our editor, Felicity Edge, and our production editor, Anita Kaufman, as well as the entire staff at Thieme Medical Publishers, New York, including: Diane Castilaw, Diane Ersepke, Chris Gausby, Marie Mitarotondo, Diane Sardini, Anne Vinnicombe, and Diana Witt.

We also acknowledge the cooperation of our chairmen for providing an excellent environment for our academic activities.

We extend our most sincere thanks to our families for their love, patience, and understanding for the many hours away from them during the editing of this book.

Patients are one group of people not usually recognized. We appreciate the opportunity to provide care for them. We learn from their diseases and misfortunes; and we strive for excellence in their care. We thank the thousands of patients who provided us with material for this work.

We are very happy to present this book to you, the readers. We invite your comments and advice for future editions, as we are already thinking about and planning for the next edition... when the time comes.

Contributors

Siobhan A. Dumbleton, M.D.
Assistant Professor of Radiology
Duke University Medical Center
Durham, North Carolina

Preston S. Fox, M.D.
Vascular/Interventional Radiology
Blue Ridge Radiology
Kingsport, Tennessee

Jeffrey E. Hull, M.D.
Chief of Interventional Radiology
Chippenham Vascular Center
Richmond, Virginia

John A. Kaufman, M.D.
Professor of Interventional
    Radiology and Surgery
Dotter Institute
Oregon Health Sciences University
Portland, Oregon

Robert D. Lyon, M.D.
Department of Radiology
St. Mary's Hospital
Milwaukee, Wisconsin

Matthew A. Mauro, M.D., F.A.C.R., F.S.I.R.
Professor of Radiology and Surgery
Vice-Chairman, Department of Radiology
University of North Carolina School
    of Medicine
Chapel Hill, North Carolina

Allen J. Meglin, M.D.
Staff Radiologist
Delaney Radiologists
and
New Hanover Regional Medical Center
Wilmington, North Carolina

William J. Miller, M.S., M.D.
Mid-Ohio Heart Clinic
Mansfield, Ohio

Janice M. Newsome, M.D.
Department of Cardiovascular
    and Interventional Radiology
Inova Alexandria Hospital
Alexandria, Virginia

Philip C. Pieters, M.D.
Radiology Associates of Richmond
and
Director, Interventional Radiology
Henrico Doctors Hospitals
and
Clinical Assistant Professor
Medical College of Virginia
Virginia Commonwealth University
Richmond, Virginia

Uma R. Prasad, M.D.
Clinical Assistant Professor
Department of Radiology
Medical College of Virginia
Virginia Commonwealth University
Richmond, Virginia
and
Southside Regional Medical Center
Petersburg, Virginia

Melinda J. Pyle, R.T., R.C.V.
Cardiovascular Interventional Technologist
Department of Special Procedures
New England Medical Center
Boston, Massachusetts

Melvin Rosenblatt, M.D.
Department of Interventional Radiology
Memorial Sloan Kettering Cancer Center
New York, New York

**Jaime Tisnado, M.D., F.A.C.R.,
F.A.C.C., F.S.I.R.**
Professor of Radiology, Cardiovascular
and Interventional Radiology,
and Surgery
Medical College of Virginia
Virginia Commonwealth University
and
Consultant Cardiovascular
and Interventional Radiologist
McGuire Veterans Administration
Medical Center
Richmond, Virginia

Kurt H. Wetzler, M.D.
Clinical Assistant Professor of Radiology
Brody School of Medicine
East Carolina University
and
Pitt County Memorial Hospital
and
Eastern Radiologists
Greenville, North Carolina

Chapter 1

Establishing (and Maintaining) a Venous Access Service

Philip C. Pieters
William J. Miller

A more appropriate title of this chapter might have been *Maintaining (and Establishing) a Venous Access Service*. Obviously, this appears backwards: One must have a catheter service before one can maintain it, but the implication is that one must make a major commitment to provide the necessary services before attempts are made at starting a venous access service. The establishment of a successful venous access service resembles the establishment of a surgical practice more than it does that of a radiology practice. A catheter service is not simply a venous access placement service (hence we chose not to title this book *Placement of Venous Catheters: A Practical Manual*). The key term is *service*. Service must be provided before, during, and after placement of catheters. The service requires expertise, especially for such a critical procedure that is so important for the long-term care of the patient. Therefore, the experts should perform these procedures. Whoever plans to perform them must have the desire and commitment to become an expert. This is not to say that one must place catheters and care for these patients all the time as a full-time job. The commitment must be made to learn as much as possible about the subject, however, and then one must be ready to be involved at all times and in all facets — before, during, and after the procedure.

To establish a good catheter service, one must provide the following:

- Expert consultation
- Clinical responsibility
- Technical proficiency
- Consistency of service

We know from personal experience the difficulties of acquiring this expertise. Information on these subjects either is scattered in numerous articles or absent. A great deal must be learned by trial and error. Nonetheless, this book will allow the reader to benefit from the experience of persons who have had active, successful services. We have attempted to explain and provide expert advice for every step of this process: consultation, placement, care of the catheter, and its removal. We hope this book will assist the reader in becoming the catheter expert.

THE EXPERT CONSULTANT

Because of the wealth of information and therapeutic options and the focused training of specialists, it now has become imperative for physicians to rely on the expertise of others. Referring physicians must place the responsibility for their patients having a functioning, well-maintained venous catheter on members of the vascular access service, either surgeons or interventional radiologists, who must be the "expert," not merely a technician who places a catheter whenever requested. The referring physicians are not aware of the different catheter options and need advice about the best option for a given patient. Therefore, the catheter expert must be familiar with the various options, their properties, flow rates, indications for use, cost, and so on. It is essential that the catheter expert not become trapped in a routine of placing the same catheters in all patients simply because of familiarity with a particular catheter. It is a disservice if the optimal catheter is not placed in a particular circumstance warranting its use. Catheter placement procedures are very important to patients; therefore, placement must be done correctly the first time it is attempted. Close communication with the referring physician is critical, both before and after procedures. Numerous questions must be answered before deciding on the best catheter and the best approach for a particular patient: What is the patient's history? Why is a catheter needed? What will it be used for? How long will it be needed? Has the patient had other procedures that might influence the choice of venous access sites (e.g., a mastectomy and axillary lymph node dissection)? Has the patient had central catheters in the past? If so, were any problems associated with the previous catheter? Only after acquiring this information from the patient, along with the patient's medical records (if available), and discussing the case with the referring physician, can the decision be made about which catheter to place and where and how to place it.

CLINICAL RESPONSIBILITY

The referring physician sends the patient to the venous access service because of the expertise this service offers and does not expect to be contacted to make decisions concerning the catheters. Obviously, if a complication occurs or if the plans change (e.g., there are venous occlusions and an alternative route of access must be used), the referring physician must be kept informed.

The purpose of these calls is to inform the physician of the game plan, not to consult about what should be done. If a complication occurs or if a patient requires prolonged observation after the procedure, the venous access service should offer to admit the patient to the service. If a case is especially complex (because of multiorgan failure) and the radiologist is not comfortable with assuming responsibility for the general care of the patient, the patient can be admitted to the venous access service, with the referring physician assuming the complex medical care as a consultant. Alternatively, referring physicians can admit patients to their service. In either case, the venous access service must closely monitor all aspects of catheter care. It is not acceptable for the service to insert catheters and then expect the referring physician to do the rest. Furthermore, the referring physician usually prefers not to fill this role. The catheter service must stand by, ready to provide emergency coverage for any catheter problems, such as infection, hematoma, vein thrombosis, hemorrhage, and to remove the catheter when necessary.

Inpatients who have had a venous catheter placed should be followed up regularly by the venous access service while in the hospital, and a brief progress note should be written daily (at least for the first week after placement). The admitting service greatly appreciates these efforts. These visits should monitor for complications, check wound healing, and ensure that the catheter is maintained in a secure position and functioning adequately. All aspects of catheter care must be done by the catheter service (e.g., orders for flushing, dressing changes). It is important for the catheter service to talk with the nurses and inquire about catheter function and any problems. As soon as problems arise, suggestions must be made to handle them. The catheter service must be the experts on dealing with complications and must be available at all times. Patients who are in the hospital for an extended time need not be seen every day but can be seen once or twice a week after the first week or so if the catheter is working well. A general rule is that a note always must be written on the chart. If a patient is seen three times a day, then three notes should be written. The referring physicians must know that the service was concerned enough to follow up often with the patient.

After the patient's discharge, the service must try to maintain contact with the patient, for example, by asking the patient to stop in for a brief office visit whenever he or she is in the facility for visits to the referring physician or for other therapies. These visits need last only a few minutes—to ask the patient whether the catheter is working well and to check the skin site. Suture removal also can be done at the appropriate time; otherwise, the referring physician can be asked to contact the catheter service if any problems arise with a catheter in any patient. If the referring physician's office is nearby, a member of the catheter service might go there while the patient is in the office. A good way to maintain contact with patients is to give the patient a business card when the catheter is placed. The patient should be given instructions on how to contact a member of the venous access service 24 hours a day. In this case, one must expect to receive and answer direct phone calls from patients with questions and concerns. The main objective should be close follow-up of patients and to be aware of complications or problems as soon as they develop. This is the only way to perform adequate quality control. By no means should the referring physician consult a second service to deal with problems arising from a catheter placed by the initial service. Likewise, the catheter service should not be consulted to deal with problems with catheters placed by other services. If this does occur, the catheter service should contact the initial service to inform them of the problems.

TECHNICAL PROFICIENCY

Obtaining the technical skills to place venous catheters is the easiest aspect of initiating a vascular access service. Litera-

ture about the techniques and methods of catheter placement abounds. Every effort must be made to learn these techniques fully. Difficulties arise when procedures do not go as planned. Solutions to many problems must be learned as one goes along because individual situations can be unique, and it is impossible to anticipate (and report) every possible scenario. We attempt to include most of the commonly encountered situations and how to resolve them. Special circumstances may not be dealt with in the literature, and the catheter service physician's problem-solving abilities and creativity can make all the difference. To maintain the highest level of expertise, continuing education of the entire team, including radiologists, technologists, physician's assistants, and nurses, is essential. Attendance and active participation at society meetings, "angio club" meetings, refresher courses, and tutorials are important and ongoing. New information is always appearing that may benefit physicians and their patients. It is also important to maintain communications with colleagues, both within one's specialty and in other specialties. Frequent discussions on subjects such as "What would you do in this circumstance?" are important sources of information.

CONSISTENCY OF SERVICE

First-class service must be provided 24 hours a day, 365 days a year. This is usually not a problem in large medical centers with several well-trained persons on staff; however, smaller practices may find it difficult to provide such around-the-clock service. Smaller groups typically have a single person who is trained to place and care for central venous catheters. Obviously, that single person cannot be available at all times to provide the necessary service. The following are suggestions on how smaller groups can provide consistently good catheter service.

- Most evening calls can be delayed until the next morning, when the catheter service physician is available. If a catheter suddenly stops working and a treatment must be given, an intravenous catheter can be started and the treatment given.

- Situations that are deemed urgent by a referring physician necessitate a call to the catheter service physician. Frequently, these problems can be handled over the phone or at least stabilized adequately until the next day.
- Educating emergency room physicians in the basics of venous catheter care can help to eliminate some calls.
- When the vascular access service physician is off or away from work, patients must be scheduled accordingly, with no elective procedures scheduled on that day. If an emergency procedure arises and there is no adequate backup within the group, the patient should be referred to another hospital or another service in the same hospital. Arrangements for another service (whether it be surgical or radiologic coverage) to provide backup for urgent procedures should be made in advance. The covering service must be one that can be trusted to provide excellent service.
- Many questions can be answered by other members of the team, provided they are well educated in catheter care. If another physician in one's group is interested in helping with the catheter service, this could be an answer to the problem; however, if this person has no formal training in the field, it is imperative that this person obtain the necessary training. This can be done by attending tutorials, conferences, and such; but, most importantly, the catheter expert must work with this person as much as possible.

MARKETING YOUR SERVICE

Once the previously discussed commitments have been made, one must change the referral pattern so that patients are referred to your service rather than to others for catheter placement and care. This can be difficult because traditionally surgeons have done catheter placement. It is not unusual for a physician to exclaim that "radiologists are placing tunneled catheters!" The key is for the catheter service to get a "foot in the door" and do such a good job that word spreads and the service builds. This is why commitment to service is so important, as has been discussed so thoroughly. If a service is to compete with another service for referring physicians' patients, it must achieve results at least as good as the other services—or better. The advantages of lower costs and more timely services will help also. Because results depend on the skills, commitments, and personality of the catheter service physicians, the objectives and solutions may vary with specific practice environments, but the following suggestions may be helpful in getting started.

Relationships with Patients

One of the most important steps in building a practice is to establish strong relationships with patients, who then will provide positive feedback to the referring physician and to other patients. Patients frequently are gathered into small communities, such as dialysis units or oncology clinics, and tend to talk among themselves and compare notes. It is desirable to have patients relate positive experiences to other patients. Word will spread, and patients will request the service.

Catheter Checks

Doing catheter checks on malfunctioning catheters placed by other services is a perfect opportunity to inform the referring physician that your service places catheters and the complication rate is much lower. For instance, a frequent complication is vein thrombosis caused by inadequate position of the catheter (i.e., the catheter tip in the subclavian or brachiocephalic vein causing thrombosis when sclerosing fluids are infused). The referring physician should know that a catheter placed under image guidance would never be left in an inadequate position.

Handling Patients with Limited Access

Challenge physicians to send their most difficult patients to the venous access service. Most early opportunities to place venous catheters in a service come from patients with limited venous access, that is, patients for whom other services have tried numerous times to obtain venous access but were unsuccessful. The referring physician and patients will be appreciative if access is obtained easily under ultrasound guidance. When the referring physician asks why access was obtained so easily, we take the opportunity to tell them that we are experts in image-guided techniques that allow virtual 100% success. This not only makes it easier to obtain access but also is easier on the patient because numerous punctures are not required to obtain venous access. The referring physician should realize that this is a desirable commodity not only for patients with difficult venous access but in any patient receiving a central venous catheter.

Timely Service

One of the major advantages of placement of catheters by radiologists is that an operating room does not have to be reserved. In most institutions, operating room time is competitive and difficult to obtain. Low-priority procedures, such as elective catheter placement, can be especially difficult or impossible to schedule and may be "bumped" for "more important" emergent procedures. Radiology has the ability to, and must, provide more timely service. We must inform the referring physicians that these procedures are a high priority to our service. Same-day or next-day service must be provided, depending on clinical circumstances. This timely service is important to referring physicians and patients and will help build the service. The service must expand and grow as the number of patients increases; otherwise, scheduling will become difficult.

Dissemination to Medical Staff

As pointed out by Katzen and Van Breda,[1] "the interventionalists cannot rely on radiological articles in clinical journals to keep their clinical colleagues aware of advances in interventional radiology." One must spread the word to everyone about the advantages of catheter placement by the venous access service. The following are suggestions to market your practice:

- Provide presentations to subspecialty groups at hospital conferences.
- Invite experts on the subject who are good spokesmen to the specialty conferences in your hospital.
- Write to referring physicians emphasizing the benefits of catheter placement in radiology and make sure they understand that you are offering this service. Samples of a letter (Fig. 1–1) and a reply card (Fig. 1–2) by Borton Scientific Education Center are provided.
- Often it is adequate to convince only one referring physician to get started. You may wish to make a pact with this physician that you will provide extraordinary services if the physician will give you the opportunity to care for his patients as the primary catheter service. Having achieved this, do an outstanding job. Eventually, word will spread, and your practice will blossom.

Dear _____:

Please find enclosed articles regarding placement of long-term central venous access catheters and ports. These articles demonstrate the growing number of options open to your patients who require these devices.

As I am sure you are aware, the indications for placement of central venous catheters have expanded considerably in recent years. An important aspect of this procedure is the need for outpatient rather than inpatient treatment of these conditions. This requires devices that are relatively free of thrombosis and infection during their long-term use.

For years, interventional radiologists have helped these patients by defining venous anatomy for difficult cases, re-opening occluded catheters, relocating malpositioned tips, and retrieving catheter fragments. Recent publications have suggested that radiologists should be involved in the initial placement of these devices. This can be accomplished without an increase in catheter-related infections or placement complications.

Currently, at many institutions, radiologists are involved in device selection, placement, management, and removal of devices. The radiology service has the ability to benefit the referring physician by providing prompt and responsive service, and benefits the patient with successful placement at lower cost. The hospital benefits as well by reducing procedure-related costs while maintaining the same reimbursement rate. The enclosed articles, which document this information, are for your review.

Please feel free to call me to discuss this information further or allow me to answer any of your questions.

Sincerely,

Figure 1–1 Sample letter to referring physicians.

Please complete and mail this card to obtain more information on radiologically

placed central venous access catheters.

Name _____

Address _____

Phone _____

Medical Specialty _____

I am interested in referring patients to Radiology for placement of:

_____Subcutaneous Ports

_____PICC Lines

_____Tunneled, External Access Catheters

_____Dialysis Catheters

Figure 1–2   Example of reply card.

SUMMARY

Placement of venous catheters should be left to the "expert." When starting a venous access service, we must ensure that we have the expertise in all aspects of catheter care, not just catheter placement. Having made this commitment, the task of initiating a venous access service can be undertaken. One way to start is to perform procedures on patients with difficult access and to make every effort to educate all potential referring physicians about the advantages of radiologic placement of venous catheters, including more accurate placement of catheters, timely service, and lower costs.[2] After winning the trust of referring physicians, it is critical that the venous catheter service uphold this commitment to excellence.

REFERENCES

1. Katzen BT, van Breda A. Developing an interventional radiology practice. *Semin Interv Radiol.* 1988;5:99–102.
2. Foley MJ. Radiologic placement of long-term central venous peripheral access system ports (PASPort): results in 150 patients. *J Vasc Interv Radiol.* 1995;6:255–262.

Chapter 2

Vascular Anatomy of the Central and Peripheral Veins

Uma R. Prasad
Jaime Tisnado
Philip C. Pieters

Central venous catheter placement is a significant and growing proportion of the interventional radiologist's workload. The use of long-term vascular access devices has increased dramatically over the last decade. Central catheters are needed for infusion of fluids and other agents, such as chemotherapeutic agents, total parenteral nutrition (TPN), and antibiotics, as well as for hemodialysis and pheresis and many other less common uses.

One important aspect for the successful and safe placement of central catheters is a knowledge of the normal anatomy of the central and other veins and their variants. A brief description of the embryologic development of the central and peripheral veins is helpful to understanding the venous anatomy because anomalies of the veins are rather common. Anatomic variants of venous drainage occur because of abnormalities in formation or regression of the primitive venous system during the embryonal development. Some veins that should regress, persist, and the converse is also true.

In general, the veins preferred for placement of central and peripheral venous access catheters are the internal jugular veins in the neck, the axillary and subclavian veins in the chest, the cephalic and basilic veins in the upper extremities, and the superficial femoral and common femoral veins in the lower extremities. When all these veins are depleted for catheterization, the inferior vena cava (IVC) can be accessed by direct translumbar or transhepatic puncture. Furthermore, other veins, such as the azygous, hemiazygous, or collateral venous channels, can be used if other accesses are no longer available.

VENOUS ANATOMY OF THE UPPER EXTREMITY

The veins of the upper extremity are organized into superficial and deep systems. The superficial system consists of the basilic vein medially and the cephalic vein laterally.

The basilic vein is the larger of these, and it courses along the medial aspect of the forearm and arm. It is formed by the junction of the common ulnar and median basilic veins. The basilic vein becomes the axillary vein at the level of the inferior border of the teres major muscle. The axillary vein courses through the axilla and becomes the subclavian vein, which joins the internal jugular vein and becomes the innominate or brachiocephalic vein. The right and left innominate veins join together in the chest and form the superior vena cava (SVC).[1–3]

The cephalic vein courses along the lateral aspect of the arm, superficial to the biceps muscle, before crossing medially between the pectoralis major and deltoid muscles to join the axillary vein. The cephalic vein is smaller than the basilic vein and turns at an acute angle just before entering the axillary vein, making catheterization of this vein more difficult. Therefore, the cephalic vein is not the first choice for placement of peripherally inserted central catheters (PICCs). When the basilic vein is not available or is occluded, the cephalic vein can be used (Figs. 2–1 and 2–2).[1-3]

The deep veins of the upper extremity course parallel to the arteries and consist of paired radial, ulnar, and interosseous veins in the forearm and brachial veins in the arm. The brachial veins join the axillary vein in the axilla. The brachial veins are the only deep veins in the arm that are large enough for central access. Their deep location and proximity to the brachial artery, however, make them less than ideal for venous access, but they can be used whenever the superficial veins are not available.

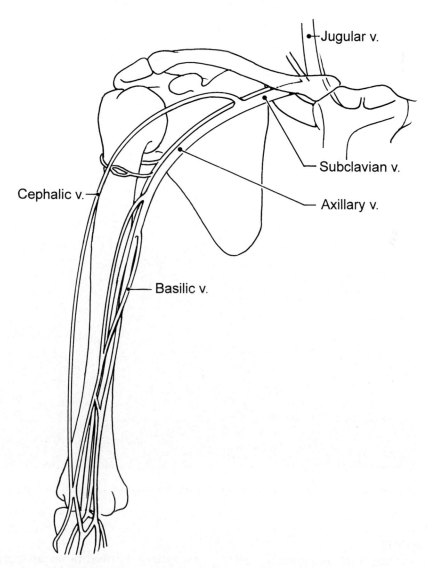

Figure 2–1 Diagram of the veins of the upper extremity. The basilic and cephalic veins and the confluence are noted.

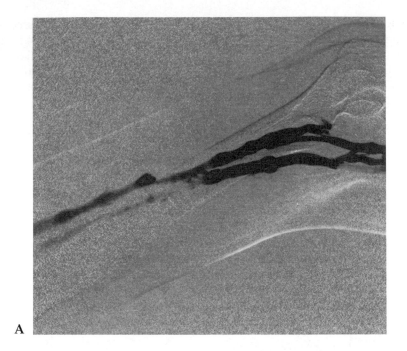

A

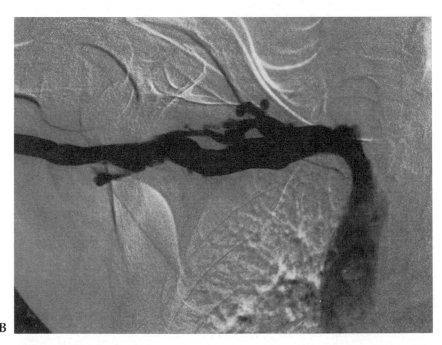

B

Figure 2–2 (A) Basilic vein in the arm. **(B)** Right axillary, subclavian, and brachiocephalic veins and superior vena cava.

HELPFUL HINTS

Variations of the venous anatomy are common. In fact, variability of size and number of veins is the rule rather than the exception. Furthermore, anatomic differences between right and left sides are common and expected, indeed.

VENOUS ANATOMY OF THE NECK

The internal jugular veins (IJVs) are continuations of the sigmoid sinuses, which drain the major intracranial sinuses. The IJVs usually are discrepant in size, with the right one often larger in diameter than the left one. The IJVs course downward and laterally in the neck, from the jugular foramen at the base of the skull to the base of the neck to join the subclavian veins in the thorax to form the brachiocephalic or innominate veins. The IJVs receive several tributaries, such as the facial, lingual, thyroidal, and other veins. The IJVs are located posterolateral to the internal carotid arteries just below the base of the skull; however, as they course downward toward the chest, the IJVs are located anterolateral to the artery. Usually, there is a valve at its junction with the subclavian vein (Fig. 2–3).[4]

As mentioned in other chapters, ultrasound guidance is preferred for access of the IJV; however, if ultrasound is not available, a "blind" puncture can be made. There are several ways to puncture the IJV, depending on the relationship of the vein to the sternocleidomastoid muscles.

- The *anterior approach* includes palpating the carotid artery and puncturing the vein just lateral to the carotid artery. The puncture traverses the belly of the sternocleidomastoid muscle.
- The *middle approach* is made at the apex of the triangle formed by the anterior and posterior bellies of the sternocleidomastoid and the clavicle. The needle is directed toward the ipsilateral nipple.
- The *posterior approach* is done posterior to the posterior belly of the sternoclei-

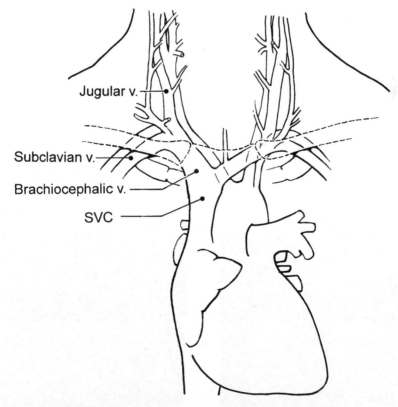

Figure 2–3 Diagram of the veins of the neck and chest. The internal jugular veins are seen joining the subclavian veins to form the brachiocephalic or innominate veins. The superior vena cava (SVC) is formed by the confluence of the brachiocephalic or innominate veins.

domastoid, in the lower neck, and the needle is directed toward the sternal notch (Fig. 2–4).

The external jugular veins (EJVs) are paired veins that drain the facial structures. They traverse the neck diagonally from posterosuperiorly to anteroinferiorly to join the proximal subclavian veins. The EJVs cross superficial to the sternocleidomastoid at the level of the bifurcation of the muscle and descend lateral to the clavicular belly of the muscle to join the subclavian veins. The EJVs can be used for relatively short-term access, but they are not used for the placement of tunneled catheters because of their small diameter and tortuous course. If the IJVs are occluded, however, the EJVs often become enlarged and can be used for long-term catheter placement.

VENOUS ANATOMY OF THE CHEST

As already described, the axillary veins are the continuation of the basilic, cephalic, and brachial veins. The medial wall of the axillary vein directly overlies the visceral pleura and lung and partially overlays the axillary artery, and it is adjacent to the medial cord of the brachial plexus. Therefore, injuries to the neural structures and the axillary artery can occur during axillary vein punctures.

The axillary vein becomes the subclavian vein at the level of the inferolateral margin of the first rib and courses medially to join the IJV to form the brachiocephalic or innominate vein. The subclavian vein courses inferiorly and ventrally to the subclavian artery, between the costoclavicular ligament and the subclavius muscle anteriorly and the anterior scalenus muscle posteriorly. Therefore, during insertion of catheters in the subclavian vein, care must be taken to ensure that a lateral rather than a medial puncture is made (laterally to the junction of the first rib and clavicle) because if the catheter is medial to or through the costoclavicular ligament, kinking or the "pinch-off" syndrome can occur.[5] The lateral approach can be done under venographic "road mapping" fluoroscopy lateral to the second or third rib. Puncturing the vein under ultrasound guidance prevents pneumothorax or inadvertent puncture of the artery.

The brachiocephalic veins (BCVs) are formed by the confluence of the subclavian and IJVs at the level of the clavicular head. The right BCV is short, coursing 2 cm before joining the left one to form the SVC. The left BCV lies ventral to the brachiocephalic arteries as they originate from the arch of the aorta. Several tributary veins drain into

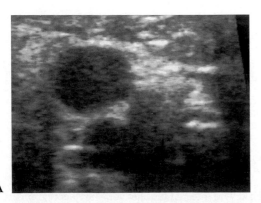 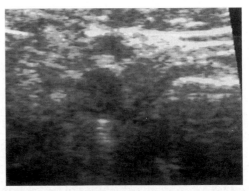

A **B**

Figure 2–4 Ultrasound guidance of the neck in transverse plane shows the right internal jugular veins without **(A)** and with **(B)** compression.

the BCVs, including the cervical, vertebral, and inferior thyroid veins superiorly and the first intercostal, supreme intercostal, and internal mammary veins and thymic vein (the vein of Keynes) inferiorly.

The SVC is formed by the junction of the BCVs at the level of the lower margin of the first costal cartilage. It measures about 6 to 8 cm in length and has no valves. The SVC enters the right atrium (RA) at the level of the third intercostal cartilage. The lower (cardiac) half of the SVC is covered by pericardium, whereas the upper half, the cephalad, is not.

The major tributaries of the SVC are the azygous arch and small pericardial and mediastinal veins.

An important central vein described here is the azygous system, which represents a separate and major drainage system of the posterior abdominal wall and thoracic walls. The azygous vein is to the right of the thoracic spine, and the hemiazygous and accessory hemiazygous veins are to the left of the thoracic spine. All join to form the azygous arch, which drains anteriorly into the posterior wall of the SVC.

The major tributaries to the azygous arch are the hemiazygous and accessory hemiazygous veins, the right superior intercostal, right posterior 5th to 11th intercostal, esophageal, mediastinal, pericardial, and right bronchial veins. The azygous system is very important because, when the central venous access sites are depleted, it can be used for central venous access (Fig. 2–5).

The most common anomaly of the central veins in the chest is the presence of a duplicated SVC, one on either side of the chest. This anomaly results from failure of the left BCV to form and a persistence of the left anterior cardinal vein. The left SVC usually drains into the coronary sinus, the right one into the RA. A duplicated SVC occurs in about 0.3% of the population and in 4.3% of people with congenital heart disease. Another uncommon anomaly is a left SVC, which occurs if

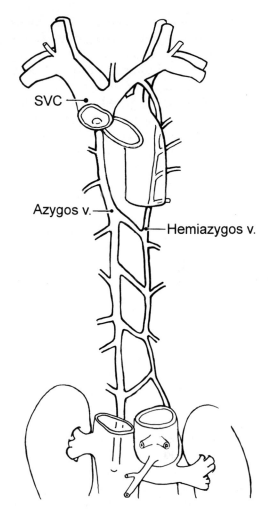

Figure 2–5 Diagram of the azygous venous system. The azygous and hemiazygous veins are shown.

the right anterior cardinal vein, the predecessor of the right SVC, regresses. The right side drainage is to the left BCV, the left SVC, and finally to the RA via the coronary sinus. A left SVC is present in about 0.3% of people.[3]

VENOUS ANATOMY OF THE ABDOMEN AND PELVIS

The lower-extremity veins and the pelvic and abdominal veins are not primary choices for venous access for long-term catheter placement; however, these veins can be alternative routes when other access sites are no longer available.

The IVC is formed at the level of L-5 by the confluence of the common iliac veins, and it drains the lower half of the human body. The IVC is a retroperitoneal vessel located to the right of the lumbar spine. The upper IVC is located in a groove on the posterior surface of the caudate lobe of the liver, and it passes through the tendinous portion of the diaphragm to enter the RA. The major tributaries of the IVC are hepatic, renal, adrenal, gonadal, inferior phrenic, and ascending lumbar veins.

Embryologically, the IVC develops from paired posterior cardinal, subcardinal, and supracardinal veins by a combination of regression, replacement, anastomoses, and alteration of directional flow. The supra-hepatic IVC is originated from the right vitelline vein. The intrahepatic IVC originates from the upper right subcardinal veins. The infrarenal portion of the IVC is formed by the subcardinal anastomoses. The renal IVC is formed by the subcardinal and supracardinal anastomoses. The suprarenal portion of the IVC is formed by the lower right supracardinal anastomoses. The posterior cardinal veins persist in part as the iliac veins. The common femoral veins are formed by the junction of the deep and superficial femoral veins at the level of the inguinal ligament and become the external iliac veins. The external iliac veins are joined by the internal iliac veins to form the common iliac veins, which drain the pelvic viscera and musculature and join to form the IVC as described.

An important anomaly of the embryologic development of the IVC is the presence of a double IVC due to persistence of both supracardinal veins. It occurs in about 2% of people. A left IVC is due to persistence of the lower left supracardinal vein rather than the right one. It is present in about 0.5% of people. It usually drains into the left renal vein.[6]

VENOUS ANATOMY OF THE LOWER EXTREMITY

The deep veins of the legs are three paired veins coursing parallel to the corresponding arteries: the anterior tibial, posterior tibial, and peroneal. The deep veins of the calf join together at the level of the proximal calf or knee to form the popliteal vein, which traverses the popliteal fossa posterolaterally to the popliteal artery. There are many anatomic variations of the popliteal vein. The popliteal vein is duplicated (*bifid*) in about 25% of people. Sometimes it is trifid or more.

The superficial femoral veins (SFVs) are the continuation of the popliteal veins at the level of the adductor hiatus. They course deep in the thigh to the groin and continue into the pelvis as the common femoral veins (CFVs). These veins are bifid in about 25% of people. Rarely, trifid SFVs can be found.

The CFV lies medially to the common femoral artery, allowing easy and safe access to this vessel without danger of arterial injury. The SFVs and deep femoral veins lie deep to the corresponding arteries (Fig. 2–6).

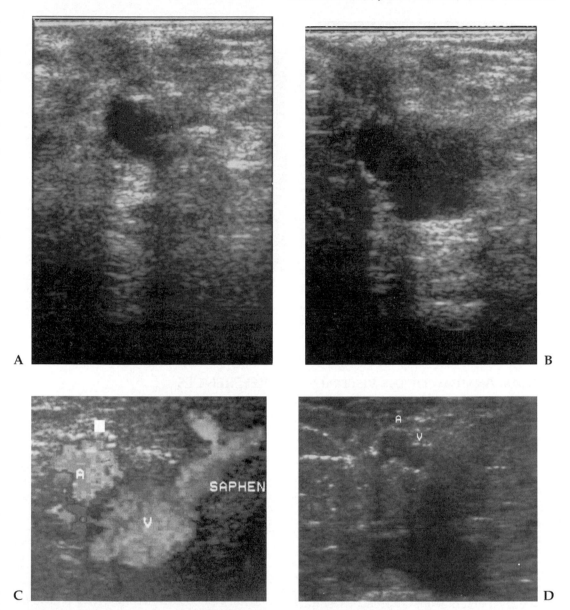

Figure 2–6 Ultrasound guidance of the common femoral region with compression **(A)** and without compression **(B)**. The vein is patent and compressible. **(C)** Doppler ultrasound of the groin to show the saphenous vein joining the common femoral vein. **(D)** Ultrasound through the thigh to show the deep location of the superficial femoral vein and artery.

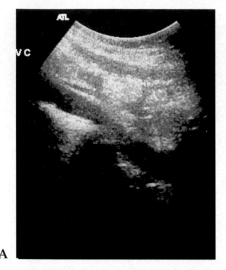
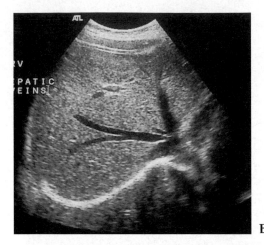

A   B

Figure 2–7 **(A)** Sagittal view of the inferior vena cava (IVC) during translumbar puncture with ultrasound guidance. **(B)** The confluence of the hepatic veins into the IVC is demonstrated during percutaneous approach for placement of a catheter in the right atrium.

VENOUS ANATOMY OF THE VISCERAL VEINS

The visceral veins include the renal veins, gonadal, adrenal, inferior phrenic, and hepatic veins, among others. The hepatic veins are important to our discussion because they can be used for central venous access when all available veins are depleted. There are usually three intrahepatic veins—right, left, and middle—joining the IVC separately or in a common trunk and draining into the intrahepatic IVC (Fig. 2–7).[3,7] These veins can be punctured under ultrasound guidance by percutaneous approach. Central catheters thus can be inserted in the RA.

SUMMARY

A basic knowledge of the venous anatomy and its common anatomical variations is important for the safe and successful placement of central catheters, PICCs, and ports.

REFERENCES

1. Ray CE, Kaufman JA. Venous anatomy for central venous access. *Semin Interv Radiol.* 1998;1:239–248.
2. Kadir S. *Diagnostic Angiography.* Philadelphia, PA: WB Saunders; 1986:541.
3. Kadir S. *Atlas of Normal and Variant Angiographic Anatomy.* Philadelphia, PA: WB Saunders; 1991:Chapters 6–9.
4. Trerotola SO, Johnson MS, Harris VJ, et al. Outcome of tunneled hemodialysis catheters placed via the right internal jugular vein by interventional radiologists. *Radiology.* 1997; 203:489–495.
5. Hinke DH, Zandt-Stastny DA, Goodman LR, et al. Pinch off syndrome: a complication of implantable subclavian venous access devices. *Radiology.* 1990;177:353–356.
6. Kidney DD, Deutsch L. Misplaced central venous catheters; venous anatomy, clinical significance, and treatment options. *Radiologist.* 1998;5:119–126.
7. Hollinshead WH. *Text of Anatomy.* 3rd ed. New York, NY: Harper & Row; 1974:75.

Chapter 3

Techniques of Venous Catheter Placement

Philip C. Pieters
Kurt Wetzler

A detailed description of the techniques involved in the placement of central venous catheters is not possible because the techniques vary widely, depending on personal preference. No two radiologists or surgeons place catheters in the same manner, step for step; however, some basic steps are invariable, including the following:

1. Preparation of the procedure room
2. Preparation of the physician
3. Preparation of the patient
4. Venous puncture and placement of the peel-away sheath
5. Creation of the subcutaneous tunnel/pocket
6. Placement of the catheter
7. Securing the catheter and closing the wound(s)

Each basic step is discussed in detail. The techniques presented are not the only "correct" techniques, but they have been successful over many years. They may stimulate discussion with the hope that the reader may develop new methods or improve the current methods that he or she employs. Techniques are constantly evolving as new information is obtained. The goal in this chapter is to present as much information about the techniques as possible so that readers can decide which methods work best for them.

PREPARING THE PROCEDURE ROOM

Procedure Room Environment

Patients are typically anxious about these procedures; therefore, the procedure room should have a warm and comfortable feel to it. Patterns on the walls will help to minimize the sterile feel of white walls. Music should be soothing to help the patient relax; however, if the patient has a strong preference for music that cannot be classified as "soothing," playing the music of the patient's choice may divert the patient's attention from the procedure and allow him or her to relax. The ceiling needs to be high enough to accommodate overhead lighting. The floor should be hard and seamless to facilitate cleaning.

The doors to the procedure room should be closed throughout the procedure. A sign should be placed on each door warning "Sterile procedure is under way: Do not enter," or something to that effect, to prevent mistaken entry into the room. Unnecessary traffic into and out of the room should be avoided. Procedure rooms typically are equipped with a high-efficiency particulate air (HEPA) filtered-air circulatory system under positive pressure with 17 to 20 air changes per hour. The air in the procedure room has a positive pressure with respect to the air in the hallways so that unfiltered air does not enter the procedure room. Air-handling systems with filtration can reduce the number of airborne microbes by reducing the number of particles to which microbes may be attached. Appropriate design of cabinetry and placement of storage space can reduce the number of times the door to the procedure room is opened during a procedure. The number of door openings, and therefore the bioparticle count, can be reduced significantly by appropriate design of the storage space.

To control the microbiology of the environment, it is important to check that surfaces are smooth, dry, and intact before use and to ensure that spillage of human secretions and excretions are cleaned promptly because these are likely to be contaminated with human pathogens. Used solutions and wet equipment are likely to encourage the growth of gram-negative bacilli and should be removed from the rooms as soon as possible. The apparent level of cleanliness is important to patient confidence. Some patients make negative comments about hospitals they consider dirty and associate this with poor care. Items not in use must be stored.

Rituals

Rituals abound in the operating room and in interventional radiology procedure rooms because the high-intensity, life-threatening situations in these areas requires control and discipline. Rigid adherence to rules that are translated into "policies and procedures" sets limits on behavior and assists in labeling actions as "correct" or "wrong."[1,2] Condon and Quebbeman[3] state that although the efficacy of many rituals has not been established, the procedures protect the patient from environmental sources of infection and are worth following for reasons of improved and disciplined behavior of the procedure room personnel.

The following procedure room rituals as listed by Gruendemann[2] may create order, consistency, cleanliness, and sterility:

- Personnel must remain in the sterile area throughout the procedure.

- Personnel who are not scrubbed must remain on the periphery of the procedure room, a distance away from sterile areas.
- A margin of safety is useful as a guide to movement and adherence to aseptic principles.
- Sterile fluids, equipment, or supplies are opened and delivered to the sterile surface without contacting the edges of the wrapper or container; only sterile articles may touch sterile surfaces.
- Tables are sterile only at and above the tabletop level.
- When a staff member is not sterile he or she must not lean or reach over a sterile field.
- Sterile drapes, towels, and covers are folded in such a way that a generous cuff is provided for handling by personnel in sterile areas.
- Once in position, sterile drapes are never moved or shifted.
- Once gowned and gloved, team members may not lower their forearms below waist level. When passing each other, personnel pass front to front or back to back.
- A sterile person first covers the near side of any unsterile surface with sterile drapes and then covers the far side.
- Movement and air currents around the sterile area are kept to a minimum.
- If there is any doubt about the sterility of an item, it is considered contaminated.

Preparing the Procedure Table

Most hospital personnel have worked in the operating room and should recall the consequences of touching or coming too close to the sterile field or to the sterile table. If one comes within 2 feet of the table, the wrath of the scrub nurse will ensue. This same mentality must prevail in the angiography suite. The table should be meticulously set up such that it is not contaminated, and once it is prepared for the procedure, only the sterile physician and assistants should touch the table. The table should stand in the center of the room and not rest against the wall or equipment.

Two-Person Technique

Preparing the procedure table should be a team effort. The procedure assistant should scrub and wear a sterile gown and sterile gloves as well as a face mask, hat, shoe covers, and glasses or mask. An assistant, also wearing hat and face mask, opens the individual packages, starting with the sterile table cover, and hands the items to the scrubbed assistant in a sterile manner. The scrubbed assistant then proceeds with organizing the tray.

One-Person Technique

On occasion, the assistant will need to prepare the room and instrument table unassisted. A sterile table cover is placed initially. The assistant (preferably wearing a sterile gown in the event that he or she rubs against the table), without sterile gloves, opens the individual packages of equipment and "dumps" on the table in an organized fashion. The assistant then should scrub, gown, and put on sterile gloves and organize the table.

Instruments

Of the many surgical instruments in use today, there are both reusable and disposable sterilizable instruments. Neither type should be the source of infection. In general, reusable, sterilizable equipment is sturdier and easier to use, although disposable instruments are adequate under most circumstances. We find that disposable instruments are more than adequate when placing most tunneled catheters; however, when performing more delicate techniques such as a running subcuticular closure of a port wound, we prefer the better-quality reusable instruments.

Needle Holder Needle holders (or needle drivers) are used to grasp and securely maintain the suture needle and to facilitate suture tying. Needle holders with flat, smooth jaws, such as the Webster and the Halsey, are less traumatic to suture material and to suture needles than are the grooves or teeth on the platforms of other needle holders, such as the Baumgartner, the Mayo-Hegar, the Derf, and the Collier needle holders. Personal preference and availability should be the deciding factor in the purchase. Comfort and control are essential, especially when doing fine work.

Forceps (Pickups) Forceps are used for handling tissue and are available with either toothed or smooth tips. Forceps with teeth are less traumatic than are smooth forceps, which tend to crush soft tissues. Commonly used forceps are the Adson forceps with teeth; they have broad handles that taper to a long narrow tip. One to three teeth are present that insert between the teeth on the opposing side of the forceps. The Brown–Adson forceps contain seven or eight interlocking teeth distributed over the length of the tip. The finer Adson forceps with teeth or the Castroviejo forceps with platforms behind their teeth are useful for manipulation of the delicate needles found with fine suture material.

Scissors Scissors depend mainly on personal preference. Commonly used scissors include the Metzenbaum and the Iris.

Scalpel Blade The scalpel blades most commonly used for placement of central venous catheters are the nos. 10, 15, and 11. The no. 11 blade is used in most central venous catheter procedures for stab incisions, such as for making a dermatotomy or short incisions at the skin exit site of a subcutaneous tunnel. The no. 11 blade is tapered with a sharp point. Longer incisions, such as for creation of a subcutaneous pocket, should be made with a no. 10 or no. 15 blade, which is wide with a convexly curved cutting edge. The incision should be made with the curved portion, not the tip of the blade.

PHYSICIAN PREPARATION

Attire

Scrubs

In the past, a radiologist would enter the room in street clothes, put on gloves and a sterile gown, and proceed. This is no longer the case. During catheter placement procedures, patients may be immunosuppressed, and introduction of an infection could be deadly. Everything possible should be done to avoid introduction of infection. Hospital scrubs should be clean and free of dust particles from the environment, which may harbor infectious agents. To ensure cleanliness, the scrubs should be put on in the hospital after arrival. No one in the procedure room should wear scrubs to or from work. Technologists, nurses, or physicians who wear personalized scrubs from home to work defeat the purpose of wearing them.

Scrubs protect the wearer from blood products. They are made of a polyester and cotton mixture and should be repellent to fluids. Blood-soaked scrubs should be changed immediately after the procedure. Scrubs should never be worn home because of the risks to personnel and family.

Shoe Covers

Shoe covers prevent contamination of the surrounding environment with blood products. The covers should be placed immediately before the procedure, and every member of the team should wear them. Anyone in the procedure room can step in a puddle of blood and track it throughout the hospital for the remainder of the day unless shoe covers are worn. The shoe cover must be removed immediately after the procedure. A bloody shoe cover tracks blood as well as a bloody shoe.

Shoe covers protect the shoes from becoming saturated with blood, which is especially important when handling the shoes. The shoestrings are especially absorbent and are handled when tying the shoes.

Surgical Mask

Since the demonstration of bacteria in droplets in the nose and mouth by Flugge in 1897[4] the face mask has been considered a necessity for reducing surgical wound infections. A 1926 study by Meleny and Stevens[5] seemed to confirm this assumption by showing a reduced infection rate when attendant personnel wear masks. Meleny[6] repudiated this finding in a subsequent 9-year prospective study, however; this study showed the infection rates to be similar with and without surgical masks. Numerous subsequent studies[7–11] also have brought into question whether masks prevent wound infections, and several of these studies suggest that face masks increase postoperative wound infection rates.[7,9] It has been suggested that the friction of the face mask against the skin of the face releases skin scales that carry bacteria, usually staphylococci.[12] The use of masks should therefore be reconsidered.

It could be argued, however, that masks do protect the operator from splashed blood products touching the mucosal surfaces of the eyes, mouth, and nose and are therefore worth wearing. Consider, however, the splash shield, which not only protects the operator from splashed blood but also eliminates friction to the skin of the face, which may release scales with pathogenic colony-forming units (CFUs). In rooms with air circulatory systems under positive pressure, which carry airborne contamination away from the center of the room toward the periphery, the splash shield should deflect a jet of air from personnel, behind his or her head, which would be carried away from the table.[13–14]

The use of surgical masks was adopted a century ago, and the practice was passed along because it seemed reasonable. The ritual of wearing a face mask continues without questioning the effectiveness of the face mask in preventing wound infections. Actual scientific studies suggest that face masks could be replaced by splash shields[15–16] without compromising the quality of care to the patient, providing savings to the medical care system (face masks cost in the range of 25¢ to 50¢ apiece) and greater comfort to personnel. The question is whether the medical community and our patients are willing to accept changes in this age-old practice.

Surgical Hat

Fallen hair from team members carry potentially pathogenic CFUs and should be excluded from the sterile field. The team members, whether sterilely scrubbed or assisting within the room, should wear hats covering all the hair on the head. Several surgical hats are available, including the large bouffant surgical cap, which should cover the hair of most personnel, although in rare instances personnel with "large hair" may require two such hats. Personnel with beards and mustaches definitely should wear face masks that cover all facial hair to prevent microbe-containing hair follicles from falling onto the sterile field.

Surgical Scrub

Sink

The sink basin preferably should be 18 to 24 inches deep, and the faucet should extend well above the basin (at least 1 foot) so that when rinsing the scrubbed, sterile hands and forearms, one does not accidentally touch the side of the basin. For the same reason, cabinets and other equipment should not be kept immediately adjacent to the sink. Foot pedals or an electric eye are very convenient for hand washing, although not absolutely necessary.

Why Scrub?

After all, surgical rubber gloves are worn, and they act as sterile barriers that provide protection against wound contamination on the hands of team members. The fact is that a large number of sterile rubber gloves become punctured during a procedure. Studies have shown gloves with holes following procedures range from 12 to 86%.[17–22] These defective gloves are a prime source of wound contamination

during procedures. Double gloving can reduce perforations and reduce the risk of wound contamination. One study showed that perforations occurred in both the inner and outer gloves in only 9% of surgical cases.[22] Although the risk of a glove being perforated and the operator carrying a virulent strain of bacteria and transferring it into the wound may be small, it is not insignificant, and the operator should scrub the hands and forearms with an antiseptic before every sterile procedure. An antiseptic is a chemical agent that reduces the microbial population on the skin.

The Skin

Human skin harbors microorganisms, providing a complex environment. The stratum corneum is the outermost surface of the skin, which comprises many layers of interposed sheaths of flat, scale-like cells composed of keratin. The cells in this layer of the epidermis are rough and contain a multitude of crevices where bacteria reside. Bacteria are most numerous near the surface of the epidermis and are less numerous in the crevices of the deeper layers of the stratum corneum. Transient bacteria, including *Staphylococcus aureus*, *Streptococcus* species, *Escherichia coli*, *Klebsiella* species, *Enterobacter* species, *Proteus* species, *Pseudomonas* species, and others, are present on the surface of the epidermis.[23] These bacteria can be exchanged easily between individuals and are removed easily with hand washing. In fact, humans continually shed the bacteria-laden cells of the stratum corneum into the environment. The bacteria in the deeper layers of the stratum corneum are called *residents* and can be removed only with a focused effort and then never completely because of the complex structure of the stratum corneum, which limits complete access of any chemical into the deeper niches. Resident flora includes gram-positive aerobes, such as *Staphylococcus epidermis* and gram-positive anaerobes. Fungi such as *Candida* species, *S. aureus*, *Klebsiella* species, and *Enterobacter* species may also be found as resident flora[23] in some individuals.

Although resident florea are ubiquitous, they are more concentrated in the axilla, groin, and scalp areas. Because they seem to be anchored firmly to the epidermal elements, they are more difficult to remove with antiseptics than are transient flora. Similarly, up to 20% live in hair follicles or in other nooks and crannies on the skin surface and therefore are not accessible to surface scrubbing. The epidermis below the stratum corneum is virtually sterile.

Cleansing Agents

Numerous antiseptic agents can greatly reduce the bacterial colony counts from the skin immediately after scrubbing. Especially in the moist environment of a sweaty hand in a plastic glove, however, the bacteria counts from the hand increase with time. The counts increase at a faster rate with agents that have only bactericidal activity compared with agents that have both bactericidal and bacteriostatic action.[24,25] These agents, however, do not create a totally sterile skin because, as noted earlier, the resident flora on the skin is not 100% accessible to these preparations. The ideal solution would be inexpensive, have a broad spectrum of bactericidal activity, and be nonirritating and nonallergenic.

Chlorhexidine gluconate (Hibiclens) is the most frequently used surgical scrub today, and it has bacteriostatic and bactericidal properties. Chlorhexidine creates a chemical bond with proteins in the stratum corneum of the skin, which is why its antibacterial action is persistent (i.e., it is also bacteriostatic).[24,26,27] This bacteriostatic action results in less rapid multiplication of bacteria on the gloved hand which, in turn, should decrease the risk of postoperative wound infection if glove puncture does occur. It has a wide range of activity against bacteria (being especially active against gram-positive bacteria and somewhat less active against gram-negative bacteria), yeasts, and viruses. The chemical binds to the negatively charged groups on the bacterial cell wall, producing irreversible

damage and death. It may cause irritation in the eyes and middle-ear damage.

Iodine solutions (Betadine) are excellent antiseptics for skin preparation because they are broad spectrum and fast acting. The formulation most commonly used for surgical scrub is iodophor, which contains 1 to 3% elemental iodine. Iodophors are a water-soluble complex of iodine conjugated with organic compounds. They have a good spectrum of activity against both gram-positive and gram-negative organisms and possess some activity against spores and fungi. The povidine–iodine preparations are similar in bactericidal effect to chlorhexidine gluconate initially; however, they lack residual activity[28] (i.e., they are bactericidal but not bacteriostatic). For short procedures (less than 1 hour), either chlorhexidine or iodophor solutions are effective and can be used.[29] For longer procedures, chlorhexidine is clearly superior and should be considered the agent of choice.[24]

Other antiseptic agents available for surgical scrub are hexachlorophene and alcohol. Hexachlorophene has a narrow spectrum of activity. It does not kill gram-negative organisms that have emerged as significant nosocomial pathogens. Alcohol has a rapid onset but no sustained action. The spectrum of activity of alcohols includes most gram-positive and gram-negative bacteria, tubercle bacillus, many fungi and viruses, including human immunodeficiency virus (HIV). Isopropyl alcohol is an excellent antiseptic and is preferred in many hospitals, although it tends to dry the skin. It is not commonly used as a hand antiseptic because it is not a detergent; therefore, it should be used on skin that is grossly clean (following hand washing with soap and water).

Length of Scrub

The concept of a good surgical scrub has undergone much refinement over the years. With the use of more effective detergents, there is an increasing tendency to shorten the scrub time. Several studies have shown no advantage of a 10-minute scrub over a 5-minute scrub[30–32] in terms of the number of bacteria remaining on the hands. The advantages of a shorter scrub time include a reduction in skin trauma and dermatitis, a saving in water consumption (it is estimated that 50 gallons of water are used in a single 10-minute scrub, and a saving in procedure time.[32] O'Shaughnessy et al.[33] recommend a 4-minute scrub for the first surgery of the day, followed by a 2-minute scrub for subsequent surgery. Interventional radiologists do not perform one sterile procedure after another, however, with nonsterile cases usually interposed. Therefore, we recommend a 4- or 5-minute scrub before each sterile procedure.[30,34]

Hand-Scrubbing Techniques

The purpose of a surgical scrub is the removal of dirt and grease as well as transient and resident flora. This is best achieved by use of a sponge brush soaked with a detergent preparation. All physicians have performed the 5-minute scrub in medical school; however, medical school may have been a few years in the past. Therefore, we will review the surgical scrub in detail. Masks, hats, glasses, thyroid shields, and lead aprons should already be in place when hand washing commences.

1. Open the scrub brush packet and saturate the sponge with water.
2. Bring to a full lather both hands and arms, up to the elbows.
3. Using the brush side of the brush/sponge, begin scrubbing every inch of skin from fingertip to elbow. Every inch of skin should be scrubbed several times.
4. Grab and squeeze the sponge in such a way that the already scrubbed hand never touches the unscrubbed hand or arm (Fig. 3–1). That is, the brush should be held in such a way that one hand never touches the other.
5. The only way to ensure that all areas of skin have been scrubbed several times is to go about the scrubbing in a systemic manner: Begin with the

fingers on the first hand, dividing each finger into four planes (Fig. 3–1). Scrub each plane of each finger five to ten times before moving onto the next plane of the finger. Pay special attention to the fingertips and under the nails. If visible dirt is under the nails, use the nail scraper.

6. The palm and dorsum of the hand must now be scrubbed.
7. Finally, the wrist and forearm are scrubbed. Again, divide the wrist and forearm into multiple planes, assuring that each plane is thoroughly scrubbed several times.
8. The process is repeated for the other hand, wrist, and forearm making sure that the first hand does not become contaminated. The systematic regimen is necessary to ensure that all areas of skin are scrubbed every time.
9. A second sponge is not used because obtaining a new sponge is highly likely to contaminate the hands.
10. Thoroughly rinse one hand, wrist, and forearm, keeping the hand elevated so that water runs down the forearm toward the elbow, not in the other direction.
11. Repeat the rinse with the other hand and arm. The two hands should not touch until they are gloved.
12. Stand at the sink momentarily to allow excess water to drip into the sink, off of the elbows.
13. Enter the procedure room with hands up, such that any residual excess water will drip off the elbow. If the hands are placed down, lower than the elbow, contaminated water from above the elbow could roll down, contaminating the forearm and hand. Obviously, do not touch anything that is nonsterile after scrubbing. If there is any question whatsoever that a nonsterile object was touched (e.g., the faucet head of the sink), rescrub.
14. A sterile towel should be obtained from the table and laid across the palm of

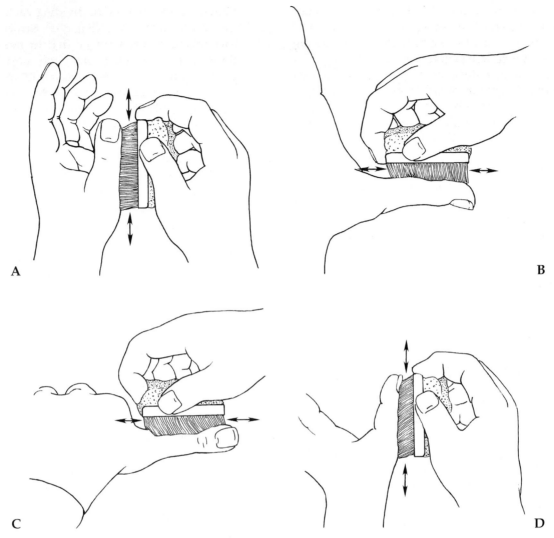

A

B

C

D

Figure 3–1 The hand holding the brush should not touch the hand being scrubbed. Divide each finger into four planes and scrub each plane of each finger five to ten times. Scrub the palm, the dorsum of the hand, the entire circumference of the wrist, and finally the forearm. Divide each part into sections and scrub each section five to ten times to ensure that every inch of skin is scrubbed multiple times.

one hand such that only one end of the towel is employed initially.

15. The other arm and hand are dried from finger to elbow so that contaminants are not brought from the elbow to the hand.

16. The other end of the towel is then laid across the already dried palm, and this end of the towel is used to dry the second hand and arm from finger to

elbow. It is important not to use the same end of the towel because of the risk of the towel becoming contaminated from drying the forearm near the elbow of the first arm.

Putting on the Sterile Gloves and Gowns
Surgical gowns must be made of waterproofed, impermeable materials. At least

the sleeves and front of the gown should be reinforced with such materials.[35]

The following is a safe way to put on sterile gloves without assistance:

1. After drying the hands and arms, grab the gown from the table, making sure not to touch the table. The gown is folded in such a way that you are grabbing the portion of the gown that will be the nonsterile inside portion.
2. Place both arms into the sleeves, allowing the gown to unfold and drop down. Work your arms into the gown by stretching your arms out, but be careful not to touch anything when stretching. Do not use one hand to pull the other sleeve up. Do not bring your hands out of the ends of the sleeves (Fig. 3–2A). The hands should be covered by the sterile sleeves.
3. Use the dominant hand to grasp the folded portion of the nondominant glove (Fig. 3–2B) (i.e., the left glove is grasped through the sleeve using the right hand in a pinching manner).
4. Now place the nondominant hand, still covered with the distal portion of the sleeve, into the glove (Fig. 3–2C). Once the fingers are covered with the glove, the sleeve can be pulled back along with the glove uncovering the fingers within the glove.
5. The gloved hand is used to pick up the glove for the dominant hand and place it on the hand in a similar manner (Fig. 3–2D). The important point is that the sleeve not uncover the hand until it is within the glove.
6. An assistant then secures the back ties or snaps of the gown. The wraparound tie of the gown is often neglected, but should always be employed. This covers the backside of the scrubbed person and decreases the likelihood of accidentally contaminating the field by rubbing up against the sterile table or patient with one's "exposed" backside.
7. If a gown must be removed for any reason (e.g., the sleeve tears), one must rescrub. There is no way to remove a gown without contaminating the hands.
8. If the first hand does not properly slide into the glove and the fingers are not all seated in the designated glove fingers, do not waste time trying to align the glove at this time. Instead, proceed to putting on the second glove. When the other hand is properly gloved, it is easy to use this hand to adjust the first glove.

PREPARATION OF THE PATIENT

Sedation

Sedation is an important aspect of any invasive procedure. The use of conscious sedation by nonanesthesiologists has helped to allow the increase in the number of minor procedures (e.g., tunneled catheters) performed out of the operating room. Appropriate conscious sedation increases patient comfort and may increase the safety and speed of a procedure by decreasing patient movement. Many patients will require several catheter-related procedures over the course of their treatment, thus making comfort an important aspect of their care.

It is important to establish a formal program for conscious sedation at every institution in which it is used. The program should be set up and run in collaboration with the anesthesia department at the institution. The Joint Commission of Accredited Healthcare Organizations (JCAHO) expects patients to receive the same quality of anesthesia throughout the hospital regardless of where it is administered and by whom. Patients can check with that institution to determine whether a program exists.

Basic elements of a conscious sedation policy should include the following:

- A basic health evaluation should be performed on all patients who might need sedation. This includes the patient's medications, allergies, cardiac and respiratory history, and any pertinent medical or surgical history.

25

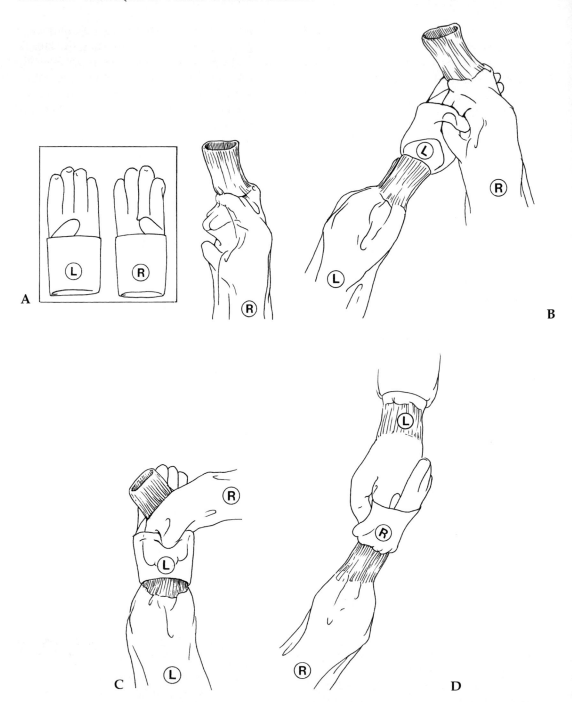

Figure 3–2 Putting on sterile gloves unassisted. **(A)** Do not bring hands out of the sleeves. **(B)** Grasp the glove (using a pinching motion through the gown sleeve) by the folded portion of the glove. **(C)** The hand, still covered by the sleeve, is slid into the glove. The hand should not emerge from the sleeve until it is inside of the glove. **(D)** The gloved hand is used to place the glove on the other hand. Again, the hand does not emerge from the sleeve until it is inside the glove.

The time of the patient's last food intake should be determined.

- The patient should not eat before sedation; this will reduce the risk of aspiration. Exact guidelines should be established, but a common practice is nothing by mouth except medications with sips of water for 6 to 8 hours before conscious sedation.

- The patient should be monitored at all times by an appropriately trained person, usually a nurse, who administers the sedation and monitors the patient. This person should be available to the patient at all times and should not be involved in other tasks (i.e., not helping perform the procedure).

- Monitoring should include oxygen saturation, blood pressure, heart and respiratory rate, level of consciousness, head position, and skin color. Respiratory compromise is a primary concern; therefore, the patient should be monitored with a pulse oximeter at all times while sedated. Supplemental oxygen should be available and used for even the slightest decrease in oxygen saturation. The patient's other vital signs should be checked and recorded periodically. The doses and times of administration of all drugs also should be recorded.

- The physicians using conscious sedation should be trained in using the administered drugs and in airway management. Drug training should include dosages, contraindications, and reversal or treatment of overdose. Airway management should include the correct use of airway positioning, ventilation bag and mask, and airway devices. The patient should be monitored until fully recovered from sedation. Discharge criteria should be established as part of the conscious sedation protocol.

- Emergency protocols should be established in case of respiratory compromise. A clearly established way to call for additional assistance (e.g., anesthesia, respiratory therapy) should be arranged and known to all involved in administering sedation.

- Emergency equipment should be available at all times. An emergency cart containing equipment for airway management and drugs for resuscitation should be readily available. The location of oxygen (source, tubing, nasal cannula, and face masks) and suction should be known to all practitioners. The equipment should be checked and restocked routinely.

A common regimen for conscious sedation involves using a benzodiazepine (BDZ) and an opiate. Specific BDZs include midazolam (the most commonly used), diazepam, and lorazepam. Midazolam has several characteristics that make it a preferred drug for conscious sedation. It is metabolized rapidly, with mental function returning to normal in about 4 hours. It frequently causes amnesia. When used with a narcotic, midazolam reduces the sympathetic response to adverse stimuli, reducing cardiac stress. Midazolam may be given as 0.5- to 1.0-mg increments administered intravenously (IV).

Narcotics provide excellent analgesia but also cause respiratory depression. Common drugs include fentanyl, morphine, and meperidine. Fentanyl has very rapid onset, with short duration of action (about 30 minutes). Repeated doses prolong its effect. Fentanyl may be given in 25- to 50-microgram increments IV.

Naloxone (Narcan) is an opiate antagonist. If oversedation leads to respiratory depression, naloxone may be given as a reversal agent. Naloxone also reverses the analgesic effects of opiates. This may result in hypertension and tachycardia if the patient is still experiencing pain. Nalaxone is given in 0.1-mg increments IV.

Flumazenil (Romazicon) is a BDZ antagonist. It may require as much as 30 minutes to take effect. If both an opiate and a BDZ have been given, treat with naloxone first. Opiates have a greater effect on respiratory drive, and naloxone takes effect more quickly than flumazenil. Flumazenil also has a shorter half-life than many BDZs. If it is used for reversal, the patient should be closely monitored because he or she may become more sedated as the effects of the flumazenil wear off. It is given in 0.1- to 0.2-mg increments IV up to 3 to 5 mg or in 0.5-mg increments if the patient is apneic.

Skin Preparation

In procedures in which indigenous contamination is not expected (such as venous catheter placement), extrinsic bacteria that contaminate the open wound cause most postoperative wound infections. Possible sources of extrinsic contamination include the skin overlying the operative site,[36,37] members of the procedure team, surgical equipment, and other items in the environment. Methods to prevent contamination from other sources, such as surgical hand scrub, wearing sterile gowns and hats, and disinfecting and sterilizing equipment have been discussed. We now discuss the preparation of the patient's skin to prevent this source of extrinsic bacteria.

Removing Hair

Multiple studies have demonstrated that shaving the skin prior to surgery increases the risk of postoperative wound infection.[38–40] The old routine of shaving the surgical site the night before surgery has been shown to be risky. Hamilton et al.[41] found the reason for the increased risk of infection. Using electron microscopy, they showed that razors cut not only hair but also the skin, leaving superficial wounds in which bacteria may multiply. If the field is shaved 24 hours in advance, the resulting exudate from abrasions becomes a breeding ground for bacteria, increasing the risk of postoperative infection. If shaving is necessary (e.g., dense hair growth makes suturing or attaching a dressing difficult),

it should be performed immediately before the procedure.

Better options than shaving are the use of clippers, which do not cause trauma to the skin, and depilatory creams. Depilatory cream does not increase the risk of infection,[39] but its use has not become widespread because of skin sensitivity to creams. The best action concerning hair removal is not to do it unless it absolutely must be done. If hair must be removed, the use of clippers is the best option.

Antiseptic Solutions

The skin is colonized by resident skin flora. These commensal organisms form part of the body's defense system and, when confined, are harmless. They are capable of multiplying, gaining nourishment from skin lubricants, burrowing into hair follicles and sweat glands, and becoming inaccessible to usual skin-cleaning methods. Some organisms, including *S. aureus*, *Micrococcus* species, *Corybacterium* species, and some gram-negative bacteria also can take residence on the skin.[23] These can cause infection when transposed to deeper tissue planes as a result of an invasive procedure. They can assume a pathogenic role and are of particular concern when foreign bodies such as catheters and ports are present. The aim of the antiseptic skin preparation is to remove transient and pathogenic organisms on the skin surface and to reduce the resident flora to a low level.[24,42,43] About 20% of the resident flora are beyond the reach of surgical scrubs and antiseptics, and therefore the skin cannot be "sterilized."[44] Bacteria harbored in the hair follicles invariably rise to the surface and contaminate the previously prepared area.

As previously discussed, several antiseptic topical agents are now available for preparation of skin. Without definitive comparative scientific studies, the consensus favors the use of an iodophor or chlorhexidine as an antibacterial agent.

Iodophors As previously discussed, iodophors are rapidly acting and have a wide range of activity against bacteria, yeasts, and viruses. These compounds, which contain 1 to 3% elemental iodine, release iodine slowly and therefore should never be wiped off immediately after application; rather, they should be allowed to remain on the skin for several minutes to obtain full effect.

Chlorhexidine Chlorhexidine has a wide range of activity against bacteria, yeasts, and viruses and, by virtue of its binding to epidermal protein, has a persistent (bacteriostatic as well as bactericidal) effect.[24] This antibacterial action increases as the number of applications increases.

Application of Antiseptic Solutions

With the patient in the proper position, preparing the field begins. The operative field must be free from contamination from hair or clothing falling onto the field. The patient should wear a surgical cap so that hair does not fall onto the field. Oxygen tubing for nasal cannula should be wrapped around the head, instead of looped around the ears, and taped to the face. The patient's gown should be pulled far away from the operative field.

To apply antiseptic solutions, 4×4 gauzes on a long clamp or disposable "lollipop" sponges can be used. The gloved hand must not be used to hold the gauzes alone because the hand most certainly will become contaminated. With the first antiseptic-soaked sponge or 4×4 gauzes, the antiseptic is rubbed onto the skin, starting at the center of the operative field, which would be the site of venous puncture and the skin exit site (or subcutaneous pocket site). From this central point, the antiseptic solution should be applied in a circular or outwardly spiraling manner (Fig. 3–3).

The edges of the field are painted last so that the contaminants from the edges are not carried to the center of the field, where the incisions will be made. This process

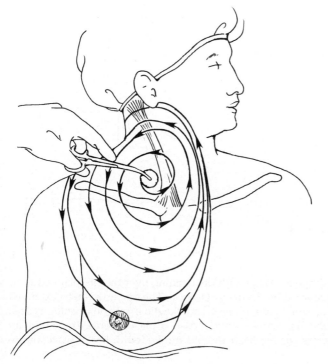

Figure 3–3 Paint the skin with antiseptic solution starting at the site of planned venous access and spiral outward from this point. Do not proceed to the center of the field if the sponge already has been used on the edge of the field. The field should be large.

should be repeated using two or three more sponges, starting in the center with each 4 × 4 or sponge and spiraling outward. It is critical that a wide area of skin be cleansed with the antiseptic solution. This wide field of preparation is necessary to prevent contamination of the central field from the edges of the operative field. For instance, surgical drapes should not be moved once they are put in place, but occasionally the drapes unavoidably shift because of patient or other motion. If a wide field of skin has been prepared, the drape that has shifted onto the central field is more likely to have migrated from an area of skin that was also cleansed with an antiseptic and will be less likely to contaminate the field. Additionally, despite well-laid plans, procedures do not always go exactly as planned. For example, a subcutaneous tunnel may need to be relocated, and it is good if the new site of the tunnel is already prepared.

HELPFUL HINT
A typical operative field for a jugular puncture, for example, should extend from the mastoid process to the nipple and from the axilla to the contralateral edge of the sternum (Fig. 3–3).

Applying the Drapes
Contamination of the catheter by skin organisms at the time of insertion is one of the causes of development of subsequent catheter-related infection. Antiseptic solutions and other methods that decrease

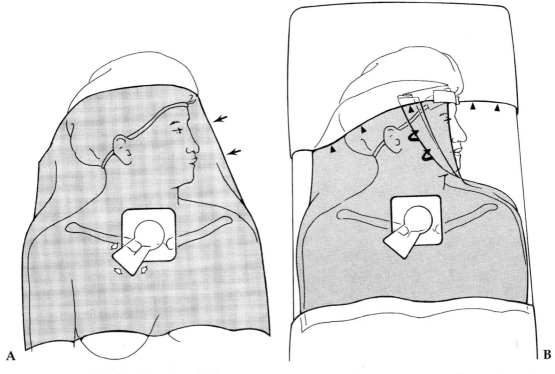

Figure 3–4 Applying the drapes. **(A)** The drape is placed with the opening over the site planned to be used for venous access. Initially, the face is covered by the drape (*arrows*). The opening can be extended by cutting away a piece of the drape with scissors (*open arrows*). The "keyhole" shape opening is seen here. **(B)** The drape has been folded off of the face (*curved arrows*). Also, a plastic sterile drape with an adhesive edge (*arrowheads*) can be taped across the forehead to hold the folded drape in place and to extend the sterile field above the head.

bacteria burden at the insertion site prevent catheter colonization and infection. Protective isolation using sterile barriers reduces nosocomial infection during catheter placement.[45-47]

Drapes come in a wide variety of shapes and sizes, with central openings that also vary in shape and size. The choice of drapes is based on personal preference and costs. For internal jugular vein punctures and subclavian vein punctures, we prefer brachial drapes, which are large enough to cover a large area, but small enough to be removed easily from the patient's face. The drape may be cut away from over the patient's face by an assistant. Another technique to remove the drape from the patient's face is to have an assistant fold the drape, exposing the face on the side contralateral from the procedure (Fig. 3–4A), with the drape still tented over the face on the side of the procedure.

HELPFUL HINT
A sterile plastic barrier with adhesive along one border can be used to drape across the forehead, taping the brachial drape into position so that it does not move or fall across the patient's face (Fig. 3–4B). This is especially useful when performing a jugular puncture while standing at the head of the table. Without the plastic barrier in place, the nonsterile top of the head and the face are too close to the sterile puncture site. In this circumstance, it would be easy for the end of the catheter or suture material to accidentally drag across the forehead or for a sterile glove accidentally to touch the top of the patient's head, thus contaminating the hand. The sterile plastic barrier also allows the physician to brush against the table without contaminating the front of the gown, which then could easily contaminate the gloves.

It is important to keep the patient's face uncovered by using one of the preceding techniques or by creating a tent under the drape. Most patients are claustrophobic to some degree, and having their face covered raises their level of anxiety. With the face uncovered, the patient is able to see the nurse nearby, who can provide moral support and comfort to the patient.

Larger drapes, such as pediatric drapes and femoral drapes (placing one of the openings at the venous access site), also can be used but may be difficult, because of the large size of these drapes, to fold away from the patient's face. Alternatively, these larger drapes can be used, and a portion of the drape cut away from the face or a tent can be created over the patient's face such that the patient can see daylight.

A large sterile barrier or femoral drape should be placed over the lower half of the body from approximately the level of the nipples to the feet. This drape allows a large working area from which to rest the end of guidewires and instruments. This drape also covers the table controls, allowing for sterile use.

After cleansing the skin, applying the drape, and obtaining venous access, gently lift the adhesive portion of the drape in the direction that you wish to create the subcutaneous tunnel (and pocket if needed). Cut a section of drape large and long enough to create the tunnel/pocket. This skin underlying the drape is still clean because the overlying drape is sterile. Ensure that the drape does not move such that a contaminated portion of the drape moves over a sterile area of the skin. Therefore, when originally placing the drape, the opening must be placed precisely at the puncture site and the drape adhesive adhered to the skin immediately. The drape should not be moved from this point onward. Care must be taken when pulling up on the adhesive to cut the drape, not to allow the drape to slide. The drape should be cut with scissors to avoid cutting the patient with a scalpel blade. We cut the drape in the shape of a keyhole (Fig. 3–4A), with the upper round portion of the keyhole being the round opening of the drape where the venous puncture was performed and the lower flared end at the skin exit site or the site where the pocket for a port will be placed. The alternative to cutting away a portion of the drape is to use a drape with a larger opening; however, it may be difficult to center the opening over the sterile area without including a nonsterile portion of the body within the drape opening. Some interventionalists place an iodophor-impregnated occlusive covering (3M) over the operative site. Incisions can be made through the covering.

When draping for translumbar and femoral venous punctures, a standard femoral drape is ideal. Place the opening over the puncture site and fix the drape adhesive to the surrounding skin. After obtaining venous access, again gently lift the adhesive portion of the drape in the direction that you wish to create the subcutaneous tunnel and cut away a keyhole portion of the drape.

Local Anesthesia

After preparing the skin and draping the patient, the skin overlying the vein to be punctured should be anesthetized. First, identify the skin site that will be punctured by palpating landmarks, by performing a preliminary localizing ultrasound, or with a venogram. Inject the lidocaine and allow the anesthetic to diffuse in the tissues for at least 30 seconds before performing the venous puncture, at which time there should be onset of anesthesia.[48] A burning pain is commonly experienced on injection of lidocaine and can make injection of a large amount of local anesthetic unpleasant to the patient. The burning pain is attributed to several factors, including an intradermal instead of subcutaneous injection, injection of anesthetic at room temperature rather than at body temperature,[49-51] pressure effect from rapid injection, the use of large needles, and the acidity of the solution.[52-54] Several precautions can be taken to make injection of lidocaine less painful: (1) always use a 25- or 27-gauge needle; (2) inject slowly to allow the anesthetic time to diffuse in the tissues and decrease the pressure effect; (3) keep lidocaine in a warmer; (4) do not start by making a large "wheal," which is very painful to the patient, instead push the

needle quickly through the dermis and inject into the subcutaneous tissue; (5) buffer the lidocaine solution (see later discussion). Other helpful steps include the following:

- Make the puncture with the 25- or 27-gauge local anesthetic needle exactly as you anticipate making the definitive puncture (i.e., go for the vein). If blood is aspirated, then you have localized the vein. Remember the exact angle and tract of the seeker needle. If blood is not aspirated, then inject lidocaine throughout this tract. The needle should be close to the vein so that you know you have anesthetized the entire tract. Never inject lidocaine if blood is aspirated.

- Always aspirate prior to the injection of lidocaine to ensure that the needle is not intravascular. Lidocaine and epinephrine have systemic toxicities and should not be inadvertently injected intravascularly. Another consideration is that there is always an artery next to the vein. We are not always careful about removing small air bubbles from the lidocaine syringe, and if the carotid artery is inadvertently punctured and an air bubble is injected, the results could be disastrous. Therefore, make sure that the needle is not in a blood vessel before injecting the local anesthetic.

- When performing a jugular puncture, do not inject a large amount of local anesthetic prior to the venous puncture. Too much local anesthetic can distort the anatomy, make it difficult to palpate the carotid artery, and may compress the jugular vein, making the venous puncture more difficult. Injection of 4 or 5 mL of lidocaine (1%) into the tract for a jugular puncture should be sufficient to numb the tract. The area can be anesthetized further after gaining access to the vein.

Buffering Lidocaine As discussed, the burning pain associated with injecting local anesthetic can be attributed to several factors, but the most important of these is the acidity of the solution being injected. Lidocaine has a pH of 5.0 to 7.0, which makes it more soluble and stable and extends its shelf life to 3 or 4 years. At the labeled pH, however, there are more charged particles, which are believed to produce the burning pain associated with injecting the solution.[55–57] Buffering the lidocaine to a pH of 7.1 to 7.4 has been demonstrated in many studies to reduce the pain of injection.[55–62] The studies have encompassed various fields of medicine, including interventional radiology,[59] foot surgery,[61] obstetrics and gynecology (Norplant System implantation)[60] and plastic surgery (liposuction).[62] The optimal concentration of buffered lidocaine as calculated by Stewart[63] can be obtained by injecting 3 mL of 8.4% sodium bicarbonate into a 30 mL vial of 1% lidocaine. That is, the mixture should be approximately 10 parts 1% lidocaine and 1 part 8.4% sodium bicarbonate. With alkalization, the shelf half-life of lidocaine is shortened, and for this reason, the mixture is prepared immediately prior to use. The rapidity of onset of anesthesia has been shown to be slightly faster with the buffered solution[48] and the duration of action is the same as the acidic solution, at least 1.5 hours.[52,58]

Lidocaine with Epinephrine Vasoconstrictors This is added to local anesthetics to decrease the amount of bleeding during an invasive procedure.[64–71] Other possible benefits of epinephrine in lidocaine are prolonged duration of anesthesia[72–75] and reduction of systemic toxicity of the anesthetic by reducing systemic absorption.

Epinephrine, however, is systemically absorbed after local injection and produces dose-dependent cardiovascular effects due to stimulation of alpha- and beta-adrenergic receptors. Stimulation of the beta-receptors occurs at lower levels of systemic epinephrine, causing increased heart rate, cardiac output, and myocardial oxygen consumption, which ultimately can lead to cardiac arrhythmias. At higher levels, alpha-receptor stimulation causes increased vascular resistance and can lead to systemic hypertension. Local toxicities also can occur with subcutaneous injection of epinephrine, including delayed healing of the wound[76] and skin necrosis.[77,78] These complications are dose related; therefore, use of the minimal concentration and minimal dose of epinephrine sufficient to provide adequate vasoconstriction to decrease bleeding should reduce the risk of toxicity. Dilute solutions of 1 to 100,000, 1 to 200,000, and 1 to 400,000 provide vasoconstriction with little difference in blood flow reduction between these concentrations.[64,66,67,72]

VENOUS PUNCTURES

General Principles

The use of small needles and wires with coaxial dilators (micropuncture sets) that allow conversion to standard guidewires is preferred for jugular and subclavian vein punctures. Using venographic or ultrasonographic guidance, traversing the pleura is unlikely, but is possible. Data comparing the rate of pneumothorax using large needles (16 to 18 gauge) and using fine needles (20 to 22 gauge) shows lower rates for the latter[79,80] during percutaneous lung biopsies. These data can be extrapolated for venous access. Also, the risk of pneumothorax increases with the number of times the pleura is transgressed. Therefore, good image guidance is very important. Smaller needles also decrease the risk of bleeding or injury to adjacent arteries if inadvertently punctured.

Also, a dermatotomy need not be made prior to skin puncture. An improperly placed dermatotomy can limit the approach and result in distortion of the skin at completion of the procedure. Therefore, it is better to make the skin puncture at the exact desired position rather than using a dermatotomy, which already has been made. Multiple dermatotomies can lead to wound and possible tunnel infections.

Making the Venous Puncture

For making the puncture, the syringe should be held with one hand only, holding the syringe within the palm of the hand and applying back pressure on the plunger of the syringe (Fig. 3–5). The other hand is used to palpate the carotid artery or hold an ultrasound probe, depending on the method employed for access. A small syringe (5 or 10 mL) with the attached needle fits nicely into the palm of the hand, and the plunger can be pulled back with the fingers at the same time.

Regardless of the technique used, always double check to ensure that the puncture is not being made through the sternocleido-mastoid muscle because dilatation of a tract through the muscle can be difficult as well as painful, and a tunneled catheter through the muscle can result in kinking of the catheter and be constant source of pain and "a stiff neck." When advancing the needle tip through the skin, resistance to puncture is felt, and care must be taken not to insert the needle too far after the "give" of the needle going through this skin. Likewise, it is common to reflexively pull back when the resistance of the skin gives way, often resulting in pulling the needle back out of the skin. This can result in unnecessary skin punctures.

Once the skin has been penetrated, back suction is applied and the needle advanced in the appropriate plane until blood is aspirated; however, frequently the needle traverses the vein through and through without blood being aspirated, because the vein is compliant and collapsible. Under ultrasound guidance, we have observed that the needle tip will often compress the vein, causing it to collapse completely before penetrating the front wall of the vein. Slightly more forward pressure can result in penetration of both the front and back walls of the vein. Therefore, suction should be applied both when advancing and withdrawing the needle. Often blood is aspirated only during needle withdrawal because the compressed vein re-expands when the through-and-through needle is pulled back and the needle tip is pulled into the lumen of the vein. If suction is not applied on withdrawal, a good through-and-through puncture of the vein will not be recognized. Furthermore, a hematoma may result, making the puncture even more difficult.

Advancing the Wire

After entering the vein, lowering the angle of the needle in such a way that the needle is more parallel with the vein will allow

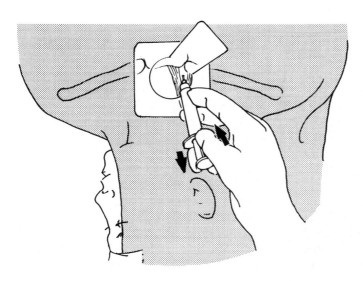

Figure 3–5 Puncturing and aspirating with one hand. The needle and syringe should be advanced and constant back pressure applied using one hand. Techniques vary, but in this example the thumb applies forward pressure on the syringe while the ring finger and small finger apply constant back pressure on the plunger. The index and middle fingers stabilize the syringe in the palm.

easier passage of the guidewire. After changing the angle of the needle, aspirate again to make certain that blood flows easily into the syringe. If blood does not flow easily into the syringe on aspiration, it is unlikely that a wire will thread into the vein. Threading a wire into a vein using the Seldinger technique is actually more difficult than threading a wire into an artery because veins are more pliable and compressible and the wire does not "track" as well. After good backflow of blood is obtained, grasp the needle hub with the other hand and carefully unscrew the Leurlock syringe (Becton Dickenson and Co., Franklin Lakes, NJ). Venous access is often lost during this step because the needle may be accidentally pushed in or pulled out while disconnecting the syringe.

HELPFUL HINT
It is difficult to hold the needle perfectly still if your hand is waving unsupported in the air. Make certain that the hand and wrist of the hand used to grasp the needle hub are securely supported by resting the wrist on the patient's forehead or chest (Fig. 3–6).

Next, attempt to advance the wire into the vein. After removing the syringe, an assistant should have the wire ready, placing the tip of the wire close to the needle hub and holding the back end of the wire. The physician should not have to move and certainly not have to turn and look for the wire. The physician simply directs the tip of the wire into the needle and advances the wire unless resistance is met. Tactile sense with the hand pushing the wire is critical. As the tip of the wire exits the needle tip, use a tapping motion with the wire to "feel" whether resistance is present (Fig. 3–6). An intraluminal wire will advance easily without resistance. If resistance is felt but the wire is nevertheless pushed in, the wire is likely not intraluminal and will curl in the subcutaneous tissues, often ruining the wire. Make small adjustments with the needle, altering the angle and possibly pulling back very slightly, all the time using a tapping motion with the wire and your tactile senses, until you feel the resistance give way and the wire advance. If, by using the tapping motion, the resistance never ceases, remove the wire and rehook

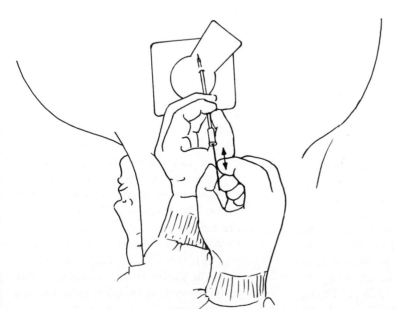

Figure 3–6 Advancing the wire. Tactile sense is used to know when to advance the wire. If resistance is met, ease advancement. Use a "to and fro" or tapping motion while making small adjustments in needle position until resistance is no longer felt. Note that the hand that is holding the needle is stabilized by resting the wrist on the patient's head.

the syringe to the needle. If no blood is aspirated at this point, advance the needle slightly and then aspirate as the needle is slowly pulled out.

HELPFUL HINTS

If the wire curls up in the subcutaneous tissue, carefully remove the wire and reconnect the syringe. Advance the needle slightly, and then aspirate as the needle is withdrawn.

If the wire curls up in the subcutaneous tissue and will not withdraw through the needle (it feels as though it is caught), do not continue pulling the wire. Instead, pull the needle and wire as a unit out of the patient. Continued attempts at pulling the wire out of the needle can result in "shearing off" a segment of wire in the patient's soft tissues.

If the wire is bent after being curled in the soft subcutaneous tissue, it still may be possible to use this wire. Have the assistant backload the micropuncture sheath onto the wire and use it as a wire introducer. This should allow one to advance the wire into the needle. If the wire is too bent or kinked, do not hesitate to get a new wire. It is sometimes better to sacrifice the cost of a new wire if it will help to get the job done. It can be extremely frustrating to puncture the vein but not be able to get the wire into the needle and ultimately lose access because of wasted time and motions. In fact, always keep an extra wire nearby so it can be dropped onto the table quickly if needed.

Ensuring a Venous Puncture

It is important to determine whether an artery or a vein of the neck has been punctured. This determination must be made prior to placement of larger dilators or catheters. Several measures (a safety checklist) are used. These measures assure that nothing larger than a micropuncture needle or dilator is placed in an artery. It is not good practice for a catheter larger than the micropuncture sheath to be in-

serted in the carotid or subclavian artery. The following steps can ensure for intravenous positioning of the needle:

- Dark red blood is aspirated; however, this can be difficult and somewhat unreliable. Dark red blood being aspirated into a syringe containing a small amount of saline may look fairly light. Differences between arterial and venous blood are not always clear, but if dark red blood is aspirated, one can feel fairly confident that the vein has been punctured.
- Venous blood has a low pressure and does not spurt; however, arterial blood does not always spurt from the small-caliber micropuncture needle. If the flow is pulsatile, it is arterial.
- Trajectory of the guidewire is an indicator of position. If the vein is entered, the wire descends on the right side of the mediastinum into the right atrium (Fig. 3–7A). The wire may go into the right ventricle and bounce around with contractions, or the wire may advance into the inferior vena cava. These wire positions definitely confirm an intravenous location of the wire. On the other hand, if the wire is intra-arterial, it usually passes down the descending thoracic aorta and should be easily recognized (Fig. 3–7B). An intra-arterial wire also may pass into the ascending aorta and bounce off the aortic valves.
- Injection of contrast through the micropuncture needle is not recommended. A small air bubble could be injected into the carotid artery. Also, it is difficult to hook up a contrast syringe, inject contrast, and observe under fluoroscopy without moving the needle tip. Extravasation of contrast into the region where a venous puncture for a long-term central venous catheter is to be made may result in inflammation causing slow healing of the wound.

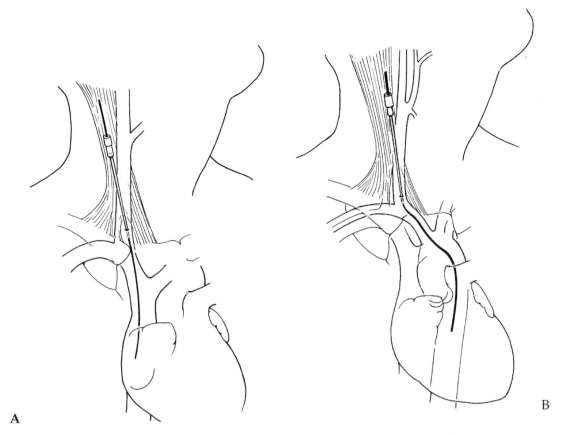

Figure 3–7 Evaluate the course of the wire. **(A)** Venous puncture. The wire descends on the right side of the mediastinum. If advanced further, the wire will pass into the right ventricle or pass below the diaphragm into the inferior vena cava. **(B)** Arterial puncture. In most cases, the guidewire will cross the aortic arch and descend the descending thoracic aorta.

- If fooled, even after using all of the above techniques, the worst that should happen is that a 4 or 5 French micropuncture sheath is placed in the artery. Always double-check the dilator for spurting arterial blood. Do not immediately cover the hub of the micropuncture sheath without confirming that this sheath lies within the vein as opposed to the artery.

Dermatotomy
HELPFUL HINTS
The dermatotomy is done after advancing the wire through the needle into the vein with a no. 11 blade held parallel to the needle. The blade is brought down the shaft of the needle so that the tip of the blade enters the same hole as the needle (Fig. 3–8).

Use only the tip of the no. 11 blade, and do not advance the blade through the skin more than 1 or 2 mm. The needle should be rocked back and forth to ensure that the dermatotomy includes the puncture site. Thereafter, remove the needle and insert the micropuncture sheaths.

The steps that follow vary, based on personal preference, but would include the following:

- Dilating the subcutaneous tract and placement of a peel-away sheath

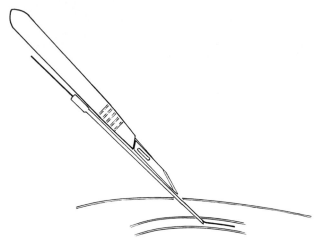

Figure 3–8 Making the dermatotomy. To ensure that the dermatotomy "connects" to the needle puncture site, advance the no. 11 blade down the shaft of the needle and enter the skin through the same skin site. The incision then is extended.

- Creating the subcutaneous tunnel (and subcutaneous pocket)
- Measuring the distance from the puncture site to the desired position of the tip for catheters that require trimming
- Advancing the catheter through the subcutaneous tunnel
- Advancing the catheter through the peel-away sheath and removing the sheath
- Securing the catheter in position
- Closing any incision(s)

These steps will be discussed later.

Internal Jugular Vein Punctures

Anatomic Considerations

The anatomy of the internal jugular vein has been described in a previous chapter, but a brief description is given again (Fig. 3–9). The internal jugular vein courses down the neck, running lateral to the carotid artery. The sternocleidomastoid muscle has origins from both the sternum and the clavicle. These two segments of the muscle join to form a larger muscle in the midneck, which then inserts into the mastoid process. The two bellies of the sternocleidomastoid muscle (the sternal and clavicular portions) create a triangle in the lower neck, with the clavicle at the base of the triangle. The internal jugular vein runs under the apex of this triangle along the posterior and medial border of the clavicular head of the sternocleidomastoid muscle, joining the subclavian vein behind the clavicle. The vein is within the carotid sheath along with the carotid artery and the vagus nerve. The vagus nerve runs between the artery and vein. The anatomy of the internal jugular vein and its relationship to the carotid artery and the sternocleidomastoid muscle are relatively constant regardless of body habitus.

Puncture Using Landmarks

Several approaches have been used for the blind (nonguided) puncture of the jugular vein, including the anterior, posterior, medial (or central), and suprasternal approaches. The medial puncture, which punctures the vein at the apex of the sternocleidomastoid muscle triangle (Fig. 3–9), is too high for placement of tunneled catheters. This can result in kinking of catheters because of the acute 180-degree turn that the tunneled portion of the catheter must make at this venous entry site. A puncture lower in the neck, the suprasternal puncture (Fig. 3–10), is preferred because a tunneled catheter essentially drapes over the clavicle with this venous entry site and rarely kinks. In reality, the usual venous puncture site is somewhat between the medial and suprasternal site.

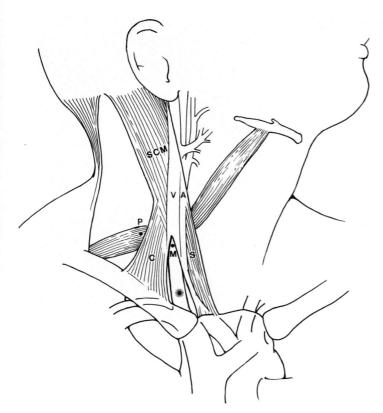

Figure 3–9 Jugular puncture anatomic considerations. SCM, sternocleidomastoid muscle; C, clavicular head of SCM; S, sternal head of SCM; A, common carotid artery; V, internal jugular vein; P, posterior puncture; M, medial puncture; *, suprasternal puncture.

Have the patient raise his or her head while you apply resistance on the face or top of the patient's head to make the sternocleidomastoid muscles more evident and more palpable. Identify the two heads of the sternocleidomastoid muscle. With the "free hand," palpate the carotid artery. The skin puncture should be made over the lateral edge of the carotid artery; however, the needle will be angled away from the carotid artery and the carotid should not be punctured. Remember to puncture the skin at the appropriate site, which should be just above the clavicle. Also, remember that the small lidocaine needle can be used as a seeker needle to localize the jugular vein. If the jugular vein is cannulated with the seeker needle, remember the skin puncture site and the angle of the needle. Again, the skin puncture is made at the lateral edge of the common carotid artery, but the needle

is angled toward the ipsilateral nipple such that the micropuncture needle should not puncture the carotid artery. It should "skim" lateral to the carotid artery. The classic definition is to insert the needle at a 30-degree angle to the skin, aiming at the ipsilateral nipple, but a more vertical approach (up to a 90-degree angle with the skin) also may be used. The more acute angle and more perpendicular approach through the skin makes it less likely to traverse the pleura and cause a pneumothorax. After puncturing the vein, the angle of the needle can be lowered to make it easier to insert the guidewire into the vein through the needle. After lowering the angle of the needle to make it more parallel with the vein, again aspirate blood to ensure that the tip of the needle still lies within the lumen of the vein.

The posterior approach into the jugular vein also may be used and provides a

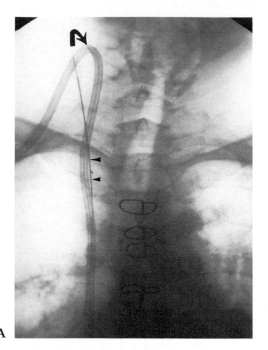
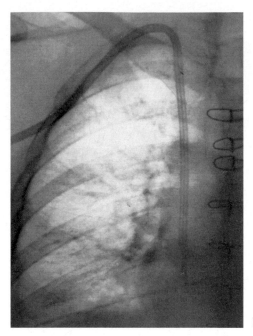

A

B

Figure 3–10 Jugular puncture too high in the neck. **(A)** Puncturing the internal jugular vein (IJV) too cephalad often results in kinking of the catheter (*arrow*). This case was complicated by thrombosis of the right IJV. A lower puncture, just above the clavicle, was performed under fluoroscopic guidance by advancing the needle until the tip hit the indwelling catheter. The guidewire is seen to be in place, adjacent to the catheter (*arrowheads*). **(B)** The malpositioned catheter was removed and the lower venous puncture was used to place a new catheter. Note how the low venous entry site allows for a more obtuse angle of the catheter in the subcutaneous tunnel.

smooth angle of the tunneled catheter into the vein. The needle passes posterior to the clavicular head of the sternocleidomastoid muscle in this approach. Locate the clavicular and sternal heads of the sternocleidomastoid by having the patient raise his or her head off the table and offering resistance. Define the lateral (posterior) border of the sternocleidomastoid muscle. The point of puncture should be approximately 4 cm above the clavicle or just above where the external jugular vein crosses the muscle (Fig. 3–9). Palpate medial to this point to verify the position of the carotid artery. Insert the needle at a 30-degree angle to the skin and advance it caudally. Aim the needle at the suprasternal notch. This is a somewhat less reliable method of puncturing the jugular vein, simply because of the longer distance that

must be traversed by the needle before the vein is entered.

Ultrasound Guidance

The use of ultrasound as a guide to puncture the internal jugular vein has made internal jugular vein cannulation a straightforward and relatively risk-free act.[81–83] Properly performed, ultrasound-guided puncture of the internal jugular vein should eliminate inadvertent puncture of the carotid artery and inadvertent puncture of the pleura. Studies have confirmed that the use of ultrasound guidance for internal jugular vein puncture has improved success rates and decreased the complications associated with venous catheter placement.[81–84] A major asset of ultrasound that should definitely decrease complications is the fact that patency of the jugular vein is verified before attempting punctures of the vein. Multiple blind attempts at cannulating a thrombosed internal jugular vein usually result in multiple inadvertent carotid punctures and possibly punctures of the pleura.

The puncture of the internal jugular vein is typically made between the two heads of the sternocleidomastoid muscle approximately 2 to 3 cm above the clavicle. This is a compromise between the medial approach and the suprasternal approach. Ultrasound is first used to ensure patency of the internal jugular vein. Both the internal jugular vein and the common carotid artery should be identified using a linear transducer in the range of 6.0 to 8.0 MHz. Confirm patency of the internal jugular vein by compressing with the transducer. Compressibility of the vein assures patency of the vein.

The technique of ultrasound-guided puncture of the internal jugular vein is one of personal preference. Most use visualization of the common carotid artery and internal jugular vein in the transverse plane although visualization of the jugular vein in the longitudinal plane also can be used. Visualization in the transverse plane has the benefit of ensuring that the visualized vessel is the jugular vein, not the carotid artery. Depending on the size of the head of the transducer, it usually allows the puncture of the vein to be closer to the clavicle.

Attempt to identify the heads of the sternocleidomastoid muscle, the internal jugular vein, and the common carotid artery all on the same image. Angle the transducer such that the center of the ultrasound image traverses between the two heads of the sternocleidomastoid muscle and the jugular vein is at the center of the image. Before performing the definitive puncture, again verify by palpation that the puncture of the skin is to be made between the sternocleidomastoid muscles and not through a head of the muscle. Perform the skin puncture at the very

center of the transducer, just above the upper edge of the transducer. Be certain not to pass through the sterile probe cover with the needle. Observe the image as the skin puncture is made. The tenting of the soft tissues at the center of the field should be visualized, and the needle itself should be visualized as it passes caudal underneath the transducer, within the soft tissues of the neck. If the internal jugular vein was properly positioned within the center of the ultrasound field, the angle of the needle should be identical to the angle of the probe except that the needle is angled more caudal. Slowly advance the needle through the soft tissues, attempting to visualize constantly the needle within the ultrasound image. Visualization of the needle can be surprisingly difficult, but one should at least see movement of the soft tissues along the tract of the needle. The ultimate goal is to visualize the needle tip entering the vein. At the very least, one should be able to visualize the needle tip compressing the internal jugular vein, in which case a brisk, short thrust then is made with the needle. Again, through-and-through punctures of the vein may occur, and back pressure must be applied as the needle is withdrawn. Once free aspiration of blood is attained, the guidewire is advanced through the needle. Correct position within the vein and visualization of the wire within the superior vena cava and right atrium should be confirmed under fluoroscopy before contamination of the sterile ultrasound cover (i.e, ensure that the wire is within the vein before giving up the sterile ultrasound probe).

Subclavian Vein Punctures

Anatomic Considerations

The axillary vein, the axillary artery, and the brachial plexus traverse the axilla within an axillary fascia. The axillary vein lies anterior to the axillary artery, and the brachial plexus runs between the artery and vein. As the vein crosses the first rib, it becomes the subclavian vein, passing anterior to the first rib and posterior to the clavicle. The subclavian artery lies posterior and slightly superior to the subclavian vein. The artery and vein are separated by the anterior scalene muscle. The anterior scalene muscle is typically 10 to 15 mm thick in the average adult, and therefore the vein and artery are separated by 1 to 2 cm at the level of the anterior scalene muscle in the average adult. More laterally, the subclavian vein and artery lie much closer together as they enter the axillary fascia together. Other anatomic relationships include entrance of the thoracic duct at the superior margin of the left subclavian vein near its junction with the internal jugular vein. The internal mammary artery arises from the underside of the subcalvian artery and passes anteriorly to a close relationship to the posterior surface of the first rib near the junction of the first rib with the sternum. Therefore, the internal mammary artery lies in contact with the posterior inferior aspect of the subclavian vein. The phrenic nerve and the pleura also lie in close contact with the posterior inferior aspect of the subclavian vein at the junction with the internal jugular vein.[85,86] As such, punctures that are too medial (close to the junction with the internal jugular vein) risk damage to the internal mammary artery, the phrenic nerve and puncture of the pleura.

Puncture Using Landmarks

Three bony landmarks are identified by palpation. The medial end of the clavicle, the achromium, and the sternal angle should be palpated. The distance between the achromium and the sternoclavicular joint is divided into thirds. At the junction between the medial third and the middle third of the clavicle, a vertical line is dropped. The needle is introduced approximately 2 cm inferior to the clavicle at this line. At that point, which is situated approximately 6 to 7 cm laterally from the sternoclavicular joint and about 2 cm below the inferior edge of the clavicle, there is a fosse about the size of the fingertip palpable in the soft tissues. This dimple separates the sternocostal and clavicular parts of the perctoralis major muscle. The needle penetrates the skin at this point and is directed medially and cephalad toward the gap between the spinous process of the 6th and 7th cervical vertebrae. Alternatively, a finger can be pressed firmly in the sternoclavicular notch, and the needle is advanced to a point slightly behind the fingertip. A shallow entry angle of the needle with respect to the sagittal plane is required (between 10 and 30 degrees). That is, the needle should be advanced in a plane that is nearly horizontal with respect to the table.[82,87,88]

Venogram-Guided Puncture

When performing puncture of the axillary or subclavian vein under fluoroscopic guidance while injecting water-soluble contrast through a peripheral IV catheter, a more lateral puncture of the vein can be performed, reducing the risk of pneumothorax or puncture of structures such as the thoracic duct or internal mammary artery.[82,89]

A peripheral IV catheter is placed in the wrist or forearm on the side where the catheter is to be placed. It is usually wise to inject a small amount of contrast before sterile preparation of the physician and patient to ensure patency of the axillary, subclavian, and brachiocephalic veins on the intended side of puncture. If the central veins are occluded, this will save the trouble of creating a sterile field only to realize that the intended vein to be punctured is occluded. This initial road map also can be used to mark the skin at the probable skin puncture site. Following preparation of the sterile field, local anesthetic should be injected into a fairly wide area at the probable skin puncture site. Local anesthesia should be given before performance of the road map because patients often move during injection of the lidocaine, which will deteriorate any stored images for road mapping. Following application of the local anesthetic, an assistant, under fluoroscopic control, injects water-soluble contrast. When there is complete opacification of the axillary and subclavian veins, the image is stored and used as a road map for the puncture of the vein. The skin puncture of the micropuncture needle is made over the axillary vein, and the needle is advanced at approximately a 45-degree angle under fluoroscopic/road map control directly at the subclavian or axillary vein. The intended site of venous puncture may vary using this technique. The traditional, landmark-guided medial puncture of the subclavian vein may be utilized. As described, however, there are advantages to a more lateral puncture, which is frequently at the level of the lateral aspect of the first rib; this is actually where the axillary vein becomes the subclavian vein.

A critical point of this technique is that the puncture of the skin should be made directly over the vein and the needle should be advanced through the soft tissues toward the intended venous puncture site, always superimposed over the vein. This ensures that the needle must traverse the vein, assuming that the needle is advanced deeply enough. If the skin puncture, for instance, is made superior to the axillary vein with the intention of puncturing the vein as it passes superolaterally across the first rib, advancing the needle tip toward the vein may result in the needle passing anterior or posterior to the vein. The relationship of the needle tip to the vein would be indeterminate when visualizing from the frontal plane under fluoroscopy. A simple analogy would be that of an airplane attempting to drop a bomb on a train (Fig. 3–11) (in this example, the airplane would be the physician, the bomb would be the needle, and the train would be the vein). There would be a much greater probability of a dropped bomb hitting the train if the plane is flying over the train in a direction parallel to the train as the bomb is dropped (Fig. 3–11A). On the other hand, there is little likelihood of a bomb hitting the train if the plane approaches the train perpendicular to the direction that the train is travelling (Fig. 3–11B). In a like manner, if the needle

enters the skin over the vein and travels in the same direction as the vein, eventually the needle must hit the vein.

In the event that peripheral IV access cannot be obtained, an intravascular device such as a catheter or a guidewire within the subclavian vein, possibly passed from a transfemoral puncture, can be used as a convenient target for puncturing the subclavian vein or axillary vein at the desired site. Again, remember to puncture the skin over the intravascular device and remain "overhead" the device at all times while passing the needle toward the desired puncture site. If road mapping is not available or if the road map images are inadequate, possibly secondary to motion of the patient, continuous injection of water-soluble contrast can be performed and the vein punctured under live fluoroscopy using the same techniques described.

Before creation of the road map image, estimate the site of skin puncture and adjust the field of view of the fluoroscopic image such that the site of venous puncture and the site of skin puncture are within the field of view but the physician's hands are out of the field of view. Obviously, this adjustment must be made before obtaining the image for road mapping.

Ultrasound-Guided Puncture

Ultrasound guidance again allows a more peripheral venous entry than the standard blind puncture using landmarks, which virtually eliminates the risk of pneumothorax and puncture of structures such as the thoracic duct and internal mammary artery.[82,90]

Using a 5 MHz to an 8.0 MHz linear transducer, the axillary artery and vein are localized. As previously described, the lateral aspect of the subclavian artery and vein and the axillary artery and vein are in close approximation as they are contained within the axillary sheath as opposed to the more medial aspect of the subclavian artery and vein, where the vessels the separated by the anterior scalene muscle. The subclavian artery and vein are localized, and while visualizing the subclavian

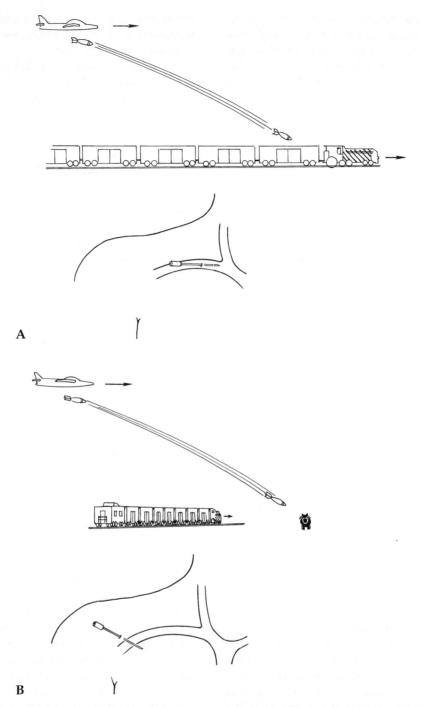

Figure 3–11 Train analogy. **(A)** The bomb has an excellent chance of hitting the train if released directly over the train by a plane flying in the same direction as the train. Likewise, the puncture should be made directly over the vein and the needle advanced parallel to the vein. **(B)** If the plane is not flying parallel to the train when the bomb is released, the bomb may hit the train but likely will drop alongside the train (on either side). Likewise, if the initial puncture is not made over the vein, the needle may hit the vein, but it is likely to pass anterior or posterior to the vein.

vein in a transverse or a longitudinal plane, perform the venous puncture. In this case, it is probably easier to puncture the vein while visualizing the vein longitudinally. Again, this allows the skin puncture to be made directly over the vein and to watch the needle as it descends directly onto the vein all under sonographic guidance. Before puncture, it must be confirmed that the vessel that is being visualized longitudinally is indeed the subclavian vein. Under ultrasound, the subclavian vein should be compressible and will vary with respirations. Typically, the transducer is placed with its medial edge against the patient's clavicle, and the subclavian vein and axillary vein are imaged in the longitudinal plane. The skin puncture site is chosen, and the micropuncture needle is advanced through the skin and advanced under real-time imaging such that the needle and vein are seen simultaneously. The tip of the needle should be seen to enter the subclavian vein or at least indent the subclavian vein. If the needle tip is indenting the subclavian vein, a short thrust is made for venous entry. Free return of blood should be obtained. The previously described checklist of safety precautions to ensure a venous puncture instead of an arterial puncture always should be performed.

CREATION OF THE SUBCUTANEOUS TUNNEL/POCKET AND PLACEMENT OF THE CATHETER

Placing the Peel-Away Sheath

After obtaining venous access and performing the dermatotomy, the next step varies with personal preference. A subcutaneous tunnel may be created at this time and the catheter pulled through the subcutaneous tunnel, or the peel-away sheath may be placed at this time. The individual steps are the same regardless of the order in which they are performed.

With the micropuncture sheath still in place, the curved clamps may be used to perform blunt dissection at the dermatotomy. Loosening of the subcutaneous tissue at the venous entry site allows easier placement of the dilators and peel-away sheath and also allows a smoother turn of the tunneled catheter as it enters the vein. If the subcutaneous tissues are not dissected at this site, the path of the tunneled catheter is restricted to the exact path taken by the tunneling device, which may or may not create an acute angle with the venous entry site. This will risk kinking of the catheter at the venous entry site.

A guidewire is advanced through the micropuncture sheath, and this guidewire is used for subsequent dilation of the subcutaneous tract and placement of the peel-away sheath. Most central venous access kits provide a 0.035 guidewire that can be used for this purpose. These wires are adequate from the right internal jugular vein approach, where the course of the dilators and peel-away sheaths are along a straight line; however, from subclavian vein approaches and from the left internal jugular vein approach, a stiffer wire is preferred. From the latter approaches, the stiff dilators are required to make sharp turns into the superior vena cava. These stiff dilators may or may not track easily over the guidewire that is provided. The larger dilators for dialysis catheters that may be as large as 14 F or even 18 F in size are especially stiff and may not track easily over the guidewire. The inherent risk is that these stiff dilators will not track over the wire but instead continue on a straight course and push through the wall of the brachiocephalic vein or superior vena cava, causing perforation of the vein and possible hemothorax. Using stiffer guidewires decreases the risk of venous perforation. An additional benefit of using a separate, stiffer guidewire is that the guidewire used is longer and can be advanced through the right atrium into the inferior vena cava. The fact that 2 or 3 feet of wire can be placed inside of the vein makes it very unlikely that the wire can be accidentally pulled out of the vein and venous access lost. Loss of venous access is much more likely when using the shorter guidewires, especially when difficulty advancing the dilators and peel-away sheath is encountered. Another trick to allow easier passage of the stiff peel-away sheath dilators over the guidewire when a curve from the subclavian vein or internal jugular vein into the brachiocephalic vein is encountered is to bend the dilator to make it slightly curved. Most dilators will maintain this curvature. The dilator must be advanced over the guidewire, with the curvature corresponding to the expected curvature of the vein. If a double curve is encountered, such as from a left internal jugular or left subclavian vein approach, after making the first turn with the curved dilator, rotate the dilator such that the curvature is in position to make the second curve. With experience, the physician will develop a "feel" for advancing the dilator to rotate in the direction desired. Essentially, the dilator will follow direction it needs to turn. Advancing a dilator through a venous curvature should be done under fluoroscopic guidance to ensure that the dilator remains co-axial with the guidewire. After placement of the peel-away sheath, the guidewire is removed, a flow valve is connected, and the dilator is flushed with normal saline.

Creating the Subcutaneous Tunnel

The subcutaneous tunnel can be created before or after placement of the peel-away sheath within the vein. The course of the subcutaneous tunnel should be planned such that the catheter, at the venous entry site, does not form an acute angle, resulting in kinking of the catheter. Subcutaneous tunnels need to be sufficiently long for lowering the risk of catheter infection. Subcutaneous tunnels should be at least 6 cm long to lower the infection rates likely because of the increased distance between the colonization at the skin entry site and the venous entry site. It is cumbersome and unnecessary to create subcutaneous tunnels of excessive length, which only serves to add to the length of the indwelling catheter. For internal jugular vein catheters, the subcutaneous tunnel can be created across the clavicle and the skin exit site 2 or 3 cm below the clavicle. Placing the skin exit site at approximately the midclavicular line or slightly more lateral usually allows for a smooth curvature of the tunnel at the venous entry site.

After carefully planning the course of the tunnel, local anesthetic is infiltrated throughout the course. It is more comfortable to the patient if the initial needle puncture for lidocaine injection is through skin, which is already anesthetized at the venous puncture site. Lidocaine then is injected in the subcutaneous tissue. An effort should be made to perform as few skin punctures as possible, using the entire length of the needle within the subcutaneous tissue with each puncture. It is not necessary to inject lidocaine into the dermis along the subcutaneous tract; this is more painful to the patient and is unnecessary. Several punctures of the skin will be necessary with the lidocaine needle, but it is possible for each puncture to be through skin, which is already anesthetized, working your way toward the skin exit site from the venous entry site. The catheter skin exit site is chosen and a stab dermatotomy performed using a no. 11 blade. The dermatotomy at the skin exit site should be made only large enough to pass the catheter cuff.

After creation of the dermatotomy, it is helpful to use a curved clamp to initiate the subcutaneous tunnel. The correct plane should be chosen such that the tunnel is through the subcutaneous tissues with an adequate amount of soft tissue between the skin and the catheter, but not so deep that muscle and bone are encounterd. The curved clamp is removed, and the tunneling device is placed through the dermatotomy and through the portion of the subcutaneous tunnel that has been initiated. The direction of the tunnel is extremely important. A common mistake is to aim the tunneling device directly toward the sheath; then the tunneling device is directed superiorly through the venous puncture site dermatotomy (Figs. 3–12A and 3–13). This can result in an acute angulation of the catheter in the transition from the subcutaneous tunnel to the venous entry site (Fig. 3–12B). To ensure a smooth angulation, the subcutaneous tunnel should be directed lateral to the venous entry site for a jugular puncture (Figs. 3–12C, D) and inferior (caudal) to the venous entry site of a subclavian puncture. As the tip of the tunneling device reaches the level of the venous puncture site, the tunneling device must be directed toward the dermatotomy. Eventually, the tip of the tunneling device is brought out of the dermatotomy. It is helpful for an assistant to place a small amount of traction or bending motion onto the peel-away sheath, to splay open the dermatotomy, allowing greater visualization of the dermatotomy.

- When tunneling to the internal jugular vein from the anterior chest wall, it is helpful to push down on the back end of the tunneling device such that the tip is elevated slightly within the subcutaneous tissue to allow passage over the clavicle.
- The tunneling device must first tunnel in a downward direction, and once over the clavicle may need to make a turn upward toward the dermatotomy. This maneuver can be difficult. Slight bending of the tunneling device can help. Also, the patient's head must be turned toward the contralateral side.
- The tunneling device must be advanced with caution to keep it in the subcutaneous plane and not too superficial, in which case one will see "tenting" of the skin. The tip of the tunneling device must not be too deep into the tissues, where it may encounter the sternocleidomastoid muscle; this would offer a great deal of resistance. Ideally, the device should pass just anterior to the sternocleidomastoid muscle within the subcutaneous tissues.

Advancing the Catheter Through the Subcutaneous Tunnel

With the tunneler entering the entry site dermatotomy and exiting the venous entry site dermatotomy, the catheter is connected to the tunneling device. Most tunnelers have screw-like threads on the tail end of the tunneling device. The tip of the catheter is pushed or twisted so that it is securely fixed to the tunneling device. The catheter should not be pushed too much onto the tunneling device, making the tip of the catheter flare outward creating a rough transition from the tunneling device to the catheter, which can get caught within the subcutaneous tunnel and dislodge the catheter from the tunneling device. The transition from the tunneling device to the catheter should be as smooth as possible. Despite precautions, the catheter can become dislodged from the tunneling device as it is pulled through the subcutaneous tunnel. The tunneling device must be advanced through the subcutaneous tunnel again, the catheter reconnected, and the procedure repeated.

HELPFUL HINTS
If the catheter continually becomes disconnected within the tunnel, the catheter tip can be secured with a suture around the tip of the catheter firmly holding the tip of the catheter onto the tunneling device. This should allow easy passage of the catheter through the tunnel. Once the tip has been brought through the subcutaneous tunnel, the suture is cut. Preferably, a stiffer suture material with "memory" should be used because if the knot is cut, the suture usually unravels easily. The 2.0 prolene sutures are ideal for this purpose. Care must be taken not to cut the catheter when cutting the suture. The tip of the catheter is disconnected and the catheter pulled through the subcutaneous tunnel. Catheters with a set length between the cuff and tip may be pulled as far as possible into the tunnel. The catheters can be pulled back easily after intravenous placement of the catheter (see below). For catheters which require

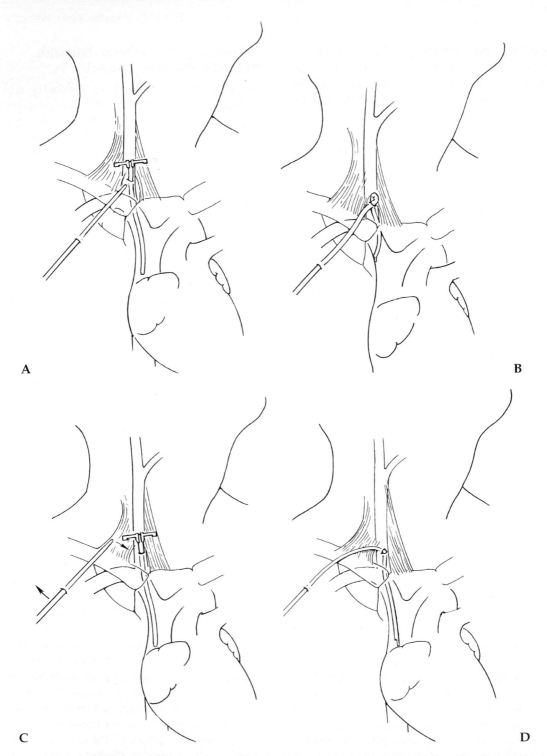

A

B

C

D

Figure 3–12 Creating the subcutaneous tunnel. Avoiding catheter kinking. **(A)** A common mistake is to tunnel directly toward the dermatotomy at the venous puncture site, **(B)** which can result in acute angulation and catheter kinking. **(C)** The tunnel should be made lateral to the venous puncture dermatotomy (or caudal for a subclavian puncture) and then brought directly medial to the dermatotomy at approximately the same level as the dermatotomy. **(D)** This allows for smooth angulation of the catheter as it enters the vein.

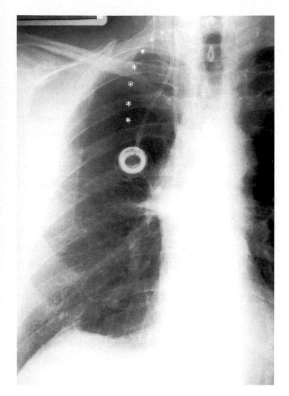

Figure 3–13 Kinking caused by improper tunneling. The subcutaneous tunnel of the portacath was created in a straight line from the subcutaneous pocket to the peel-away sheath at the venous entry site, resulting in kinking of the catheter caused by the acute angulation created by the tunnel. The subcutaneous tunnel should have been created more lateral and then toward the venous entry site (*asterisks*) to create a tunnel with less angulation at the entry site.

trimming, the Dacron cuff should be positioned approximately 1 cm from the exit site and the catheter trimmed. If the Dacron cuff is placed too close to the skin exit site, the resultant inflammation and granulation caused by the Dacron fibers can cause erythema at the exit site. The Dacron cuff should not be placed too far into the tunnel; to do so will make removal of the catheter very difficult.

Measuring Catheter Length

Catheters of a set length from tip to the cuff must be chosen beforehand, dependent on the expected length from the access site. Many other catheters require trimming of the length so the catheter tip will be positioned in the desired location. Several techniques are described to measure catheter length:

- After inserting the peel-away sheath, place the tip of the guidewire at the desired location in the lower superior vena cava or right atrium under fluoroscopy. Clamp the wire at the hub of the peel-away sheath (Fig. 3–14A). Pull the guidewire back and, under fluoroscopy, mark the venous entry site on the skin, aligning the tip of the guidewire with the venous entry site (Fig. 3–14B). Clamp the guidewire at the hub of the peel-away sheath again. The distance between the two clamps is the distance between the venous entry site and the desired location of the catheter tip. With the catheter in the desired position (with the Dacron cuff near the skin exit site), cut the catheter to the desired length. Place one clamp at the dermatotomy and lay the catheter along the wire, cutting the catheter to the length of the second clamp.
- Dilators used to dilate the subcutaneous tract are usually the same lengths as the dilator within the peel-away sheath. Place the tip of the peel-away sheath dilator at the desired location of the catheter tip within the superior vena cava or right atrium (Fig. 3–15). Subtract the distance between the hub of the peel-away sheath dilator and the skin from the total length of the second dilator (Fig. 3–15). Simply place the tip of the dilator at the venous entry site and pinch the dilator at the level of the hub of the peel-away sheath dilator. The remaining length of the dilator is the distance between the venous entry site and the junction of the superior vena cava and the right atrium. Trim the catheter accordingly.

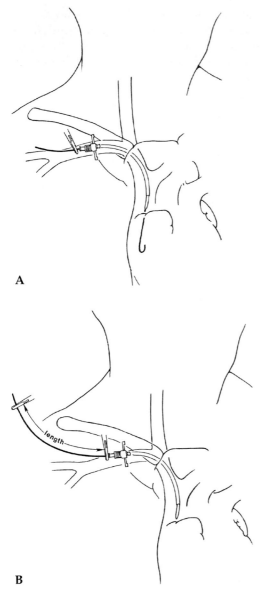

Figure 3–14 Measuring catheter length with a guidewire. **(A)** Place the guidewire tip at the appropriate level, where the final position of the catheter tip is desired, and place a clamp on the wire at the dilator hub. **(B)** Pull the wire back until the tip is at the level of the venous puncture dermatotomy and place a second clamp on the wire at the dilator hub. The distance between the two clamps equals the distance from skin entrance site to the junction of the right atrium and superior vena cava. After pulling the catheter through the subcutaneous tunnel and through the venous puncture dermatotomy, the catheter should be trimmed to this length.

- After trimming the catheter, lay the catheter on the patient's chest in the approximate position in which it will be inserted. Mark the location of the catheter tip on the chest wall. This is a rough estimate of what the length of the catheter will be once it is intravascular. Adjustments to the catheter length can be made at this time. Regardless of the technique used, it is important to remember that there may be significant changes in catheter position when the patient assumes the upright position.[91] This change in position is usually minimal for the jugular approach, but it can be significant for the subclavian vein approach, especially in obese women. Therefore, in such circumstances, the catheter tip is placed in the midatrium, assuming that the catheter will be pulled back when the patient is upright and the tissues of the chest wall drop with gravity.

Advancing the Catheter Through the Peel-Away Sheath

Both catheters that have to be trimmed and those that have a preset length should be pulled further through the tunnel before inserting the catheter through the peel-away sheath. That is, do not position the cuff at the desired location at this time; rather, pull the cuff further into the tunnel. The catheter can be pulled back once it is in the right atrium and the peel-away sheath has been removed. There are two advantages to this maneuver:

- The catheter can be easily pulled back and its tip placed at the desired location. If the length has been accurately measured, the cuff will be within approximately 1 cm of the skin exit site. If the length is inaccurate, it is best to place the tip rather than the cuff at the desired location.
- Pulling the catheter back often removes kinks at the venous entry site (Fig. 3–16).

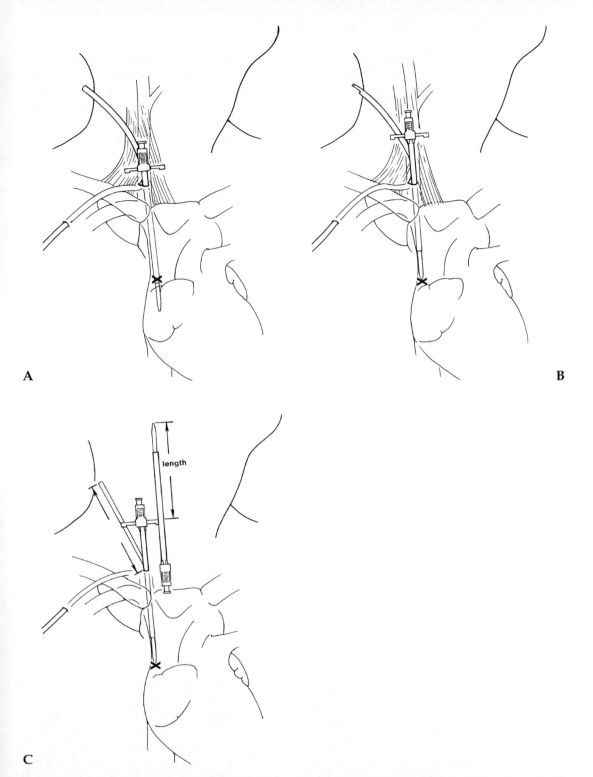

A

B

C

Figure 3–15 Use of a dilator to measure catheter length. **(A)** After pulling the catheter through the subcutaneous tunnel, **(B)** pull back the peel-way sheath until the tip of the sheath dilator is at the desired level of the catheter tip. **(C)** Subtract the exposed length of the sheath dilator from the overall length of a second dilator. The remaining length of the second dilator is the length to trim the catheter (from the venous puncture dermatotomy).

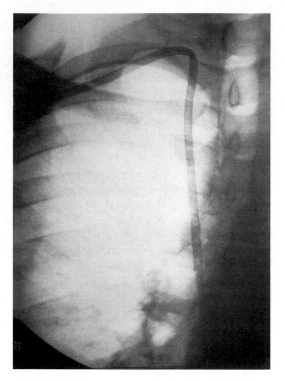

Figure 3–16 Kinking after advancing the catheter through the peel-away sheath. This catheter is kinked despite an adequate tunnel path. The kink was created when pushing the catheter into the peel-away sheath. Pulling the catheter back can remove the kink. Therefore, the catheter initially should be advanced farther than desired into the right atrium, and when the catheter is pulled back (to remove the kink), the tip will end in the desired location.

With the tip of the catheter in one hand, hold the handles of the peel-away sheath with the other hand. Have the assistant remove the dilator and quickly advance the catheter into the peel-away sheath. Before removing the dilator, make sure that the patient's intrathoracic pressure is high enough that air will not be sucked, which would cause serious air embolus. Have the patient take a deep inspiration, perform the Valsalva maneuver, or hum. The patient must be alert and able to follow commands. If the intrathoracic pressure is sufficiently high, there may be a gush of blood out of the peel-away sheath immediately after removal of the dilator. The catheter must be ready to be immediately inserted into the peel-away sheath as quickly as possible. The patient may breathe as soon as part of the catheter is within the peel-away sheath enough to occlude the lumen. Advance the catheter through the peel-away sheath. The catheter may kink as the final portion of the catheter is pushed into the sheath. This kink is removed when the catheter is pulled back (as described previously). It is easier to advance the catheter when the catheter is positioned behind the peel-away sheath instead of in front of it. An assistant should hold the catheter at the venous entry site, ensuring that the catheter is not pulled out

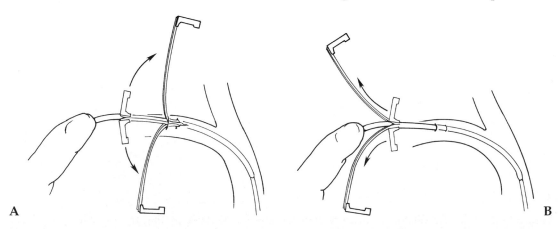

A   B

Figure 3–17 Removing the peel-away sheath. **(A)** If the handles are pulled in a purely lateral fashion, the sheath can dissect down to the vein, tearing a larger opening at the venous puncture site and causing bleeding. **(B)** The two handles should be pulled upward and lateral at the same time. The tearing portion of sheath should remain external to the body.

along with the peel-away sheath. The tension on the two handles must be equal because if one side is pulled faster than the other, the sheath will twist and clamp down on the catheter, possibly pulling the catheter out along with the sheath. Be certain not to pull the two handles of the sheath in a purely lateral direction because to do so may cause dissection down to the vein and bleeding around the catheter (Fig. 3–17A). The two handles of the sheath should be pulled backward and slightly lateral with the pressure applied against the assistant's fingers (Fig. 3–17B). There should be very little bleeding around the catheter. The catheter then is pulled at the skin entry site and adjusted under fluoroscopy.

The "Two-Stiff-Glide" Technique for Kinked Peel-Away Sheaths

Peel-away sheaths that must make an acute angle, such as from the left internal jugular vein or either subclavian vein approach, may kink (Fig. 3–18A). This will be recognized when advancing the catheter through the peel-away sheath; the catheter advances to the point of the kink of the sheath but no further (Fig. 3–18B). Long, curved peel-away sheaths are now available (in 9 F and 10 F sizes), which minimize this problem in placement of smaller catheters. This problem is especially pronounced with large dialysis catheters from a left internal jugular vein approach. In this case, insert the catheter into the peel-away sheath as far as possible (to the kink). Then advance stiff glidewires through each lumen of the dialysis catheter (Fig. 3–18C). It may be difficult to advance the guidewire through an acutely turned catheter that is not fully advanced into the vein and with a sharp loop at the venous entry site; however glidewires usually can traverse such a loop. Make sure that while advancing the glidewire, the catheter does not straighten out and get pulled out of the peel-away sheath. Advance the glidewire through the tip of the catheter and through the kinked portion of the sheath, into the right atrium. Ideally, both glidewires should be advanced as far as possible down the inferior vena cava to prevent losing access. The operator then pushes the catheter into the peel-away sheath while the assistant removes the peel-away sheath (Fig. 3–18D). Once the peel-away sheath has been pulled back far enough that it no longer is kinked at the curve, the catheter will advance over the glidewires into the superior vena cava and right atrium (Fig. 3–18E). The glidewires assure the venous access is not lost and allows easier tracking of the catheter. The stiffness of the glidewire also straightens the tortuousness of the veins.

CLOSING WOUNDS

Wound Healing

The sequence of events occurring from a full-thickness incision of the skin to a mature, remodeled scar is described because these events underlie the complications that may arise from skin incisions. Patients seem to judge the ability of the interventional radiologist based on three criteria: (1) Was the procedure painful? (2) Does the catheter work as expected? (3) How does the scar look? Assuming the patient has been comfortable during the procedure and that the catheter functions well, the cosmetic appearance of the wound(s) is an important final consideration and is, in fact, the only criterion that is permanent. Therefore, it is prudent to take time for careful closure of wounds using a refined suturing technique that will not leave unsightly scars in any patient.

Bridgens[92] describes wound healing as "a biologic process in which disrupted tissue surfaces attempt to restore their original integrity by proliferation of fibroblasts and elaboration of structurally stable collagen fibers." The best results are obtained by ensuring close apposition of the divided edges of tissue, where the clinician can make enormous differences in the healing outcome.

53

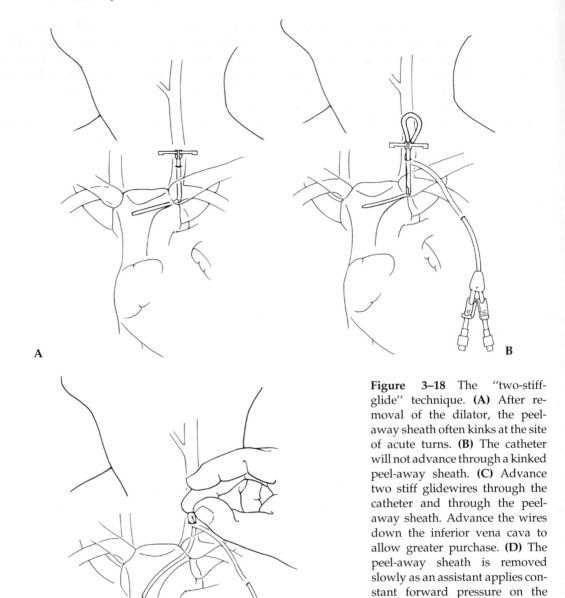

A

B

E

Figure 3–18 The "two-stiff-glide" technique. **(A)** After removal of the dilator, the peel-away sheath often kinks at the site of acute turns. **(B)** The catheter will not advance through a kinked peel-away sheath. **(C)** Advance two stiff glidewires through the catheter and through the peel-away sheath. Advance the wires down the inferior vena cava to allow greater purchase. **(D)** The peel-away sheath is removed slowly as an assistant applies constant forward pressure on the catheter. **(E)** When the peel-away sheath is pulled back far enough that the kink is no longer present, the catheter easily advances over the wires and is pushed into the vein. The wires now can be pinned and the catheter easily advanced over the wires and placed in final position.

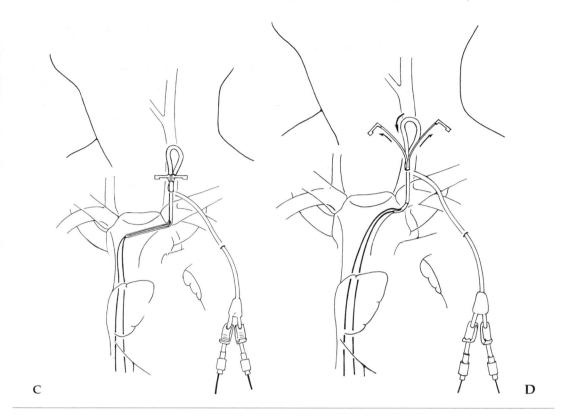

C   D

Normal wound repair occurs through a series of interactive phases progressing in an orderly and timely fashion. If any of these phases are prolonged or disordered, the repair process is deemed to be *chronic.* Causes of delayed wound healing include the following:

- Reinjury due to trauma or pressure (crushed vasculature)
- Vascular disease (venous, lymphatic, or arterial)
- Nutritional deficiency
- Compromised immune system
- Metabolic disorders (e.g., diabetes or gout)
- Infection (local or systemic)

There are three stages in wound healing: inflammation (or lag), proliferation (or fibroblastic), and maturation.[92,93] The first phase begins at approximately 12 hours, peaks at 36 hours, and resolves by the fifth day. This phase is basically an inflammatory reaction to the trauma, with phagocytosis of necrotic tissue, fluid, and bacteria as an attempt to repair the injury. Neutrophils and macrophages react with lymphocytes to stimulate fibroblast activity. Platelet-derived growth factor (PDGF), a protein produced by the activated platelet, is a critical part of the early stage of inflammation and is essential in the initiation of the wound repair process. Neutrophils decrease the bacterial count at the incision site and minimize local infection.

During the proliferative or fibroblastic phase, which takes place during days 5 to 15, fibroblast proliferation is the central activity. Fibroblasts arrive and replicate and synthesize collagen, glycoproteins, and mucopolysaccharides. The wound gains strength rapidly during this phase. During this phase, epithelium also migrates over the wound base. The wound is usually considered healed once it is covered with epithelium, which migrates across the granulation tissue surface, proliferates, and differentiates to form the outer layer, the stratum corneum.

The maturation phase may last several months and represents further organization, remodeling, and interweaving of collagen fibers and is essentially a balance between manufacture of new collagen and destruction of old collagen. The scarring mechanism appears to overcompensate (to protect against dehiscence) but, in time, collagen remodeling normalizes the scar. These phases make up a continuous process. Any disruption or prolongation of a phase will affect subsequent ones and adversely affect the course of events, which weakens the overall tensile strength of the scar.[94] As an example, if an immunocompromised patient is unable to mount a normal inflammatory response, phagocytosis of necrotic tissue may be delayed, and subsequent phases also may be delayed. The ultimate result may be a delayed healing and possibly decreased tensile strength of the wound. At the other extreme, an increased inflammatory reaction can prolong the lag phase as well, delaying subsequent phases of healing and resulting in a weakened wound. As such, care must be taken during the procedure to minimize trauma to the tissue so that the resulting inflammatory response is minimized and wound healing progresses without delay.

Suture Materials

Surgical sutures are sterile filaments used to approximate tissue edges until wound healing provides the wound with sufficient strength to withstand mechanical stress. The decision of which suture materials to use should be based on knowledge of factors such as the biologic, physical, and chemical characteristics of the sutures. The "ideal" suture would consist of inexpensive material that is easy to tie, holds the knot securely with excellent tensile strength, creates minimal tissue reaction, does promote bacterial growth, and, most importantly, causes no adverse effects on healing.

The characteristics of suture material are as follows.

- *Tissue reactivity* depends on the biologic properties of the suture material and is the degree of foreign body inflammatory response by tissue to the material. In general, natural materials (catgut, silk) are much more reactive than the synthetic materials (nylon, polypropylene). Greater tissue reactivity can result in an increased risk of wound infection with delayed healing.
- *Tensile strength* is the force required to break a suture, divided by the cross-sectional area of the suture. It varies with the diameter of the suture as well as the material itself. Stainless steel has the highest tensile strength of all suture materials, followed by the synthetic materials, and the materials with the least tensile strength are the natural fibers (e.g., silk).
- *Knot-holding ability* is the force necessary to cause a knot to slip. All other factors being equal, certain suture materials do hold knots better than others. The knot-holding ability of a given suture material is directly proportional to the friction of the suture material although other factors also pertain. The more slippery the suture material is, the easier it is to move through the tissues, but the more likely it is that the resulting knot will slip.
- *Configuration* may be monofilament (single-stranded) or multifilament (several strands are braided or twisted together). This refers to the construction of the suture material. Generally, braided sutures handle and tie more easily but can lead to increased infection due to the potential of harboring organisms between the filament strands.
- *Elasticity* is the inherent ability of the suture to regain its original strength after stretching (*strain*). A highly elastic suture material (*compliant*) has the

ability to allow for tissue swelling, and can be stretched so as not to cut into the swollen tissue. The opposite of compliant would be a suture material that is stiff.

- *Plasticity* is the ability for suture material to retain its new length and form after being stretched. Terms used to describe plasticity are *ductile* versus *brittle*.
- *Workability* is the ease of handling of the suture for knot tying. Silk is the standard to which all other materials are compared because of its exceptional handling characteristics.
- *Memory* is the suture's ability to return to its former shape after it has been deformed with tying and is related to the suture's elasticity and plasticity. More memory results in less knot security. Suture materials with a large amount of memory, such as prolene, will be stiff with poor workability. These high-memory sutures require increased number of ties to ensure that the knot does not slip. Materials with low memory, such as silk, are easy to handle (have high workability) and rarely become untied.
- *Color* Suture materials are often colorless but may be dyed either black or blue. If the suture will be left in place

and not removed, a colorless suture will be less conspicuous and will avoid unsightly show-through. Colored sutures allow easy visualization when a suture will be removed.

- *Suture diameter* The United States Pharmacopoeia has specified the system for a measurement of the diameter of suture material. The sutures used most commonly in catheter placement are the sizes 2.0, 3.0, and 4.0.

Absorbable Sutures

The United States Pharmacopeia (USP)[95] defines an *absorbable suture* as a sterile strand of material that is prepared from collagen derived from healthy mammals or a synthetic polymer that is capable of being absorbed by living mammal tissue. Absorbable sutures will lose most of their tensile strength within 60 days after being placed below the skin surface. More recently developed absorbable sutures are synthetic; these have superior mechanical properties compared with surgical gut,[96–101] including superior tensile strength, knot security, and handling properties. The biologic characteristics of these materials are also superior in that they incite far less tissue reaction and inflammation (Table 3–1). Absorbable suture materials include:

Table 3–1 Absorbable Sutures

Suture	Raw Material	Strength Half-Life (days)	Handling	Knot Security	Tissue Reaction
Surgical gut (plain)	Submucosa sheep intestine	4	Fair	Poor	Moderate–severe
Surgical gut (chromic)	As above, treated with chromic salts	7	Fair	Poor–moderate	Moderate
Dexon	Glycolic acid, braided	14	Good	Good–excellent	Low
Vicryl	Copolymer of lactide and glycolide	14	Good	Good–excellent	Low
Maxon	Monofilament, glycolic acid	28	Fair–good	Good	Low

- *Surgical Gut* is used infrequently today and was produced from the intestines of sheep or cattle. These sutures have poor tensile strength and poor knot stability and elicit an increased tissue reaction.
- *Polyglycolic Acid* (*Dexon*), a synthetic material, was introduced in 1970 as a polymer of glycolic acid. The tensile strength is good, with approximately 50% tensile strength remaining at 2 weeks. The material is totally degraded by hydrolysis at 90 days. The chief advantage of Dexon is the decreased inflammatory reaction.
- *Polyglactin 910* (*Vicryl*), introduced in 1974, is a braided copolymer lactide and glycolide with a lubricant coating, which allows less drag or friction. As with Dexon, this material is hydrolyzed and has decreased tissue reaction. Vicryl is absorbed slightly more quickly than Dexon, usually within 60 days. The material has a high tensile strength and comes in dyed or white material.
- *Polydioxanone* (*PDS*) was developed in 1980 and is a polymer of polydirinone. PDS has a prolonged tensile strength, with 58% of the original tensile strength present at 4 weeks. There is complete absorption of this suture material within tissues at 180 days. The material is stiffer, less pliable,

and more difficult to tie, but it also elicits a minimal tissue response.
- *Polytrimethylene Carbonate* (*Maxon*) is a synthetic monofilament with prolonged tensile strength such as with PDS but with improved handling over PDS. The tensile strength at 14 days is 81% and it is 59% at 4 weeks. There is complete absorption by 180 days. Again, minimal tissue reaction is elicited.

Nonabsorbable Sutures

By USP definition, *nonabsorbable sutures* are strands of material that are resistant to degradation by living mammalian tissue. The natural fibers, silk and cotton, consistently incite more tissue reaction than their synthetic counterparts and are responsible for the greatest incidence of infection.[96,102] The synthetic sutures cause significantly less tissue reaction, and those made of polypropylene are especially inert (Table 3–2). Nonabsorbable sutures include:

- *Silk* is a natural suture material from natural protein filaments spun by silk worm larvae. The material is usually dyed black for better visibility. Silk is the standard for having the highest workability, handling extremely well, and the easiest suture material to tie. The major disadvantages of silk are

Table 3–2 Nonabsorbable Sutures

Suture	Raw Material	Handling	Strength	Knot Security	Tissue Reaction
Cotton	Twisted cotton fibers	Good	Fair	Good	Severe
Silk	Braided silk fibers	Excellent	Good	Excellent	Moderate–severe
Ethilon	Monofilament nylon	Good	Excellent	Fair	Low
Dermalon	Monofilament nylon	Good	Excellent	Fair	Low
Prolene	Monofilament polypropylene	Fair–good	Excellent	Fair	Minimal
Ethibond	Braided polyester	Good	Excellent	Fair–good	Moderate

the very low tensile strength and the greater tissue reactivity of this material. Also, because silk is a braided multifilament, the risk of infection is increased.

- *Nylon* was first introduced in 1940 and was the first synthetic nonabsorbable suture. Nylon is widely used because of its minimal tissue reactivity, relatively high tensile strength, and relatively low cost. The disadvantages of nylon are its stiffness and high memory, which require an increased number of knot throws.
- *Polypropylene* (*Prolene, Surgilene*) are plastic sutures that are formed by the polymerization of propylene; they are flexible monofilaments with fair to good tensile strength, although not as strong as nylon. This smooth monofilament results in little drag and is easy to pull through tissues. The material is also very ductile (high plasticity) and compliant (high elasticity). These materials are especially inert, eliciting little tissue response, and are highly resistant to bacterial contamination. These materials have been described as the ideal skin closure material.
- *Polyesters* (*Dacron, Ethibond, and Mersilene*) are braided polyfilaments. They handle well and have high tensile strength, higher than nylon or prolene.

Knots

Square Knot

The most common knot used is the square knot, which will provide 80 to 90% of the tensile strength of an intact suture. Each strand of the square knot begins and ends on the same side of the knot. Because of this symmetry, it tends to tighten and remains secure when tension is applied equally to both strands. If the knot is not placed flat or if tension on the strands is uneven, the square knot twists into a half hitch knot, which slides and is extremely unstable (Fig. 3–19A).

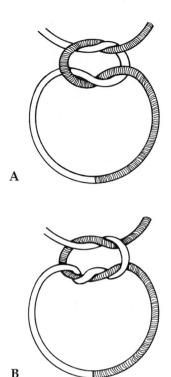

Figure 3–19 **(A)** The square knot. **(B)** The surgeon's knot.

Surgeon's Knot

This knot is similar to the square knot with the exception that the knot is started with a double throw instead of a single throw (single loop). The initial double throw provides increased friction to hold the wound together until the second throw can be placed (Fig. 3–19B).

Knot Tying

Two-Hand Tie

The two-hand tie technique is the most commonly used suture-tying technique. It allows creation of symmetrically tied knots, which are extremely stable (Fig. 3–20).

1. The process of tying the knot is performed using only the thumbs and index fingers of the two hands. The third, fourth, and fifth fingers are used only to pin the suture against

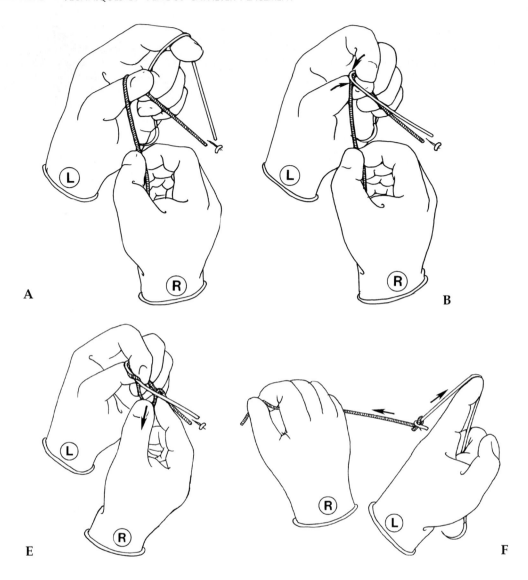

the palm of the hand and create tension on the suture. The needle end of the suture is draped over the index (second) finger, which is bent in a C-shape, and the suture is pinned against the palm by the bent third to fifth fingers to create tension on the suture (Fig. 3–20A).

2. The free end of the suture is wrapped around the left thumb so that it passes over the palmar surface of the tip of the thumb and then passes over the medial aspect of the thumb

(the surface of the thumb between the thumb and index finger) and finally the dorsal aspect of the thumb at approximately the level of the interphalangeal joint of the thumb. The free end of the suture is held by pinching the right thumb and index finger (Fig. 3–20B).

3. The left index finger opposes the thumb, forming an "o"; the needle end of the suture is allowed to slide down the lateral aspect of the index finger onto the thumb. The thumb

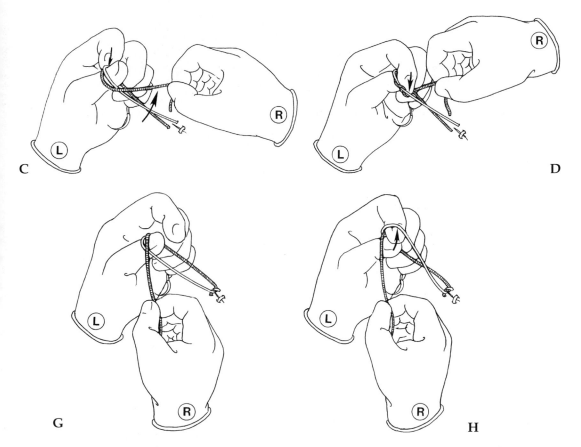

Figure 3–20 Two-hand tie (see text for step-by-step instructions). **(A)** The needle end of the suture is draped over the index finger and the suture is pinned against the palm to create tension on the suture. **(B)** The free end of the suture is held by pinching the right thumb and index finger. **(C)** The needle end of the suture is allowed to slide down the lateral aspect of the index finger onto the thumb. **(D)** Tension is maintained on the needle end of the suture by pinning it against the palm. **(E)** Tension is maintained on the needle end of the suture. Steps A to E could be repeated to create a surgeon's knot. **(F)** Tension is pulled on both ends of the suture, and the knot is laid down flat. **(G)** Tension is maintained by the second throw of the knot. **(H)** The left index finger opposes the left thumb such that the distal thumb is surrounded by a loop of suture. (*Figure continues on page 62.*)

now is encircled by the two ends of the suture: the needle end crossing the nail and the free end crossing on the dorsal surface (Fig. 3–20C).

4. The right hand brings the free end of the suture into position so that it can be pinched between the left thumb and index finger. The free end of the suture is pinned between the left thumb and index finger. Tension is maintained on the needle end of the suture by pinning it against the palm

with the third to fifth fingers and its position on the nail of the thumb is maintained (Fig. 3–20D).

5. In a rocking motion, while maintaining opposition of the left thumb and index finger, the free end of the suture is pulled down through the loop of suture, which was previously created around the thumb.

6. When the free end has been pulled through, the right hand lets go of the free end.

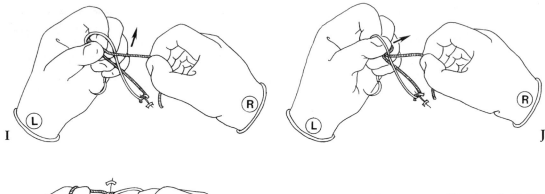

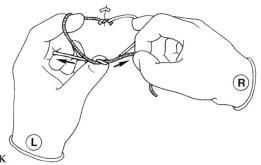

Figure 3–20 (*Continued*) **(I)** The free end of the suture is brought into position to be pinched between the left thumb and index finger. **(J)** The free end of the suture is brought through the loop. **(K)** Tension is applied to both ends of the suture and the knot is slid down onto the first throw of the knot.

7. The free end, which has now been pulled through the loop, is again grabbed by the right hand between the thumb and index finger. Tension is maintained on the needle end of the suture (Fig. 3–20E). **At this point, steps A–E can be repeated to create a surgeon's knot.**

8. Tension is pulled on both ends of the suture, and the knot is laid down "flat" on the skin (Fig. 3–20F).

9. The second throw of the knot is initiated by looping the needle end of the suture over the nail (dorsal aspect) of the left thumb and then pinning the suture against the palm of the left hand with the left third to fifth fingers. This tension is maintained throughout the second throw (Fig. 3–20G).

10. The free end of the suture is laid on the palmer aspect of the left thumb, and tension is maintained by the right hand.

11. The left index finger opposes the left thumb so that the distal thumb is surrounded by a loop of suture. The needle end is looped around the nail (dorsal) aspect of the thumb, and the free end is looped around the palmer aspect of the thumb (Fig. 3–20H).

12. The loop of suture slides onto the distal phalanx of the left index finger (Fig. 3–20I).

13. The right hand brings the free end of suture into position to be pinched between the left thumb and index finger.

14. In a rocking motion, the thumb rocks upward through the loop of suture, bringing the free end through the loop.

15. The free end is released temporarily by the right hand (Fig. 3–20J).

16. After being pulled through the loop, the free end is again grabbed by the right hand.

17. Tension is applied to both ends of the suture and the knot is slid down onto the first throw of the knot (Fig. 3–20K).

18. The ends of the suture should be held in control at all times. The left hand always has control of the needle end

of the suture, and the right hand has control of the free end of the suture. This may be reversed for someone who is left-handed.

Instrument Tie

1. The needle end of the suture is pulled through the tissue such that only a short free end is left.
2. The needle end is pulled taut, and the needle driver is positioned directly over the wound and placed against the needle end of the suture, which then is wrapped once or twice around the needle driver (Fig. 3–21A).
3. The needle driver then is opened and used to grab the short end of the suture (Fig. 3–21B).
4. The suture, which was wrapped around the needle holder, is slid down the needle driver and the free end of the suture, pulling it through the loop (Fig. 3–21C).
5. Keeping the free end of the suture grasped with the needle driver and tension on the needle end of the suture being provided by the left hand, the two ends are pulled across the wound so that the loops lie flat against the wound without any bunching.
6. For the second throw, the needle end of the suture is again held with tension, and the needle holder is pressed against it but on the opposite side of the suture (i.e., the needle holder is pushed against the nonwound side of the suture).
7. The suture is looped around the needle holder once, which should be in the opposite direction of the first loop (Fig. 3–21D).
8. The needle holder is opened and the short, free end of the suture is grasped with the needle holder (Fig. 3–21E).
9. Again, the loop around the needle holder is slid down and the free end of the suture is pulled through the loop (Fig. 3–21F).

10. For the third tie, the suture is wrapped around the needle holder once in the original direction, and the short end is grasped and pulled through. Tension should be kept on the first throw to prevent slippage. Three to six throws are usually required depending on the friction coefficient and memory of the suture material used.
11. The knot should be tied as to lie flat against the skin surface with perfect opposition of the wound edges. There should not be significant tension or tightness on the two edges. Increased tension on the wound edges risks wound edge strangulation and possible necrosis.

Suturing Techniques

Basic Principles

- The suturing needle can be subdivided into the fine point, flattened body and the swage, which is the attachment to the needle and is the broadest point of the needle.
- The needle holder always should be clamped onto the midbody of the needle, approximately one half to three fourths of the way from the tip to the swage. Do not clamp onto the rounded swage, which can lead to twisting of the needle in the needle holder.
- The needle should be positioned within the needle holder at the end of the jaws. This allows for greater accuracy and precision in suturing.
- The needle holder may be grasped in the hand in one of two ways: the first is with the thumb and the middle or ring finger through the loops of the instrument. The index finger should be extended and rest on the arms of the instrument with the tip of the index finger at or near the fulcrum of the instrument. None of the fingers is inserted past the first knuckle to allow for maximum dexterity and rotation. The second way is to palm the instrument, which involves pla-

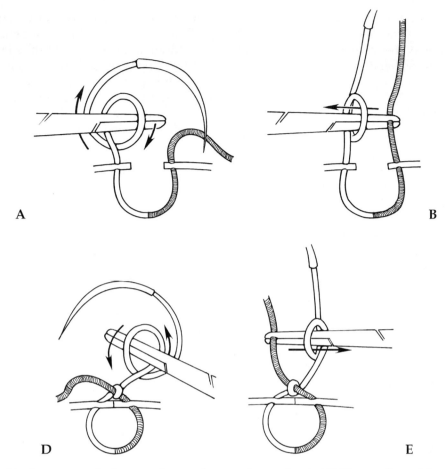

Figure 3–21 Instrument tie (see text for step-by-step instructions). **(A)** The needle end is pulled taut and then is wrapped once or twice around the needle driver. **(B)** The needle driver is used to grab the short end of the suture. **(C)** The wrapped suture is slid down the needle driver and the free end of the suture, and pulled through the loop. **(D)** The suture is looped around the needle holder once, which should be in the opposite direction of the first loop. **(E)** The needle holder is opened and the short free end of the suture is grasped with the needle holder. **(F)** The loop around the needle holder is slid down and the free end of the suture is pulled through the loop.

cing both loops of the instrument within the palm and the second, third, fourth, and fifth fingers curled over the loops, grasping the instrument in a fist-like manner (Fig. 3–22). The index finger is extended over the arms of the instrument with the tip of the index finger at or near the fulcrum of the instrument.

• The needle always should penetrate the surface of the skin or tissue perpendicularly (Fig. 3–23). The needle tip is the sharpest point, and it allows easiest passage through the skin or other tissues. The needle should be rotated only after the initial perpendicular penetration.

• Stabilize the hand on the patient so that with the suddenness of the penetration of the needle tip through the skin, the operator does not reflexively withdraw the needle.

Simple Interrupted Sutures

There are several advantages to using the simple interrupted suture, not the least of

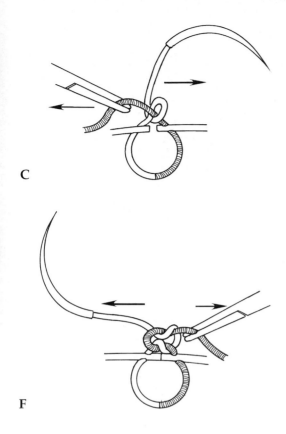

C

F

surface. With inversion of skin edges, healing occurs below the surface and a slight trough will occur along the suture line.

HELPFUL HINTS
Using minimally reactive sutures such as polypropylene, suture marks are reduced. The sutures also should be removed as soon as possible, usually around 7 days to reduce suture marks.

Vertical Mattress Suture
The advantages of this technique are that it ensures eversion of the skin edges and closes gaps below the skin surface; however, because this technique leaves four suture holes, it should be used only when these indications exist. Applications in a catheter service may include closure of the wound following removal of a port where there is a large dead space with overhanging epidermal edges (Fig. 3–24).

Initially performing a wide interrupted suture 5 to 10 mm from the wound edges creates the vertical mattress suture. The needle puncture sites should be of equal

which is ease of use. This stitch also can be performed quickly. In addition, the simple interrupted suture is useful for making minute adjustments to the wound edges for proper alignment. This stitch has greater security than a running stitch. The principal disadvantage of the stitch is the railroad track scarring that results.

The needle enters the skin at a 90-degree angle approximately 1 to 2 mm from the wound edge. After penetration, the needle should be redirected to proceed in a slightly oblique direction away from the wound edge to the desired depth. The needle tip then is directed across the wound, to the other side of the wound, where its course should follow a mirror image of the first side. This creates a flask-like shape of the loop. Because there is a greater amount of tissue being pushed together deeply, eversion of the wound edges results, which is desirable. Eversion of wound edges is important because it allows wound healing to occur evenly with regard to the skin

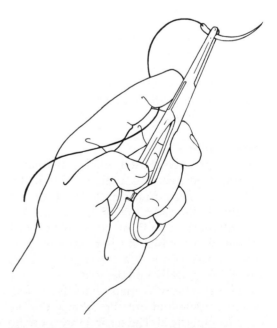

Figure 3–22 Palming the needle holder.

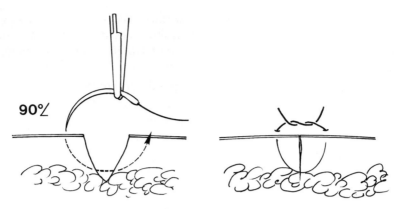

Figure 3–23 Simple interrupted suture. The skin is punctured 1 to 2 mm from the wound edge. The needle point always should be perpendicular to the tissue being punctured. In a circular motion, the needle is directed across the wound and should exit the skin 1 to 2 mm from the wound edge. A square knot or surgeon's knot is tied in an attempt to evert the wound edges.

distance from the wound edges. A flask-like configuration of the loop is again desirable. This closes any dead space under the skin surface. After exiting the skin, the needle is reinserted on the same side but closer to the wound edge. The second puncture occurs within the first loop and should be within 1 to 2 mm of the wound edge. A flask-like configuration of the second loop again is performed, and the stitch is completed on the opposite side in the epidermis.

Horizontal Mattress Suture
This stitch is usually used to secure large flaps. Use in catheter placement should be nil. The primary purpose of this stitch is to reduce tension across wound closures under significant tension.

Buried Sutures
Buried sutures are used when a two-layer closure is needed. Absorbable suture material is used. The purpose of these sutures are to bring the incision together, allowing the second more superficial layer to be used primarily for cosmetic, not tension, purposes. Because this is a "strength" suture, 2-0 or 3-0 typically will be used.

The first throw is made into the subcutaneous tissue and out the dermis, that is, deep to superficial. The second throw on the other side of the incision is made from the

dermis to the subcutaneous tissue, that is, superficial to deep. The resulting knot then is placed away from the incision.

Running Subcuticular Suture
The running subcuticular suture removes almost all suturing from the epidermis and with it the possibility of any suture tracks in the final scar. It is one of the most difficult sutures to place, but properly placed, it results in a most elegant closure. When absorbable sutures are used, such as Vicryl or Dexon, the suture may be left in place.

Techniques: Initiating the Stitch (Corner Stitch) The running subcuticular stitch may be initiated in several ways:

1. Puncture the skin several millimeters from the apex of the wound (Fig. 3–25 A,B), bringing the needle out of the apex at the subcuticular layer (the shallow dermis). A knot is then tied at the end of the suture, which exits through the skin puncture site. This particular initial stitch should be used when a permanent suture such as Prolene is being used and will be removed when the wound has healed.

2. Take a deep bite of subcutaneous tissue at the apex of the wound, and bring the

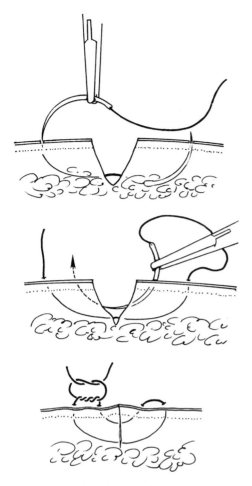

Figure 3–24 Vertical mattress suture. Puncture 5 to 10 mm from the wound edge and advance the needle across the wound, exiting 5 to 10 mm from the wound edge. Puncture on the same side that the needle exited, 1 to 2 mm from the wound edge. Advance the needle back through the wound and exit 1 to 2 mm from the wound edge. A square knot or surgeon's knot is tied.

needle out of the subcuticular layer at the apex of the wound. A short tail is left, and a knot is tied using an instrument tie (Fig. 3–25 C,D). Make sure that the knot is not tied too snuggly so that the subcutaneous tissue is not torn. This technique can be used when an absorbable suture material is used.

3. The initial puncture of the subcuticular layer is performed approximately 5 mm from the apex of the wound, bringing

the needle out at the apex of the subcuticular layer (Fig. 3–25 E,F). The subcuticular layer is again punctured at the apex bringing the needle out on the opposite side of the wound, an equal distance from the apex as the initial puncture. An instrument tie is performed closing the apex. Care must be taken to ensure that the initial knot does not slip, allowing gaping of the wound at this end of the wound. The short tail of the suture is cut close to the knot.

The Running Stitch Regardless of how the stitch was initiated, the result is a needle and suture secured at one end of the wound, exiting from the wound through the subcuticular layer, near the apex. The needle then is passed from one side of the wound to the other in the shallow dermis (subcuticular) layer, taking a horizontal bite on each side and continuing down the length of the wound, backtracking slightly with each pass across the wound (Fig. 3–26 A, B). With each bite, the needle is brought out within the wound, grasped with the forceps and pulled through.

HELPFUL HINTS
- **The smaller the bite with each pass, the better the wound approximation.**
- **Remember to puncture the subcuticular layer perpendicular with the needle tip, turning the needle only after penetrating the tissue.**
- **The needle (and therefore the suture) should pass through the mid-dermal layer. The needle should be passed parallel to the skin, maintaining the same depths throughout the bite.**
- **The subcuticular layer can be more easily seen by everting the skin edge with forceps (Fig. 3–26A). The skin must be grasped gently with the forceps, however, to minimize tissue trauma.**
- **After pulling through the needle and suture, have an assistant apply slight tension to the suture, holding the**

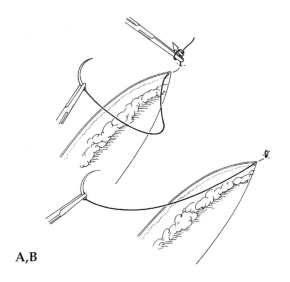

A,B

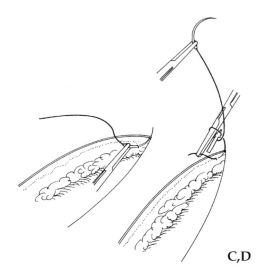

C,D

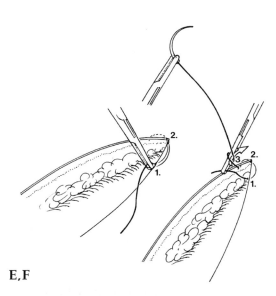

E,F

Figure 3–25 The corner stitch. Methods of initiating a running subcuticular stitch. **(A,B)** Puncture the skin 2 to 4 mm from the apex of the wound, bringing the needle out of the subcuticular layer at the apex. Instrument tie the tail of the suture. **(C,D)** Puncture the subcutaneous tissue within the wound, bringing the needle out of the subcuticular layer at the apex. Instrument tie and cut the tail of the suture at the knot. **(E,F)** Puncture the subcuticular layer approximately 5 mm from the apex of the wound (*1*). Advance the needle through the subcuticular layer, bringing the needle out of the subcuticular layer at the apex (*2*). Again puncture the subcuticular layer at the apex (*2*) and advance the needle through the subcuticular layer on the opposite side of the wound, bringing the needle out approximately 5 mm from the apex (*3*). It is important that the two ends of the suture exit the tissue an equal distance from the apex (i.e., segment 1 to 2 is equal to segment 2 to 3). An instrument tie is performed, and the tail is cut at the knot.

previously sutured portion of the wound closed under tension and holding open the remaining wound. This allows better visualization of the wound edges.
- Do not "backtrack" with punctures such that the subcuticular bites are interlocked.
- Brace your hand with the needle holder on the patient by resting your wrist or your small finger on the patient. This allows more precise puncture and more control of the needle.

Ending the Stitch There are two methods of ending the running subcuticular stitch:

1. Do not pull the suture completely through after taking the last bite. Leave a long loop, which will be used to tie

a knot, using either the two-hand tie or an instrument tie (Fig. 3–26B). Before tying the final knot, be sure to apply tension on the looped end such that the entire running subcuticular stitch is under slight tension, closing the wound completely. The suture is ended by tying it to the last loop that has been placed (Fig. 3–26C). Using the looped end and the needle end of the suture, a knot is tied (Fig. 3–26D). The loop end then is cut, close to the knot, leaving the needle end of the suture. The needle then is used to take a deep bite into the subcutaneous tissue, bringing the needle out 5 to 10 mm beyond the apex of the wound (Fig. 3–26E). This should pull the knot into the wound and bury the knot. The suture then is cut at the skin level. This technique may be used when using an absorbable suture.

2. If nonabsorbable sutures are used, as the distal end of the wound is reached, the needle is passed out from the wound, exiting at 5 to 10 mm from the apex of the wound. Tension is applied to the suture to close the gaps in the wound. The suture is wrapped around the needle holder twice, and the suture is clamped approximately 5 mm above the skin level, forming a loop. The looped portion of the suture is pushed down to the skin, creating a knot. The instrument tie then is continued.

Securing the Catheter in Place

There are two major methods of securing catheters into place. Most catheter kits include wings, which may be sutured to the catheter and then sutured to the skin. Alternatively, a suture may be tied to the skin, looped around the catheter, and tied to the catheter, securing the catheter into place.

Using the Provided Wings
The wings must fit snugly over the catheter. Making sure not to pull the catheter, the wings are gaped open and placed over the catheter. It is better to position the wings close to the skin exit site so that the catheter can not be accidentally pulled during dressing changes. Two stitches are tied on either side of the wings with the sutures within the provided grooves of the wings. After securing the wings to the catheter, the wings are sutured to the skin. A simple interrupted suture is tied. There is no need to (and it is undesirable to) tie this stitch tightly to the skin because to do so can result in difficulty in removing the stitch and pain to the patient when the stitch is eventually removed. Instead, create a loop by first tying a knot with a clamp or dilator on the skin. After tying a knot, the suture then is passed through the hole in the wing and another square knot is tied. Disadvantages of using the provided wings include that two additional needle punctures are made, causing additional scarring. Also, four knots must be tied, which is time-consuming. Finally, the tension of the sutures on the catheter (holding the wings to the catheter) is critical, and it is slightly more difficult to judge how snuggly the loop is being tied with the wings in place as opposed to tying the stitch directly to the catheter.

Tying the Suture Directly to the Catheter
A suture, after being tied to the skin, can be looped directly around the catheter and a knot tied, securing the catheter into place. Using this technique, the skin suture may be used to close the skin exit site snuggly around the catheter (Fig. 3–27A,B) in a "pursestring" manner.

After tying this knot to the skin, the two ends of the suture are looped around the catheter twice. A two-hand tie technique is used to tie a surgeon's knot or square knot (Fig. 3–27 C,D). Again, tension on the knot and loop is critical. The advantage of this technique is that one can visualize how snuggly the suture is being tied to the catheter. The knot should be tied such that the suture loop barely indents the catheter. Always test the catheter after tying this knot to ensure that adequate flow rates still can be obtained. After tying the initial surgeon's knot or square knot the two ends

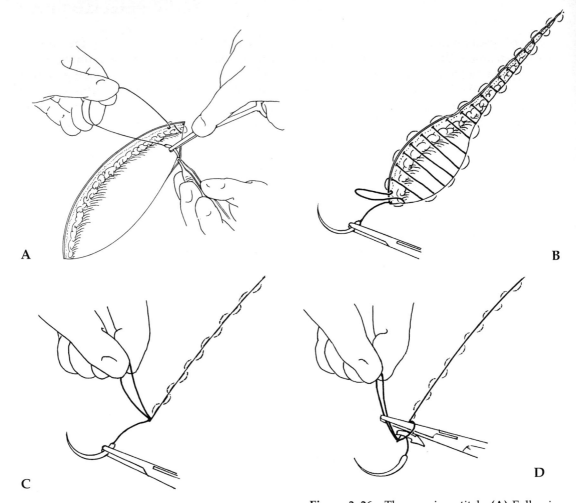

A

B

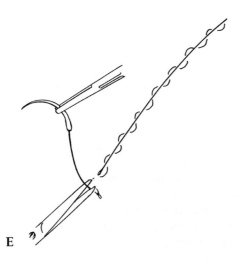

C

D

E

Figure 3–26 The running stitch. **(A)** Following the corner stitch, begin taking alternating bites on each side of the wound. The needle should enter the tissue in the subcuticular layer, advance through this layer, and exit from this layer (parallel to and always at the same depth from the skin surface). Equal bites should be taken each time, and opposing exit and entrance sites should align. **(B)** Continue alternating from side to side until the other apex of the wound is reached. When the final bite is taken, bringing the needle out of the apex, do not pull the suture completely through, leaving a loop, which will be used for the final corner stitch. **(C)** Apply tension on the loop to tighten the stitch and oppose the two edges of the wound. **(D)** Use the needle end of the suture and the loop to instrument tie a knot. The loop (but not the needle end of suture) is cut near the knot. **(E)** The needle then is passed through the wound, taking a bite with the needle exiting the skin at a distance of 2 to 5 mm from the wound apex. The suture is pulled to bury the knot and then cut at the skin.

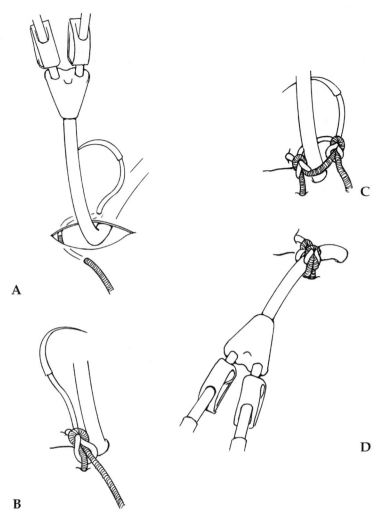

Figure 3–27 Securing the catheter. **(A)** The catheter is lifted off the skin. The initial puncture with the needle is made directly inferior to the skin exit site and the needle is brought out of the lateral aspect of the incision. The needle again is advanced through the lateral aspect of the incision and brought out of the skin directly superior to the skin exit site. **(B)** The suture is pulled through such that the two ends of the suture are of equal length. The needle can be cut off at this point. A square knot or surgeon's knot is tied using the two-hand technique. The resulting knot should "pursestring" the incision around the catheter. **(C,D)** The two ends of suture are wrapped around the catheter, and a surgeon's knot is tied. After tying this initial knot, the two ends of suture can be wrapped around the catheter again and another surgeon's knot tied.

of the suture again are wrapped around the catheter, and another knot is tied.

HELPFUL HINTS
Should one determine that a knot is too tight and must removed, use a scalpel to cut the knot, not the loop around the catheter. When using a suture with "memory," such as Prolene, cutting the knot will allow the knot to unravel and untie. Cutting the loop over the catheter endangers cutting the catheter.

REFERENCES

1. Crow S. It's second nature to me now. *Today's OR Nurse.* 1990;12:6–8.
2. Gruendemann BJ. Surgical asepsis revisited. *Today's OR Nurse.* 1990;12:10–14.
3. Condon RE, Quebbeman EJ. Preparing the operating room. In: Wilmore DW, Brennan FM, Harken AH, Holcroft JW, Meakins JL, eds. *Care of the Surgical Patient,* Vol 2. New York, NY: Scientific American; 1988:82–85.
4. Flugge C. Uber Luftinfection. *2 Hyg* 1897; 25:139–224.
5. Meleny FL, Stevens FA. Postoperative haemolytic streptococcus wound infections and their relation to haemolytic streptococcus carriers among the operating personnel. *Surg Gynecol Obstet.* 1926; 43:338–342.
6. Meleny FL. Infection in clean operative wounds: a nine year study *Surg Gynecol Obstet.* 1935;60:264–275.
7. Orr NWM. Is a mask necessary in the operating theater? *Ann R Coll Surg Engl.* 1981;63:390–392.
8. Mitchell NJ, Hunt S. Surgical face masks in modern operating rooms: a costly and unnecessary ritual? *J Hosp Infect.* 1991;18: 238–242.
9. Tunevall TG. Postoperative wound infections and surgical face masks: a controlled study. *World J Surg.* 1991;15:383–387.
10. Jepsen OB, Pers C, Lester A, Jensen A. Importance of surgical masks for perioperative asepsis. *Ugeskr Laeger.* 1993;155: 1990–1942.
11. Ruthman JC, Hendrickson D, Miller RF, Quigg DL. Effect of cap and mask on infection rates in wounds sutured in the emergency department. *Illinois Med J.* 1984;165:397–399.
12. Letts RM, Doermer E. Conversation in the operating theater as a cause of airborne bacterial contamination. *J Bone Joint Surg Am.* 1983;65:357–362.
13. Belkin NL. The surgical mask: is it still necessary? *Surgery.* 1997;122:641–642.
14. Jones MA, Johnson JC, French MLV, Hart JB, Ritter MA. Unidirectional airflow and surgical facemask exhaust system in the prevention of airborne surgical infection. *Am J Surg.* 1972;124:49–51.
15. Beck WC. The surgical mask. *The Guthrie J.* 1993;62:97–98.
16. Ritter MA, Eitzen H, French ML, Hart JB. The operating room environment as affected by people and the surgical facemask. *Clin Orthop.* 1975;III(section II): 147–150.
17. Konig M, Bruha M, Hirsch HA. Perforation of surgical gloves in gynecologic operations and abdominal caesarian section. *Geburtshilfe Frauenheilkd.* 1992;52:109–112.
18. McLeod GG. Needlestick injuries at operations for trauma: are surgical gloves an effective barrier? *J Bone Joint Surg Br.* 1989; 71:489–491.
19. Devenish EA, Miles AA. Control of *Staphylococcus aureus* in an operating theater. *Lancet.* 1939;1:1088–1094.
20. Miller JM, Collier CS, Griffith NM. Permeability of surgical rubber gloves. *Am J Surg.* 1972;124:57–59.
21. Russell TR, Roque FE, Miller FE. A new method for detection of the leaky glove: a study on incidence of defective gloves and bacterial growth from surgeons hands. *Arch Surg.* 1966;93:245–249.
22. Cole RP, Gault DT. Glove perforation during plastic surgery. *Br J Plast Surg.* 1989;42:481–483.
23. Leclair J. A review of antiseptics. *Today's OR Nurse.* 1990;12:25–28.
24. Dahl J, Wheeler B, Mukherjee D. Effect of chlorhexidine scrub on postoperative bacterial counts. *Am J Surg.* 1990;159: 486–488.
25. Brown TR, Ehrlich CE, Stehman FB, Golichowski AM, Mandura JA, Eitzen HE. A clinical evaluation of chlorhexidine gluconate spray as compared with iodophor scrub for preoperative skin preparation. *Surg Gynecol Obstet.* 1984;158:363–366.
26. Aly R, Maibach HI. Comparative antibacterial efficacy of a 2-minute surgical scrub with chlorhexidine gluconate, povidone-iodine, and chloroxylenol sponge-brushes. *Am J Infect Control.* 1988;16:173–177.
27. Faogali J, Fong J, George N, Mahoney P, O'Rourke V. Comparison of the immediate, residual and cumulative antibacterial effects of Novaderm R, Novascrub R, Betadine Surgical Scrub, Hibiclens, and liquid soap. *Am J Infect Control.* 1995;23:337–343.
28. Craig CP. Preparation of the skin for surgery. *Today's OR Nurse.* 1986;5:17–20.
29. Ritter MA, French ML, Eitzen HE, Gioe TJ. The antimicrobial effectiveness of operative-site preparative agents: a microbiologi-

cal and clinical study. *J Bone Joint Surg Am.* 1980;62:826–828.

30. Tucci VJ, Stone AM, Thompson C, Isenberg HD, Wise L. Studies of surgical scrub. *Surg Gynecol Obstet.* 1977;145:415–416.

31. Dineen P. An evaluation of the duration of the surgical scrub. *Surg Gynecol Obstet.* 1969;129:1181–1189.

32. Galle PC, Homesley HD, Rhyne AL. Reassessment of the surgical scrub. *Surg Gynecol Obstet.* 1978;147:215–218.

33. O'Shaughnessy M, O'Malley VP, Corbett G, Given HF. Optimum duration of surgical scrub time. *Br J Surg.* 1991;78:685–686.

34. Wheelock SM, Lookinland S. Effect of surgical hand scrub time on subsequent bacterial growth. *AORN J* 1997;65:1087–1092, 1094–1098.

35. Leonas KK, Jinkins RS. The relationship of selected fabric characteristics and the barrier effectiveness of surgical gown fabrics. *Am J Infect Control.* 1997;25:16–23.

36. Garibaldi RA, Skolnick D, Lerer T, et al. The impact of preoperative skin disinfection on preventing intraoperative wound contamination. *Infect Control Hosp Epidemiol.* 1998;9:109–113.

37. Sebben JE. Sterile techniques and the prevention of wound infection in office surgery. Part II. *J Dermatol Surg Oncol* 1990;1:38–48

38. Seropian R, Reynolds BM. Wound infections after postoperative depilatory versus razor preparation. *Am J Surg* 1971;121:251–252.

39. Cruse PJE, Foord R. A five-year prospective study of 23,649 surgical wounds. *Arch Surg.* 1973; 107:206–209.

40. Alexander JW, Fischer JE, Boyajian M, Palaiquist J, Morris MJ. The influence of hair-removal methods on wound infections. *Arch Surg* 1983;118:347–351.

41. Hamilton HW, Hamilton KR, Lone FJ. Preoperative hair removal. *Can J Surg.* 1977;20:269-275.

42. Lowbury EJL. Skin preparation for operation. *Br J Hosp Med.* 1973;10:627–634.

43. Lowbury EJL, Lilly HA, Bull JP. Disinfection of the skin of operative sites. *BMJ.* 1960;2:1039–1044.

44. Selwyn S, Ellis H. Skin bacteria and skin disinfection reconsidered. *BMJ.* 1972; 1:136–140.

45. Raad II, Hohn DC, Gilbreath BJ, et al. Prevention of central venous catheter-related infections by using maximal sterile barrier precautions during insertion. *Infect Control Hosp Epidemiol.* 1994;15:231–238.

46. Klein BS, Perloff WH, Maki DG. Reduction of nosocomial infection during pediatric intensive care by protective isolation. *N Engl J Med.* 1989;320:1717–1721.

47. Melmel LA, McCormick RD, Springman SR, Maki DG. The pathogenesis and epidemiology of catheter-related infection with pulmonary artery Swan-Ganz catheters: a prospective study using molecular subtyping. *Am J Med.* 1991;91(suppl 3B): 197–205.

48. Parham SM, Pasieka JL. Effect of pH modification by bicarbonate on pain after subcutaneous lidocaine injection. *Can J Surg.* 1996;39:31–35.

49. Davidson JA, Boom SJ. Warming lidocaine to reduce pain associated with injection. *BMJ.* 1992;305:617.

50. Williams HO. A study of pH of dental local anesthetic solutions [letter.] *Br Dent J.* 1985;158:119.

51. McKay W, Morris R, Mushlin P. Sodium bicarbonate attenuates pain on skin infiltration with lidocaine, with or without epinephrine. *Anesth Analag.* 1987;66: 572–574.

52. Christoph RA, Buchanan L, Begalla K, Schwartz S. Pain reduction in local anesthetic administration through pH buffering. *Ann Emerg Med.* 1988;17:117–120.

53. Morris RW, Whish DKM. A controlled trial of pain on skin infiltration with local anesthetics. *Anaesth Intensive Care.* 1984;12: 113–114.

54. Hilgier H. Alkalinization of burpivacaine for brachial plexus block. *Reg Anesth.* 1985; 10:59–61.

55. Bartfield JM, Gennis P, Barbera J, et al. Buffered versus plain lidocaine as a local anesthetic for simple laceration repair. *Ann Emerg Med.* 1990;19:1387–1389.

56. Bartfield JM, Homer PJ, Ford DT, et al. Buffered lidocaine as a local anesthetic: an investigation of shelf life. *Ann Emerg Med.* 1992;21:16–19.

57. Bartfield JM, Ford DT, Homer PJ. Buffered versus plain lidocaine for digital nerve blocks. *Ann Emerg Med.* 1993;22:216–219.

58. Martin AJ. PH-adjustment and discomfort caused by the intradermal injection of lignocaine. *Anesthesia* 1990;45:975–978.

59. Matsumoto AH, Reifsnyder AC, Hartwell GD, Angle JF, Selby JB Jr, Tegtmeyer CJ. Reducing the discomfort of lidocaine administration through pH buffering. *J Vasc Interv Radiol.* 1994;5:171–175.

60. Nelson AL. Neutralizing pH of lidocaine reduces pain during Norplant system insertion procedure. *Contraception.* 1995;51: 299–301.

61. Friedman HE, Jules KT, Springer K, Jennings M. Buffered lidocaine decreases the pain of digital anesthesia in the foot. *J Am Podiatr Med Assoc.* 1997;87:219–223.

62. Klein JA. Anesthesia for liposuction in dermatologic surgery. *J Dermatol Surg Oncol.* 1988;14:1124–1132.

63. Stewart JH, Chinn SE, Cole GW, Klein JA. Neutralized lidocaine with epinephrine for local anesthesia. *J Dermatol Surg Oncol.* 1990;16:842–845.

64. Siegel RU, Vistnes LM, Iverson RE. Effective hemostasis with less epinephrine. *Plast Reconst Surg.* 1973;51:129–133.

65. Siegal RU, Vistnes LM. Epinephrine requirements for effective hemostasis in local anesthetics. *Surg Forum.* 1972;23:514–516.

66. Millay DJ, Larrabee WF. Carpenter RL. Vasoconstrictors in facial plastic surgery. *Arch Otolaryngol Head Neck Surg.* 1991;117: 160–163.

67. Wilmink H, Spauwen PHM, Hartman EHM, Hendriks JCM, Koeijers VF. Preoperative injection using a diluted anesthetic/adrenaline solution significantly reduces blood loss in reduction mammoplasty. *Plast Reconstr Surg.* 1998;102:373–376.

68. Verma SK, Henderson HP. A prospective trial of adrenaline infiltration for controlling bleeding during surgery for gynaecomastia. *Br J Plast Surg.* 1990;43:590–593.

69. Brantner JN, Peterson HD. The role of vasoconstrictors in control of blood loss in reduction mammoplasty. *Plast Reconstr Surg.* 1985;75:339–341.

70. Grubb W. A concentration of 1:500,000 epinephrine in a local anesthetic solution is sufficient to provide excellent hemostasis. *Plast Reconstr Surg.* 1979;63:834–836.

71. Hirshowitz B, Eliachar I. Effective haemostasis with local anaesthesia in nasal surgery. *Br J Plast Surg.* 1972;25:335–341.

72. Liv S, Carpenter RL, Chiu AA, McGill TJ, Mantell SA. Epinephrine prolongs duration of subcutaneous infiltration of local anesthesia in a dose-related manner. *Reg Anesth.* 1995;20:378–384.

73. Tverskoy M, Cozacov C, Ayache M, Bradley EL, Kissin I. Postoperative pain after inguinal herniorraphy with different types of anesthesia. *Anesth Analg.* 1990;70: 29–35.

74. Ejlersen E, Anderson HB, Eliasen K, Morgensen TA. A comparison between pre- and post-incisional lidocaine infiltration on post-operative pain. *Anesth Analg.* 1992;74:495–498.

75. Dahl JB, Moiniche S, Kehlet H. Wound infiltration with local anesthetics for postoperative pain relief. *Acta Anaesth Scand.* 1994;38:7–14.

76. Bodvall B, Rais O. Effects of infiltration anaesthesia on the healing of incisions in traumatized and non-traumatized tissues. *Acta Chir Scand.* 1962;123:83–91.

77. Wu G, Calamel PM, Shedd DP. The hazards of injecting local anesthetic solutions with epinephrine into flaps. *Plast Reconstr Surg.* 1978;62:396–403.

78. Dunlevy TM, O'Malley TP, Postma GN. Optimal concentration of epinephrine for vasoconstriction in neck surgery. *Laryngoscope* 1996;106:1412–1414.

79. Berquist TH, Bailey PB, Cortese DA, et al. Transthoracic needle biopsy. Accuracy and complications in relation to location and type of lesion. *Mayo Clin Proc* 1980;55: 475–481.

80. Sinner WN. Complications of percutaneous transthoracic needle aspiration biopsy. *Acta Radiol.* 1976;17:813–828.

81. Denys BG, Uretsky BF, Reddy PS. Ultrasound-assisted cannulation of the internal jugular vein: a prospective comparison to the external landmark-guided technique. *Circulation.* 1993;87:1557–1562.

82. Mauro MA, Jaques PF. Radiologic placement of long-term central venous catheters: a review. *J Vasc Interv Radiol.* 1993;4:127–137.

83. Schnabel KJ, Simons ME, Zevallos GF, et al. Image-guided insertion of the Uldall tunneled hemodialysis catheter: technical success and clinical follow-up. *J Vasc Interv Radiol.* 1997;8:579–586.

84. Randolph AG, Cook DJ, Gonzales CA, Pribble CG. Ultrasound guidance for placement of central venous catheters: a meta-analysis of the literature. *Crit Care Med.* 1996;24:2053–2058.

85. Moosman DA. The anatomy of infraclavicular subclavian vein catheterization and its complications. *Surg Gynecol Obstet.* 1973; 136:71–74.

86. Lechner P, Anderhuber F, Tesch NP. Anatomical bases for a safe method of subclavian venipuncture. *Surg Radiol Anat.* 1989;11:91–95.

87. Aubaniac R. Nouvelle voie d'injection ou de poncture veineuse: la voie sousclaviculaire. *Sem Hop Paris.* 1952;28:3445–3450.

88. Jaques PF, Campbell WE, Dumbleton S. Mauro M. The first rib as a fluoroscopic marker for subclavian vein access. *J Vasc Interv Radiol.* 1995;6:619–622.

89. Page AC, Evans RA, Kaczmarski R, Mufti GF, Gishen P. The insertion of chronic indwelling central venous catheters (Hickman lines) in interventional radiology suites. *Clin Radiol.* 1990;42:105–109.

90. Gualtieri E, Deppe SA, Sipperly ME, Thompson DR. Subclavian venous catheterization: Greater success rate for less experienced operators using ultrasound guidance. *Crit Care Med.* 1995;23:692–697.

91. Nazarian GK, Bjarnason H, Dietz CA, Bernadas CA, Hunter DW. Changes in tunneled catheter tip position when a patient is upright. *J Vasc Interv.* 1997;8:437–441.

92. Bridgens NK. A comparative study of surgical suture materials and closure techniques. *J Am Osteopath Assoc.* 1983; 82(suppl 9):715–718.

93. Bolton L, van Rijswijk L. Wound dressings: meeting clinical and biological needs. *Dermatol Nurs.* 1991;3:146–161.

94. Howes EL. The strength of wounds sutured with catgut and silk. *Surg Gynecol Obstet.* 1933;57:309–317.

95. *United States Pharmacopeia XX.* Rockville, MD: The US Pharmacopial Convention. 1980;390–410.

96. Postlethwait RW, Willigan DA, Ulin AW. Human tissue reaction to sutures. *Ann Surg.* 1975;181:144.

97. Van Winkle W, et al. Effect of suture materials on healing skin wounds. *Surg Gynecol Obstet.* 1975;140:7–12.

98. Laufman H, Rubel T. Synthetic absorbable sutures. *Surg Gynecol Obstet.* 1977;145: 597–608.

99. Forrester JC. Suture materials and their use. *Br J Hosp Med.* 1972;12:578–592.

100. Macht SD, Krifex TJ. Sutures and suturing: current concepts. *J Oral Surg.* 1978;36: 710–712.

101. Postlethwait RW. Long-term comparative study of non-absorbable sutures. *Ann Surg.* 1970;171:892–898.

102. Peacock EE, Van Winkle W. Repair of skin wounds. In *Wound Repair.* Philadelphia, PA: WB Saunders; 1976; 117–130.

103. Edlich RF, Panek PH, Rodeheaver GT. Physical and chemical configuration of sutures in the development of surgical infection. *Ann Surg.* 1973;177:679–688.

Chapter 4

Central Venous Catheters: Materials, Designs, and Selection

Matthew A. Mauro

Currently, a wide array of central venous access devices is available, for a variety of indications, and in a multitude of sizes, shapes, lengths, and configurations to meet the demands of current medical practice.[1] Despite their apparent differences, all central venous access devices are alike in that they are placed within the central venous circulation, typically in the superior vena cava (SVC), inferior vena cava (IVC), or right atrium (RA).

CATHETER MATERIAL

Virtually all current central venous catheters (particularly long-term catheters) are made of silicone rubber or polyurethane. These two materials have different properties and handling characteristics. Intravascularly placed silicone rubber has been used safely since the 1970s. Silicone is a soft, biocompatible material that has been placed within the vascular system by open cutdown for many years. This soft material, which has a high coefficient of friction, makes manipulations with standard stainless steel guidewires extremely difficult. These features, combined with nontapered tips, require the use of peel-away sheaths for percutaneous insertions. The difficulties in guidewire manipulation were minimized by the introduction of relatively stiff hydrophilic guidewires, which now are used routinely for catheter placement. Although silicone typically is used in long-term devices, temporary or short-term devices

also currently are made of silicone. These temporary silicone devices have tapered tips and stiffening cannulas for percutaneous insertion without the use of hydrophilic guidewires or peel-away sheaths.

Polyurethane is a newer material that is stronger and stiffer than silicone. The stronger material allows thinner walls and larger lumen diameter while maintaining the same outer diameter of the catheter. A polyurethane catheter may have a comparable inner-diameter lumen with a smaller outer diameter. Polyurethane has a lower coefficient of friction and can be used with conventional stainless steel guidewires. A large polyurethane catheter with nontapered tips still may require peel-away sheaths; however, over-the-wire insertions of smaller polyurethane catheters are possible. Although the polyurethane material is stiff, it softens within the body, making it suitable for long-term use within the vascular system.

TIP CONFIGURATION

Catheters are available in one of three basic tip configurations: end-hole, valved tip, and staggered tip[2,3] (Fig. 4–1). End-hole catheters are the standard tip design that can be trimmed at the tip to fit the patient's anatomy without changing the design. Single-, dual-, or triple-lumen catheters are available with end-hole design. The valved-tip catheter has a closed blunt tip with valved slits just proximal to the tip. These slits allow blood to be withdrawn and

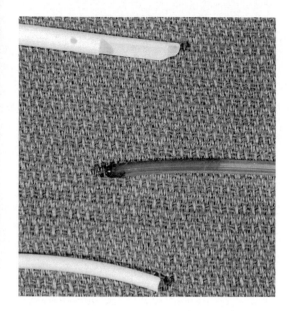

Figure 4–1 Tip configurations of central catheters. *Top:* Staggered tip. *Middle:* Valved tip. *Bottom:* End-hole tip.

solutions to be infused, but they will not allow blood to enter the lumen when not in use.[4] Single- or dual-lumen catheters are available with the valved-tip configuration. The advantage over the simple end-hole catheter design is that the valved-tip catheter does not require routine heparinization to prevent catheter thrombosis. Because of the valved tip, however, these catheters cannot be trimmed at the tip during placement. Therefore, to modify the catheter length to fit anatomy, valved-tip catheters usually have a removable connection, which allows the catheter to be trimmed at the hub. Staggered-tip, dual-lumen catheters are specially designed for therapies that require rapid simultaneous aspiration and infusion with limited admixture (e.g., pheresis, hemodialysis).[5] These catheters cannot be trimmed at the tip because it would defeat the purpose of staggered configuration. Although available with removable hubs, these catheters more commonly have fixed hubs made in a variety of lengths. In practice, fixed-length, staggered-tip catheters can be modified at the tip by trimming and recreating the staggered configuration,

but this would alter the volume of the intracatheter heparinization solution needed and is not recommended.

CENTRAL VENOUS ACCESS DEVICES

Central venous access devices can be classified initially into two categories: (1) short-term (temporary) and (2) long-term (permanent) devices. The latter can be further subdivided into (1) peripherally inserted central catheters (PICCs); (2) chest-wall external catheters, which can be either tunneled or nontunneled; and (3) subcutaneous ports, which can be implanted either in the chest wall or in the extremities.

Short-Term Central Venous Catheters

These catheters usually are placed at the bedside when immediate central access is needed. Most commonly, these catheters are made of polyurethane and are available with single, dual, or triple lumen with tapered end-hole tips. Sizes range from 5 to 14 French (F). They are inserted with standard Seldinger over-the-wire techniques and are intended for short-term (days to weeks) in-hospital use. More recently, 11.5 and 14 F silicone, dual-lumen pheresis/hemodialysis catheters have become available; these have a tapered end-hole and a stiffening cannula to facilitate over-the-wire insertion.

Long-Term Central Venous Catheters

Peripherally Inserted Central Catheters
As the name indicates, PICCs are inserted through a peripheral vein of the upper extremity (basilic, cephalic, brachial, antecubital), and the tip is placed in the central circulation[6] (Fig. 4–2). It is therefore a true central venous catheter. PICCs are available in 2 to 7 F with single or dual lumen. PICCs are external, nontunneled catheters and require tape or suture fixation. These catheters are convenient for home use for an intermediate period—from several weeks to

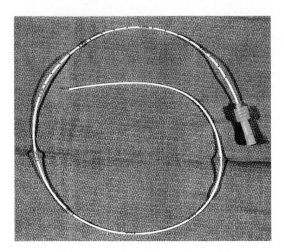

Figure 4–2 Peripherally inserted central catheter.

3 to 6 months. Although PICCs can remain functional for longer than 6 months, their small diameter and fragility somewhat limit their longevity.[1] Advantages of the PICC include a lower procedural complication rate, patient preference, and the potential of cost-effective bedside placement by special nursing personnel. Disadvantages are their small diameter (restricted flows, fragility, poor radiopaque quality) and the need for an intact upper-extremity venous anatomy. Their small caliber also may lead to less reliable transfusion and phlebotomy.

Silicone and polyurethane PICCs can tolerate flow rates ranging between 0.4 and 7.0 mL per second and 0.6 to 10.2 mL per second, respectively. The 5 F silicone PICC and the 4 and 5 F polyurethane PICCs routinely tolerate flows greater than 4 mL per second.[7]

Chest-Wall External Catheters
Nontunneled These catheters usually are made of silicone, are nontapered, and are intended for intermediate-length home therapy (weeks to months). Their longevity is similar to that of PICCs, but they are placed via the central veins.[8] They are available in single-lumen 5 F and dual-lumen 7 F varieties (Hohn Catheter, Bard Access Devices, Salt Lake City, UT)

(Fig. 4–3). Because they are made of silicone and are nontapered, insertion is more difficult than with conventional acute-care central catheters. Stabilization is with tape or suture.

Tunneled Tunneled external chest wall catheters are the "traditional" and initial long-term central venous access devices. They are available with single, dual, or triple lumen; made of silicone or polyurethane material; and with end-hole, valved-tip, or staggered-tip configurations[2,3] (Fig. 4–4). Sizes range from 3.5 to 21 F for use in the pediatric population and adult hemodialysis populations, respectively. The devices have a tissue ingrowth cuff attached to the shaft that is positioned within the subcutaneous tunnel, which is made between the original venous access puncture site and the catheter exit site.[9] The subcutaneous tunnel provides long-term catheter stabilization and protection from infection. The cuff incites a desmoplastic tissue response within 4 to 6 weeks that stabilizes the catheter, allowing long-term use of the device, intended for months to years. Some catheters are available with an "antimicrobial" cuff (Vitacuff; Vitaphore, Menlo Park, CA) that is positioned just proximal (closer to the skin exit site) to the tissue ingrowth cuff.[10]

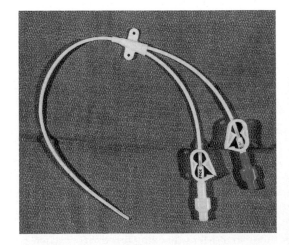

Figure 4–3 Dual-lumen nontunneled Hohn catheter.

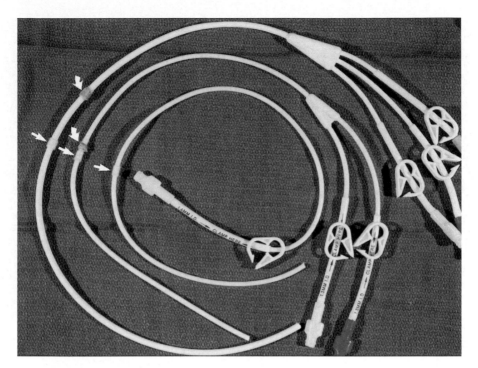

Figure 4–4 Tunneled chest-wall silicone catheters. *Outer:* Triple-lumen catheter. *Middle:* Dual-lumen catheter. *Inner:* Single-lumen catheter. Note tissue ingrowth cuff (*white arrows*) and Vita cuff (*curved arrows*).

This second cuff is intended as a temporary stabilizer and antimicrobial barrier. Some recent evidence suggests that this silver-impregnated cuff causes a local cytotoxic effect on fibroblasts and actually may delay fibrous tissue ingrowth.[11]

Pheresis/dialysis catheters are a special type of externally tunneled chest-wall devices. The pheresis and dialysis processes require simultaneous aspiration and infusion of blood while limiting admixture. The pheresis process requires approximately 125 cc per milliliter; dialysis requires 400 to 450 cc per minute through each lumen. Therefore, catheters designed for high-flow dialysis also can be used for the lower-flow pheresis procedures. Several configurations of dialysis catheter configurations are now available, including (1) standard dual-lumen, staggered-tip, end-hole catheter; (2) two individual (twin) single-lumen catheters, each with an end hole and multiple side holes; and (3) a single dual-lumen cath-

eter in which the distal catheter may be split apart, each lumen an end hole and multiple side holes[5,12,13] (Fig. 4–5). The single dual-lumen catheters (types 1 and 3) are placed by using a single venotomy and a single subcutaneous tunnel. The twin catheter system (type 2) requires either a large single venotomy or, more commonly, two different adjacent venotomies and two parallel subcutaneous tunnels with the potential advantage that each catheter more reliably allows higher flow rates.[14] On the other hand, the insertion procedure is longer and more traumatic because two separate punctures and tunnels are required. The single split catheter (type 3) attempts to provide the flow advantages of a twin catheter system while requiring a single venous puncture and subcutaneous tunnel.

Subcutaneous Ports

The conventional port developed by Nierderhuber in 1982 consists of a reservoir

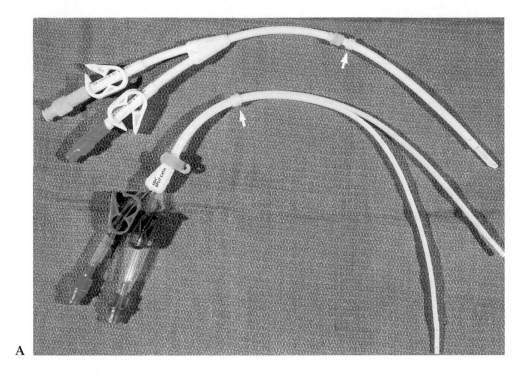

A

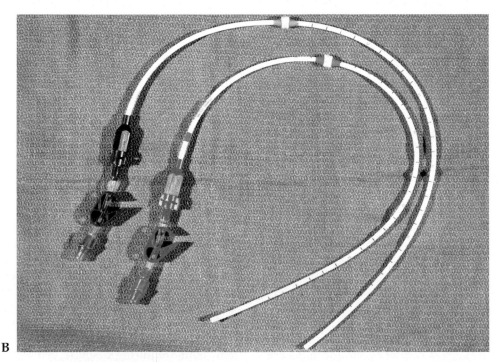

B

Figure 4–5 Dialysis catheters: **(A)** *Top:* Dual-lumen staggered tip catheter. *Bottom:* Split Ash catheter. Note the separated distal lumens. Each catheter has a tissue ingrowth cuff (*white arrows*) attached to the catheter. **(B)** Twin catheter system. *Outer:* Venous catheter. *Inner:* Arterial catheter.

of stainless steel, titanium, or plastic connected to a polyurethane or silicone catheter.[15] Ports can be implanted within the subcutaneous tissues on the chest wall, arm, or forearm.[16–19] Stainless steel ports produce severe magnetic resonance (MR) and computed tomographic (CT) imaging artifacts and now are implanted only rarely in the chest wall. Titanium ports produce only local MR distortion. Plastic ports produce little, if any, CT or MR image distortion. The catheter and port reservoir either are pre-attached at the factory or require attachment during the insertion procedure with a locking mechanism. Single- or dual-chamber ports are available with end-hole, valved, or staggered tips.

The implanted ports are covered by intact skin and need to be accessed with special noncoring needles that penetrate the overlying skin and the compressed silicone septum.[3] The septum of a standard-sized port can accommodate approximately 2000 and 4000 punctures with 20- and 22-gauge needles, respectively. The septum of smaller-diameter and thinner- extremity or pediatric ports accommodates fewer punctures before septum fatigue occurs. Ports are now available in a multitude of sizes designed for different implantation locations (chest wall, extremity). Typically, the larger ports have larger attached catheters. The choice of the appropriately sized port is important for both appearance and function. A port that is too large protrudes from the body and produces excess tension of the suture line. A port that is too small is difficult to palpate and to access successfully using a needle.

A nonreservoir port is available that allows direct access with an Angiocath, which directly enters the attached catheter. The port is made of stainless steel and is connected to a polyurethane catheter (Cath-Link 20, Bard Access Systems). The port has three concentric silicone rings that are traversed by the Angiocath to enter the attached polyurethane catheter directly. Thus, solutions are infused directly into the catheter without a reservoir to minimize the risk of inadvertent needle dislodgment and potentially harmful extravasation of solutions. Access techniques differ from conventional ports and require special training (Fig. 4–6).

Ports are easier and less expensive to maintain than externally tunneled catheters, requiring minimal skin care and only once-monthly heparinization, compared with three-times-weekly heparinization for most tunneled catheters. Ports are more expensive than external catheters, but they are cost effective when in place longer than 6 months. Furthermore, ports are preferred by active patients and by patients concerned with cosmetic appearance.[2,3]

DEVICE SELECTION

Multiple factors to be considered before selecting the appropriate venous access device include type or purpose, frequency and length of therapy, patient comfort and activity, ability to care for the device, and personal preference (physician, nurse, home health care, patient). Pheresis or dialysis requires large-bore, dual-lumen, tunneled chest-wall catheters. Currently, no peripherally inserted catheters are available that can provide the high flow rates for these therapies. Frequent (daily) use favors an external device, whereas infrequent use (weekly to monthly) favors a subcutaneous port. Intermediate use (weeks to months) favors nontunneled chest-wall external catheters, PICCs, and tunneled chest-wall external catheters. Long-term use (many months to years) favors tunneled chest-wall external catheters and subcutaneous ports. Ports become more cost effective when in place for longer than 6 months. Catheter longevity is related to length of therapy and size of the device. Ports are more durable than external catheters because of the lack of exposed parts that withstand mechanical trauma. PICCs are small and prone to mechanical damage. Although the larger chest-wall catheters are more durable than PICCs, they too undergo mechanical damage at the hub (Table 4–1).

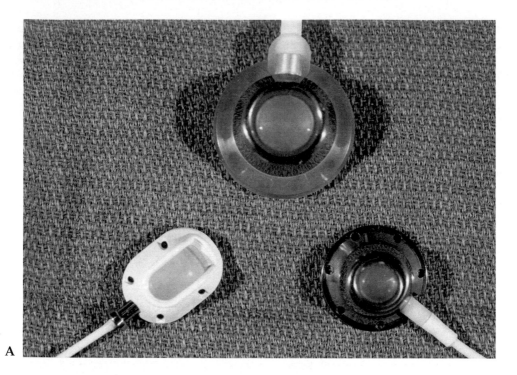

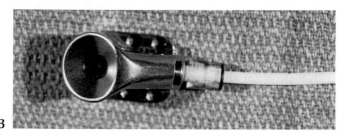

Figure 4–6 Subcutaneous ports. **(A)** Conventional reservoir ports. *Top:* Standard port. *Lower left:* Extremity port. *Lower right:* Low-profile port. **(B)** Nonreservoir port.

Table 4–1   Choice of Devices

Device	Duration
Peripherally inserted central catheter	Weeks to months
Nontunneled external chest-wall catheter	Weeks to months
Tunneled external chest-wall catheters	Months to years
Subcutaneous ports (extremity, chest wall)	Months to years

Multilumen catheters have higher infection rates than do single-lumen catheters and are used only when multiple simultaneous therapies are needed.[20] Single-lumen catheters are used for single therapies or multiple nonsimultaneous therapies. Blood-product transfusions and blood drawings can be better achieved with catheters larger than 3 or 4 F.[21]

Debate about the advantages of chest-wall versus extremity ports continues. Advantages of extremity ports include patient preference (cosmetic), lower subclavian vein thrombosis rates, and smaller size. Advantages of chest-wall ports include patient preference, easier insertion, and more reliable access. Personal preference influences this decision but should not be the overriding consideration. The selected port must accomplish the intended treatment plan. The preferences of the physician are secondary to those of the caregiver and patient. The interventional radiologist should be able to insert any device in any location. Nursing and home health care personnel will be accessing and caring for these devices on a constant basis. For example, nurses may feel uncomfortable accessing extremity ports and may prefer chest-wall ports. A port that is difficult to access is frustrating to both the nurse and the patient and may prevent therapy from taking place. Discussions with the patient should take place before the port is placed. Once the incision is healed, ports allow full patient activity and are particularly well suited for active patients.[16,17] Active patients also prefer PICCs above the elbow rather than at or below the elbow.[22] Incapacitated patients are candidates for subcutaneous ports, which require minimal skin care when not in use. Some patients are frightened by needles to access the port and are more comfortable with external catheters. Some patients also may have aversion to chest-wall or extremity port placements. Usually, more than one device will meet the needs of therapy and maintenance personnel; so the patient should participate in the decision.

SUMMARY

Successful results are obtained by using the most appropriate central venous access device that will accomplish the intended treatment plan. The interventional radiologist must be knowledgeable about all the available devices. Once the treatment plan is outlined by the referring physician, the interventional radiologist must select the device that will satisfy the wishes and needs of the referring clinician, the nurse, and the patient. A venous access service requires open discussions with nursing and home health care personnel—the people who will be accessing and caring for the devices. Finally, if the treatment plan can be accomplished by using a variety of devices or insertion locations, the patient should be openly consulted.

REFERENCES

1. Renner C, Knutson P, Lawson T. Vascular access in home care: current trends. *Infusion.* October 1996;11–24.
2. Mauro MA, Jaques PF. Radiologic placement of long-term central venous catheters: a review. *J Vasc Interv Radiol.* 1993;4:127–137.
3. Denny DF. Placement and management of long-term central venous access catheters and ports. *Am J Radiol.* 1993;161:385–393.
4. Delmore JE, Horbelt DV, Jack BL, Roberts DK. Experience with the Groshong long-term central venous catheter. *Gynecol Oncol.* 1989;34:216–218.
5. Trerotola SO, Johnson MS, Harris VJ, et al. Outcome of tunneled hemodialysis catheters placed via the right internal jugular vein by interventional radiologists. *Radiology.* 1997; 203:489–495.
6. Gardella JF, Cardella K, Bacci N, Fox PS, Post JH. Cumulative experience with 1,273 peripherally inserted central catheters at a single institution. *J Vasc Interv Radiol.* 1996; 7:5–13.
7. Rivitz SM, Drucker EA. Power injection of peripherally inserted central catheters. *J Vasc Interv Radiol.* 1997;8:857–863.
8. Openshaw KL, Picus D, Hicks ME, Darcy MD, Vesely TM, Picus J. Interventional radiologic placement of Hohn central venous catheters: results and complications in 100 consecutive patients. *J Vasc Interv Radiol.* 1994;5:111–115.
9. Robertson LJ, Mauro MA, Jaques PF. Radiologic placement of Hickman catheters. *Radiology.* 1989;170:1007–1009.
10. Maki DG, Cobb L, Garman JK, Shapiro JM, Ringer M, Helgerson RB. An attachable silver-impregnated cuff for the prevention of infection with central venous catheters: a prospective, randomized multicenter trial. *Am J Med.* 1988;85:307–314.
11. Hemmerlein JB, Trerotola SO, Kraus MA, Mendonca MS, Desmond LA. *In vitro*

cytotoxicity of silver-impregnated collagen cuffs designed to decrease infection in tunneled catheters. *Radiology.* 1997;204:363–367.

12. Mauro MA, Jaques PF. Insertion of long-term hemodialysis catheters by interventional radiologists: the trend continues. *Radiology.* 1996;198:316–317.

13. Tesio F, DeBaz H, Panarello G, et al. Double catheterization of the internal jugular vein for hemodialysis: indications, techniques, and clinical results. *Artif Organs.* 1994;18: 301–304.

14. Canaud B, Beraud JJ, Joyeux H, Mion C. Internal jugular vein cannulation using 2 Silastic catheters: a new, simple and safe long-term vascular access for extracorporeal treatment. *Nephron.* 1986;43:133–138.

15. Niederhuber JE, Ensminger W, Gynes JW, et al. Totally implanted venous and arterial access system to replace external catheters in cancer treatment. *Surgery.* 1982;92: 706–712.

16. Morris SL, Jaques PF, Mauro MA. Radiology-assisted placement of implantable subcutaneous infusion ports for long-term venous access. *Radiology.* 1992;184:149–151.

17. Simpson KR, Hovsepian DM, Picus D. Interventional radiologic placement of chest wall ports: results and complications in 161 consecutive placements. *J Vasc Interv Radiol.* 1997;8:185–195.

18. Foley MJ. Radiologic placement of long-term central venous peripheral access system ports (PAS port): results in 150 patients. *J Vasc Interv Radiol.* 1995;6:255–262.

19. Kaufman JA, Salamipour BS, Geller SC, Rivitz AM, Waltman AC. Long-term outcomes of radiologically placed arm ports. *Radiology.* 1996;201:725–730.

20. Early TF, Gregory RT, Wheeler JR, et al. Increased infection rate in double lumen versus single lumen Hickman catheters in cancer patients. *South Med J.* 1990;83:34–36.

21. Angle JF, Matsumoto AH, Skalak TC, O'Brien RF, Hartwell GD, Tegtmeyer CJ. Flow characteristics of peripherally inserted central catheters. *J Vasc Interv Radiol.* 1997;8: 569–577.

22. Polak JF, Anderson D, Hagspiel K, Mungovan J. Peripherally inserted central venous catheters: factors affecting patient satisfaction. *Am J Roentgenol.* 1998;170:1609–1611.

Chapter 5

Peripherally Inserted Central Catheters and Ports

Preston Fox
Jaime Tisnado
Philip C. Pieters

PERIPHERALLY INSERTED CENTRAL CATHETERS

Venous Anatomy

A review of the upper extremity venous anatomy will be helpful before discussing peripherally inserted central catheters (PICCs) and subcutaneous arm ports. In the upper extremity, there are superficial and deep veins. The superficial veins are the basilic vein, cephalic vein, and median cubital vein. The main deep veins correspond to the arteries, including the radial, ulnar, and interosseous veins in the forearm; the brachial veins in the arm; and the axillary vein in the axilla. In the upper extremity, the superficial veins are important for catheter or port placement. In the arm, the sites most often used for peripheral line placement are, from medial to lateral, the basilic vein, the brachial veins, and the cephalic vein. The basilic vein is relatively superficial and usually is the largest in the arm. Because of these two anatomic facts, the basilic vein is the optimal site for PICC or port insertion. The puncture of the basilic vein is easy because of its caliber and its shallow location under the skin. Furthermore, because the luminal diameter is larger, the rate of catheter-related thrombosis is low.

The brachial veins often are paired and located deep in the soft tissue, adjacent to the brachial artery and in close proximity to the median nerve. Therefore, the brachial veins are less desirable than the basilic vein for PICC insertion. The deep location can lead to catheter kinking if the angle of puncture and catheter introduction is too steep. Furthermore, if the operator does not palpate the brachial artery while using contrast-guided fluoroscopy for venipuncture, one could inadvertently puncture the unopacified artery as the needle travels to enter the brachial vein; however, the brachial veins still may be a good location for PICC insertion. Ultrasound-guided puncture of the brachial veins allows direct visualization of the brachial artery to ensure that the artery is not traversed during puncture.

The cephalic vein is located lateral in the arm and is also superficial. The cephalic vein courses over the biceps muscle and may make an acute caudal turn at the shoulder as it enters the axillary vein in the deep pectoral groove. The location of the cephalic vein over the biceps muscle may result in excessive movement of the catheter during arm flexion and extension, causing discomfort and limiting arm motion as well as kinking of the catheter. In addition, the caudal turn at the shoulder may result in the catheter entering the axillary vein in a peripheral direction rather than centrally during insertion. This may be a problem during insertion without fluoroscopy and may be time consuming and require additional manipulation to redirect the catheter into the superior vena cava (SVC).

The cephalic vein is also the smallest of the arm veins; therefore, a greater incidence of thrombosis can be expected after PICC insertion.

Additional factors to consider in selecting the optimal insertion site include the presence of acute or chronic thrombus in the target vein, soft-tissue inflammation, induration or hematoma from prior intravenous (IV) sites, or failed IV placements. Overall, the basilic vein is the optimal site for PICC, followed by the brachial veins and the cephalic vein. If the patient has chronic renal insufficiency and is a candidate for an upper-extremity graft or an arteriovenous fistula, PICC lines should be avoided.

Indications and Contraindications

The primary indication for PICC placement is short- to intermediate-term central venous access, that is, from approximately 2 to 8 weeks. PICCs are used for antibiotic therapy, hyperalimentation (total parenteral nutrition, or TPN), chemotherapy, fluid administration, and pain-control medication administration. Important considerations prior to PICC placement are the duration of therapy, type of medication (viscosity), frequency of administration, and number of medications needed. Insight into these questions mandates proper selection of either a single- or dual-lumen catheter, thus keeping the patient and physician well served by the venous access service. If questions arise concerning the clinical need or application of the PICC, a brief discussion with the referring physician often clarifies issues and saves headaches.[1,2]

In general, PICCs have optimal application in the 2- to 8-week period. Some PICCs, however, last much longer, up to a year, with meticulous care.

Dual-lumen PICCs are used in cases where multiple drugs or simultaneous infusions are needed. Single-lumen PICCs allow greater flow rates than dual-lumen PICCs because of their larger inner lumen and thus are preferred for hyperalimentation (TPN) or more viscous infusions. The *Poiseuille law* states that the flow rate is directly proportional to the fourth power of the radius and inversely proportional to the viscosity of the fluid infused as well as to the length of the catheter. Hence, the greatest flow rates will be achieved in the catheter with the largest luminal diameter (single-lumen PICCs), shortest length, and least viscous infusate. Unfortunately, a catheter intended for infusion of TPN should have a lumen dedicated only to TPN and should not be used for other infusions or blood draws. Therefore, if a single-lumen catheter is placed for TPN, other venous access often is required.[3]

The PICCs have significant advantages over short-term centrally placed catheters because there is no risk of pneumothorax and very little risk of bleeding, even in thrombocytopenic patients or patients taking anticoagulants. In addition, PICC insertion success rates are higher than 98%; they are cost effective, practical, and avoid considerable pain and discomfort for patients with poor peripheral veins in whom multiple punctures may be needed to start an IV which will last only several days.[1,2] Furthermore, many chemotherapeutic agents are irritant or caustic to peripheral veins and therefore are better tolerated if given centrally. Patients needing relatively short duration of treatment do not require placement of a longer-term tunneled catheter. PICCs also may have a lower incidence of central venous stenosis relating to central catheters because of the small diameter of the catheter and because an axillary or subclavian vein puncture is not needed.

Contraindications to PICC insertion include phlebitis or cellulitis at the insertion site. A relative contraindication may include central venous stenosis or occlusion. In such cases, the contralateral arm can be used for insertion, or the PICC may be placed to the SVC via a collateral vein using a 0.018-inch hydrophilic wire to negotiate the venous channels and advance the catheter into the right atrium (RA). Other relative contraindications may include a prior mastectomy on the side of planned insertion or that a dialysis graft or arteriovenous (AV) fistula might be needed in the future in the arm.

Insertion Techniques

It is essential that the patient's medical record be reviewed before the procedure is performed to ensure that a PICC, rather than other central catheters, is the optimal choice for central venous access. As discussed already, the duration of the therapy must be short to intermediate in length (2 to 8 weeks) for PICC placement. Otherwise, a tunneled catheter or port is better if the patient is likely to have a repeated and long-term need for venous access (e.g., cystic fibrosis, human immunodeficiency virus). Also, a review of the medications and dosing regimen is important to determine whether multiple simultaneous infusions will require a dual-lumen PICC or whether a single lumen will suffice. This review should include knowing what is going to be infused through the catheter. Hyperalimentation (TPN) is more viscous than saline. The more viscous the infusate, the larger the lumen needed; so a single-lumen catheter may be preferable. If the fluids to be infused are caustic, such as chemotherapeutic agents, the tip placement needs to be in the high-flow SVC or the RA. If only saline is to be given, it will be tolerated easily in a more peripheral position of the catheter tip. A prior history of allergic-like reaction to radiographic contrast material necessitates placement of the PICC using CO_2 or ultrasound guidance. On occasion gadolinium can be used as a contrast agent. A brief review of operative and progress notes for prior central catheter placements, cardiac pacer placement, or a known history of central venous stenosis or thrombosis will avoid confusion or embarrassment and allow choosing the best arm for insertion.

After a quick chart review, we inspect the patient's chest and arms. If a prior subclavian catheter insertion site is discovered, the ipsilateral arm should be avoided because of the risk of subclavian stenosis.

Also, chest-wall vein collaterals may be present on one side as warning signs of subclavian or brachiocephalic vein occlusion. We also examine the arms for phlebitis or cellulitis from prior IV sites or infiltrated IVs. If no adverse conditions exist in either arm, the nondominant arm is preferable for placement of PICC.

Several techniques for PICC insertion are effective. These include fluoroscopically guided venous puncture using iodinated contrast material or CO_2, ultrasound-guided venous access with fluoroscopic insertion, or bedside insertion, which requires taking a chest radiograph to check tip position. In our experience, fluoroscopic venous puncture with contrast material is quicker than ultrasound guidance and also allows visualization of most of the veins and thus the opportunity to choose the optimal vein and site for insertion. Therefore, this technique is discussed in greatest detail.

A 22-gauge IV is started in a forearm, wrist, or hand vein. A 23- or 25-gauge butterfly needle can be used if the veins are not suitable for cannulation with an Angiocath. The practice of injecting a contrast agent through a butterfly needle should be discouraged, however, because of the increased risk of infiltration. The initial contrast injection should be performed under fluoroscopic control while observing the needle to ensure that the contrast is not extravasating. In our opinion, if an Angiocath cannot be placed, the next best option is to place the PICC under sonographic guidance rather than to place a butterfly needle for contrast injection. The IV is connected to extension tubing, which will allow injection of contrast material without disrupting the sterile field. The location of the port for the IV tubing should be planned in advance, prior to preparing the sterile field, so that a last-minute search for the port under the sterile field will not be necessary.

The patient is placed on the angiographic table with the arm abducted, resting on an arm board. The image intensifier is positioned over the midarm so the insertion site is visualized as well as the shoulder and chest when the table is moved. The arm then is raised and held by the circulating nurse and is prepped from axilla to below the elbow with 2% chlorhexidine or Betadine solution (Purdue, Fredrick, Norwalk, CT). The entire circumference of the arm should be painted from the axilla to below the elbow with each sponge, and the axilla should be painted last with each sponge. This process of painting the arm and the axilla should be repeated three times. Sterile towels (or a sterile sheet) are placed under the prepped arm, and a sterile tourniquet is placed as high as possible on the arm. The arm then is lowered with the palm of the hand supinated to expose the medial aspect of the arm. The basilic vein is optimally exposed for puncture with the arm in this position. The distal arm and hand are covered with sterile towels, as are the axilla and chest region. A sterile angiography drape is placed over the patient's body with a sterile image-intensifier cover placed as well. This leaves the upper arm uncovered for the procedure. The junction of the proximal and midhumeral region is placed under the image intensifier, and iodinated contrast material or CO_2 is injected by the circulating nurse to opacify the basilic, brachial, and cephalic veins. It is helpful to compress the forearm gently to "pump" contrast material from the forearm to the arm, giving more complete opacification of the arm veins.

HELPFUL HINTS

Do not tie the tourniquet until the vein has been opacified. Perform fluoroscopy while contrast is injected. When the veins are opacified, step off of fluoroscopy, tie the tourniquet, pick up the needle, and then resume fluoroscopy. Continue the slow injection of contrast during this process. This method allows better opacification of the vein because the unopacified blood is pushed out of the vein before the tourniquet is tied. This method also decreases the pressure within the vein and probably decreases the amount of extravasation into the surrounding soft tissues. If the tourniquet is tied before contrast injection, unopacified blood becomes "trapped" in the vein; as iodinated contrast is forcefully injected until there is enough mixing of opacified blood with unopacified blood to visualize the vein, the pressure within the vein is increased to a point that any puncture in the vein—even a single wall puncture—may result in extravasation of contrast.

A 21-gauge, 4-cm-long needle is used to perform a single wall puncture of the basilic vein at the junction of the proximal third and middle third of the arm. It is helpful to magnify the image—even to an extreme level—when attempting to puncture the vein under fluoroscopic guidance (Fig. 5–1). Precise positioning of the needle is easier when the target appears larger. Also, the collimators should be closed so that the needle tip is in the field of view but not the hand holding the needle (Fig. 5–2A). The needle is guided exactly parallel to the basilic vein at approximately a 30- to 45-degree angle and advanced under fluoroscopic observation as it enters the anterior wall of the vein. As discussed in Chapter 3, "Techniques of Venous Catheter Place-

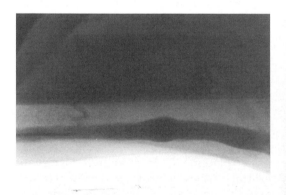

Figure 5–1 Venographic guidance. The field is maximally magnified to give optimal visualization of the vein. The field of view is centered so that the needle is seen, but the operator's hand is out of the field. The needle is parallel and perfectly superimposed over the vein.

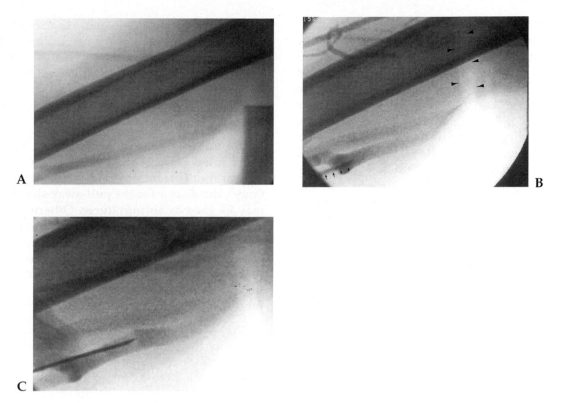

Figure 5–2 Venographic guidance techniques. **(A)** The tourniquet should not be tied until contrast material is present in the target veins. Slow contrast injection is continued while the tourniquet is tied. This technique prevents markedly elevated pressures in the target vein, which could cause extravasation. **(B)** The tourniquet (*arrowheads*) has been tightened, and the target veins are well visualized. The needle (*small arrows*) should puncture the skin directly over the vein and should be advanced toward the vein remaining superimposed over the vein at all times. **(C)** The needle is advanced until the needle tip compresses the vein. This is seen as a halo around the needle tip, which represents compression of the vein with displacement of contrast within the compressed segment of vein. To perform a single wall puncture and minimize extravasation, the needle should be advanced a minimal distance (1 to 2 mm) in a sharp jabbing motion.

ment," always puncture the skin directly over the vein with the entire needle superimposed over the vein (on a parallel course over the vein) (Fig. 5–2B). The hand used to perform the venous puncture must be in a stable position, not floating and wagging in the air. With the forearm and wrist resting on the patient's forearm, the needle should be held like a pencil. The needle tip will indent the vein wall as it enters the lumen. The needle is advanced slowly until the needle tip is seen to compress the vein. The contrast material actually will be seen clearing out from the needle tip as the needle compresses the anterior and posterior walls

of the vein together (Fig. 5–2C). A slight forward jab of the needle usually results in puncture of the anterior wall of the vein. The vein should be punctured in the midline to facilitate passage of a 0.018-inch guidewire, which then is advanced to the level of the subclavian vein. With the tourniquet tied, the pressure within the vein is great enough that blood will return through the needle and constant aspiration with a 5 mL syringe is not necessary. If imaging indicates that the needle has entered the vein but no "flashback" is seen, then the syringe should be connected and aspirated while slowly withdrawing the needle.

HELPFUL HINTS
Advancement of the wire is especially difficult in peripheral veins because of the relatively small caliber of the veins and the fact that the walls of the veins are pliable and not supported (i.e., they "roll"). Tactile sense is critical when advancing the wire through the needle into the vein. If the needle tip is in the center of the vein, there is a smooth transition as the wire passes from the needle into vein and very little resistance is felt. If the needle tip is against the wall of the vein, or not in the vein at all, resistance to advancing the wire will be felt. When resistance is encountered, the wire must not be pushed forcefully.

Advancement should be done in the following steps:

1. Lower the angle of the needle, relative to the skin surface, bringing the angle of the needle and wire more in line with the angle of the vein lumen. As the needle angle is lowered, continually test for passage of the wire using a gentle tapping motion with the wire (i.e., gently pulling the wire in and out and tapping the tip of the wire against the wall of the vein). If there is a decrease in resistance to pushing the wire, it has likely entered the vein lumen. This should be confirmed by fluoroscopy.
2. If lowering the angle of the needle does not allow successful passage of the wire into the vein, remove the wire, increase the angle of the needle to approximately 30 degrees, advance the needle tip 2 to 3 mm, reattach the syringe to the needle, and slowly withdraw the needle until blood is aspirated.
3. If these maneuvers do not allow successful placement of the guidewire into the vein, release the tourniquet, remove the needle and hold pressure to minimize the amount of contrast extravasation and hematoma formation. After hemostasis has been obtained, venographic guidance can be attempted again, although this segment of vein will likely

be compressed by hematoma or narrowed due to spasm. In most instances, another vein will need to be used for access, or possibly a more central segment of the same vein can be used.

HELPFUL HINTS
If the guidewire becomes deformed because it has curled within the soft tissues (which results from pushing against resistance), the dilator for the pull-away sheath may be used as an introducer. Otherwise, if the wire is too deformed, a new guidewire should be used for subsequent attempts at cannulating the vein. It is easy to move the needle tip out of the vein lumen while attempting to place a deformed wire into the needle.

Release of the tourniquet allows visualization of the central veins. The circulating nurse flushes the IV used for injection of contrast with 20 to 30 mL of saline to clear the vein and to prevent contrast-induced thrombophlebitis. Local infiltration of 1% lidocaine with sodium bicarbonate is performed at the puncture site and approximately 3 cm distally, where the PICC hub will be sewn in place. Generally, the initial puncture is relatively painless, and the puncture is easier without prior infiltration of lidocaine. With the guidewire in place, a 2-mm dermatotomy is made, and a peel-away sheath, ideally 0.5 F larger than the PICC, is placed. The existing guidewire then is used to measure the length to the SVC–RA junction, and the PICC then is cut to the measured length (Fig. 5–3). Under fluoroscopic guidance, the tip of the guidewire is placed at the junction of the SVC with the RA, and the guidewire is bent or the wire clamped at the hub of the peel-away sheath dilator. After the wire is removed, it can be used to measure the catheter, keeping in mind that the measured distance (from wire tip to clamp) is actually 1 to 2 inches longer than the distance of skin entrance site to SVC–RA junction (accounting for the length of the dilator hub, outside of the skin). Alternatively, marker wires may be in-

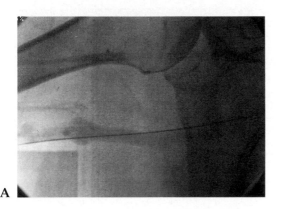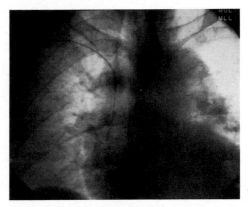

A B

Figure 5–3 Measuring length for a peripherally inserted central catheter (PICC). **(A)** Under fluoroscopic guidance, the guidewire is advanced through the central veins into the superior vena cava (SVC). **(B)** The guidewire is placed with its tip at the SVC-right atrium junction. The guidewire is either bent or clamped where it exits the peel-away sheath. The length of wire between the clamp (or bend) and the wire tip is the desired length of the PICC.

cluded in kits and allow for measurement without removal of the wire.

The dilator of the peel-away sheath is removed, and the PICC is inserted. Often the PICC will advance smoothly to the SVC–RA junction; otherwise, the 0.018-inch guidewire may be used inside the PICC for added rigidity. If difficulty arises, the PICC may be inserted tracking over the guidewire to the SVC–RA junction. Some kits include a 0.018-inch wire stylet as a stiffener for insertion.

HELPFUL HINTS
Occasionally, a central venous stenosis will be encountered such that the 0.018-inch guidewire passes the stenosis, but the PICC will not track over the wire through the stenosis. A maneuver that occasionally allows passage of the catheter through the stenosis is to remove the wire from the PICC and forcefully inject saline through the PICC using a 5- or 10-mL syringe and, at the same time, attempt to advance the catheter. Often the catheter will spurt through the stenosis in a flow-directed manner. Why does it work? We are not certain, but perhaps the sudden increase in intraluminal pressure allows a slight increase in diameter of the stenosis, allowing the flow of blood to carry the catheter tip through the stenosis.

Occasionally, severe central venous stenoses or occlusions are encountered. These lesions may need to be angioplastied using the usual methods (Fig. 5–4) by using the access already gained for PICC insertion. If a central occlusion is present and cannot be recannulated, the PICC may be left with the catheter tip proximal to the occlusion (Fig. 5–5), but the catheter should be used as if it were a peripheral IV and not a central venous catheter. Infusion of sclerosing materials, such as TPN or chemotherapy, will result in further thrombosis of the vein. Once the tip of the catheter is in place, the peel-away sheath is removed as the PICC hub is held in place. It is important not to peel away the sheath against the skin but rather retract and split it outside the skin to prevent enlarging of the puncture site and bleeding. Pressure is applied to achieve hemostasis, and the hub is sewn in place with nonabsorbable monofilament suture.

HELPFUL HINTS
It is better not to suture the hub directly to the skin; rather, make a 1-cm throw through the skin followed by a nonsliding square knot. Then sew the hub to this knot rather than to the skin. After taking a bite through the skin, tie a square knot or surgical knot by placing a clamp or dilator on the skin (i.e., the clamp is between the

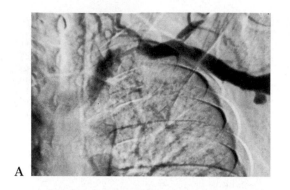
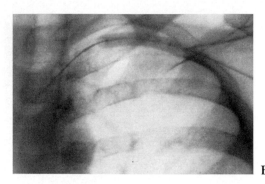

A

B

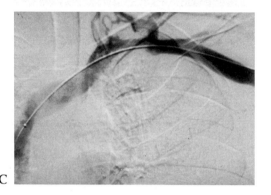

C

Figure 5–4 Venous angioplasty during placement of a peripherally inserted central catheter (PICC). **(A)** The left basilic vein was successfully punctured using ultrasonographic guidance, but the guidewire could not be advanced through the central veins. A venogram was performed that demonstrated a severe stenosis of the subclavian vein with formation of collaterals. **(B)** A vascular sheath was placed, and a glidewire was used to recannulate the stenosis. Angioplasty was performed with a 10-mm balloon. **(C)** Excellent results were obtained postangioplasty, allowing placement of the PICC. The vascular sheath was exchanged for a peel-away sheath, and the PICC was placed.

skin and the knot). The suture then is advanced through the hole of the hub wing, and another knot is tied. This technique protects the integrity of the skin and is more comfortable for patients.

The line is flushed and locked with 100 U/cc of heparin solution. Three milliliters of heparin solution is used for single-lumen PICCs and 2 mL per port for dual-lumen PICCs. Gauze is placed and then is covered with a bio-occlusive dressing. Several sterile gauzes can cover these, and the arm is wrapped with 2-inch Co-Flex (Androver, Salisbury, MA) for slight pressure to the insertion site. Co-Flex is an elasticized self-adherent bandage, which does not stick to the skin, does not injure the skin, and is

easily removed and changed. A needleless connecting hub to the PICC can be used.

Also, PICCs can be inserted with CO_2 injection or ultrasound guidance. In patients with renal insufficiency or allergy to iodinated contrast, CO_2 is an excellent alternative to iodinated contrast. Approximately 30 mL of CO_2 is injected under fluoroscopic observation. The venous puncture and insertion techniques are the same. If no peripheral IV placement is possible, ultrasound guidance is used (Fig. 5–6). A 7- or 10-MHz transducer with color flow is optimal for visualization of arterial or venous anatomy. The veins are readily distinguished from arteries by their compressibility. Ultrasound is performed in the

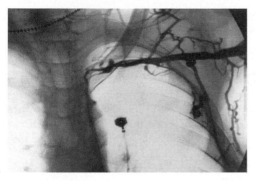 A

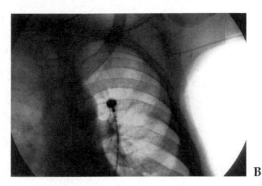 B

Figure 5–5 Peripherally inserted central catheter (PICC) placement in patients with central venous occlusion. **(A)** The guidewire could not be advanced into the right atrium during PICC placement. A venogram was obtained that demonstrated occlusion of the left innominate vein. **(B)** Attempts at recannulating the occluded innominate vein were unsuccessful. A PICC was placed with catheter tip in the axillary vein. Such a catheter, placed proximal to a central venous occlusion, should be considered a peripheral line, not a central line. This catheter would be adequate for hydration and a select few medications, but it should not be used for infusion of sclerosing materials, such as total parenteral nutrition or chemotherapeutic agents.

transverse plane to localize and identify the basilic vein in the midarm. It is important always to localize the brachial artery to avoid inadvertent puncture of this vessel. The puncture then is performed either in the longitudinal or transverse plane with visualization of the needle tip. A tourniquet above the intended puncture site is used to make the puncture and introduction of the guidewire easier. Fluoroscopic guidance is used for length measurement and tip placement. Ultrasound guidance has the advan-

tages of avoiding a peripheral IV, avoiding contrast, and identifying adjacent structures, such as the brachial artery, muscles, and median nerve. The latter advantage is particularly important when puncturing the brachial vein.

The duration of PICCs is dependent on meticulous routine care. After each infusion, the line should be flushed with 10 mL of saline and locked with 2 mL of 100 U/cc of heparin solution. If the PICC is not in use, it should be flushed every 3 to 4 days with

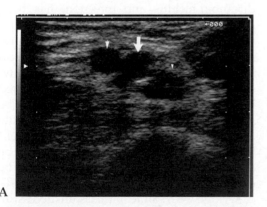 A

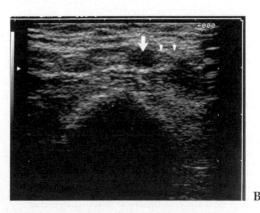 B

Figure 5–6 Ultrasound guidance for peripherally inserted central catheter (PICC) placement. **(A)** Ultrasonography of the arm typically shows the brachial artery (*white arrow*) flanked by the brachial vein and by the basilic vein (*arrowheads*). **(B)** With compression, the veins collapse (*arrowheads*), confirming patency, whereas the artery (*arrow*) does not compress.

Table 5–1 Data in Single-Lumen Peripherally Inserted Central Catheters

Manufacturer	Outer Diameter (F)	Inner Diameter (in. or gauge)	Material	Length	List Price ($)	Comment
Arrow (Reading, PA)	4	0.032	Polyurethane	56	60	High flow rates, small OD
800-523-8446	5	16 gauge	Polyurethane	70	70	High flow rates
Bard (Salt Lake City, UT)	4	18 gauge	Silicone	60	75	Groshong catheter with valved tip
800-545-0890	5	17 gauge	Polyurethane	65	70	open ended
Boston Scientific (Boston, MA)	5	0.030	Polyurethane	60	64	High flow rates, good durability
800-225-3238		0.040				
Cook (Bloomington, IN)	3	0.018	Silicone	50	52	Good durability, excellent insertion kit
800-457-4500	4	0.023	Silicone	60		
	5	0.030	Silicone	60		

F, French; OD, outer diameter.

the same regimen. PICCs never should run dry at the end of an infusion to prevent thrombus formation. Routine cleansing of the insertion site with hydrogen peroxide or Betadine and placement of sterile dressing are important. The injection site must be kept dry during bathing and at all times to prevent infection. Using these measures, infection rates as low as 0.13 per 100 catheter days have been reported.[4]

Many excellent single- and dual-lumen PICCs are available. These are listed in Tables 5–1 and 5–2, respectively.

Comments

The technical success of PICC insertion is as high as 98%, as shown by several studies.[1,2] Technical failures are usually secondary to inability to cannulate a vein, most commonly in the pediatric neonatal population. PICCs can be maintained with a low infection rate of 0.13 per 100 catheter days.[4] The most common failures include thrombosis, kinking at the insertion site, and dislodgment. Thrombosis may be secondary to

inadequate flushing or allowing the catheter to run dry during infusion. Kinking at the insertion site is usually due to a steep angle of the initial venous puncture or placement at a site of excessive motion, such as the elbow. Dislodgement can be prevented by careful suturing technique and by an elasticized bandage.

A complication rate of 4.6%, including thrombophlebitis and infection, has been reported.[1,2] Thrombophlebitis requires removal and, if extensive thrombosis is present, anticoagulation may be needed. Local infection will resolve with removal; however, if bacteremia is present or if continued IV access is needed, a new PICC can be placed at an alternative site, ideally the contralateral arm. The catheter tip should be cultured, and blood culture should be obtained. A thrombosed PICC may be cleared by gently flushing with a 3- to 10-cc syringe with saline. If this is unsuccessful, then 5000 U of urokinase (Abbott Laboratories, Chicago, IL) or 1 mg of tissue plasminogen activates (tPA) may be injected and left in place for 20 to 60 minutes. If these

Table 5–2 Data in Dual-Lumen Peripherally Inserted Central Catheters

Manufacturer	Outer Diameter (F)	Inner Diameter (in. or gauge)	Material	Length	List Price ($)	Comment
Arrow (Reading, PA) 800-523-8446	5	0.022/0.01	Polyurethane	58	72	High flow rates, fixation device may compress catheter
Bard (Salt Lake City, UT) 800-545-0890	5	19 gauge/ 20 gauge	Silicone	57	115	Groshong catheter with valved tips high flow
	6	18 gauge/ 18 gauge	Polyurethane	65	90	open ended
Boston Scientific (Boston, MA) 800-225-3238	5	0.031/0.02	Polyurethane	60	78	High flow, hub clamp may crimp catheter
	6	0.037/0.02	Polyurethane			
Cook (Bloomington, IN) 800-457-4500	5	0.018	Silicone	60	68	Good durability, low flow through small lumen
	6	0.026	Polyurethane	60	68	

F, French; OD, outer diameter.

maneuvers fail, a 0.018-inch hydrophilic guidewire can be inserted to dislodge thrombus or to exchange the PICC. If the preceding maneuvers are ineffective, replacement in the contralateral arm or exchange over a guidewire is necessary.

Summary

PICCs are of great help to patients with poor peripheral venous access as well as those in need of short- to intermediate-term central venous access. PICCs avoid the discomfort of many unsuccessful IV attempts and the occasionally disastrous pneumothorax from central line placement.

ARM PORTS

Peripherally placed ports allow intermittent venous access for months to years. They are implanted subcutaneously, have a lower risk of infection than PICCs, are easily inserted, and avoid the risks associated with chest-implanted ports, such as pneumothorax. Placement in the medial aspect of the proximal arm renders them inconspicuous relative to chest ports, and the lower profile allows for smaller incisions and less scarring and protrusion. Patients who may benefit include those with cystic fibrosis, HIV, breast and other cancers, and lymphomas.

Insertion Techniques

Prior to the procedure, 1 gm of ceftazidime, or 1 gm of vancomycin if the patient is penicillin-allergic, is given for prophylaxis. The basilic vein in the middle or proximal aspect of the arm is the optimal insertion site. Venous access is obtained as with PICCs. A central venogram is obtained through the sheath to ensure central venous patency, prior to opening and wasting an expensive device. The subcutaneous tissues and skin medial, lateral, and distal to the

95

puncture site are anesthetized with 1% lidocaine with sodium bicarbonate. A 2- to 3-cm skin incision is made with a no. 15 blade to include the puncture site. A subcutaneous pocket is created about 0.5 cm under the skin by blunt dissection to accommodate the port that is chosen. Two 3-0 nonabsorbable monofilament sutures are placed on the medial and lateral sides of the pocket to secure the port in place. Some prefer to use absorbable sutures or no sutures. The pocket is flushed with saline, and any bleeding is controlled. The port and catheter are flushed, and the catheter is advanced over a hydrophilic wire through the sheath to the SVC–RA junction. The sheath is removed with the wire in place to prevent catheter migration. The catheter tip is checked and the wire removed. Hemostasis is achieved at the vein entry site with manual pressure, and the catheter is flushed with heparinized saline and clamped. The catheter is cut and connected to the port, and the port is secured in place with the previously placed sutures. The retaining sutures must be placed before insertion of the port because of difficulty suturing with the port already in the pocket. The port and catheter are checked for appropriate aspiration and flushed with 2 or 3 mL of 100 U/cc heparin solution. The port and catheter are checked fluoroscopically for kinking or poor port orientation prior to skin closure. The pocket is flushed again to remove clots and tissue and the skin closed with a running sub-cuticular stitch using 4-0 absorbable suture. The site is dressed with 4 × 4 gauze, a bio-occlusive dressing, and a Co-Flex bandage or accessed for infusion with a 20- or 22-gauge Huber needle.

Summary

Technical success for arm port placement has been shown to be 100%.[5] In addition, the rates of venous thrombosis, catheter fracture, and infection are very low. Infection rates of 2.5% were reported with no incidence of venous thrombosis.[5] In general, port or catheter thrombosis may be successfully treated by instillation of urokinase, tPA or Retarase with the same protocol as for PICCs. Subcutaneous arm ports offer long-term central venous access with excellent cosmetic results and no risk of pneumothorax.[6]

REFERENCES

1. Cardella JF, Fox PS, Lawler JB. Interventional radiologic placement of peripherally inserted central catheters. *J Vasc Interv Radiol.* 1993;4:653–660.
2. Cardella JF, Cardella K, Bacci N, et al. Cumulative experience with 1,273 peripherally inserted central catheters at a single institution. *J Vasc Interv Radiol.* 1996;7:5–13.
3. Angle JF, Matsumoto AH, Skalah TC. Flow characteristics of peripherally inserted central catheters. *J Vasc Interv Radiol.* 1997;8:569–577.
4. Raad I, Davis S, Becker M, et al. Low infection rate and long durability of non-tunneled silastic catheters: a safe and cost-effective alternative for long-term venous access. *Arch Intern Med.* 1993;153:1791–1796.
5. Kahn ML, Barboza RB, Kling GA, et al. Initial experience with percutaneous placements of the PAS ports implantable venous access device. *J Vasc Interv Radiol.* 1992;3:459–461.
6. Andrews JF, Walker-Andrews SC, Ensminger WD. Long term venous access with a peripherally placed subcutaneous infusion port: initial results. *Radiology.* 1990;176:45–47.

Chapter 6

Tunneled Catheters and Chest Ports

Jeffrey E. Hull

DETAILED DESCRIPTION OF OPTIONS

About 400,000 long-term central venous access catheters are placed annually in the United States. These catheters include tunneled right atrial catheters and subcutaneous ports. Originally, these catheters were placed in the operating room and more recently in the radiology suite.[1-6] Major concerns regarding their placement are: (1) selecting a suitable access site, (2) avoiding complications of placement, (3) obtaining satisfactory final catheter position, and (4) preventing infection.[1-9] This chapter describes placement technique and problems, delayed complications of central catheters and their treatment, and results of radiologic placement.

Catheter Selection

Catheter selection is based on: (1) patient needs (including comfort and ability to care for the catheter), (2) catheter function, and (3) cost.

Patient Needs

Choosing a long-term central catheter requires familiarity with the devices available and their relative advantages and disadvantages. Patient comfort and ability to care for a catheter are important considerations in choosing a catheter. Both debilitated and active patients are good candidates for subcutaneous port catheters. These ports require minimal maintenance and are less likely to interfere with daily activities when not in use. Tunneled external catheters are best for patients requiring large double- and triple-lumen catheters if they are able to care for them. Some properties of catheters are described in the following sections.

Catheter Function

Tunneled Catheters
These catheters are suited for intermediate (i.e., less than 6 months) and long (i.e., more than 6 months) duration access because of their ease of placement and atraumatic access. The external catheters are ideal for multiple and repetitive access and have an advantage over ports in these patients. An example is patients undergoing bone marrow transplant. These patients need frequent access and are often thrombocytopenic. External catheters are without the risk for port pocket bleeding due to thrombocytopenia.[10]

Peripherally Inserted Central Catheter Lines
Peripherally inserted central catheter (PICC) lines can be substituted for tunneled catheters and ports in many patients. A PICC line can used for up to 6 to 9 months, and, when placed at the bedside, costs the same as three intravenous (IV) placements (John Cardella, personal communication). Any patient expected to have more than three IV catheters during a hospitalization or home treatment is a candidate for a PICC line. One advantage of the PICC line is decreased risk of placement complications of pneumothorax. Subclavian access frequently causes thrombosis or stenosis of

the subclavian vein. PICC lines may reduce these complications.

Subcutaneous Ports

Patients requiring less frequent use of their access device for a long term (i.e., more than 6 months) are candidates for subcutaneous ports. Subcutaneous ports are more difficult to place because of the need to create a subcutaneous pocket for the injection port. The ports come in a variety of sizes and configurations, including dual-lumen ports and small ports that are placed in the arm.[11] External catheters need to be flushed as often as once a day and have dressing changes every 3 days. Subcutaneous ports need to be flushed only once a month, and dressing changes are not required after the first week post placement. Patients who are unable to care for an external catheter are candidates for subcutaneous ports because of the minimal maintenance that is required. Active patients are also candidates for ports because they do not interfere with daily activities, such as exercise, bathing, and swimming.

Several studies suggest that ports have lower infection rates compared with external catheters.[12–19] Other studies[16,20] and the only prospective randomized study in the literature,[21] however, have shown no significant difference in infection rates between ports and catheters. There are no conclusive data showing a lower infection rate with subcutaneous ports at this time.

Cost and Maintenance

The overall cost of long-term central venous access is time dependent. The purchase price and placement-related costs of ports are higher than external catheters. Ports cost twice the price of an external catheter. On the other hand, the quantity of maintenance supplies required for external catheters is greater than that for ports. Overall, the cost of maintaining a port is less than that of an external catheter, with the break-even point in terms of cost occurring at 6 months.[15,22]

Low-maintenance cost has been reported with the Groshong catheter (Bard Access, Cranston, RI, U.S.A.) relative to other tunneled right atrial catheters.[1,5] The Groshong catheter has a slit valve at its tip and needs to be flushed only once a week with saline as opposed to daily flushes with heparinized saline for nonvalve tip catheters. The decreased need for flushing reduces maintenance cost and is more convenient for patients.[1] A recent study showed that these cost benefits are overshadowed by costly problems with line dysfunction.[23]

DESCRIPTION OF CATHETERS

Tunneled Catheters

The tunneled catheters are made of silicone or polyurethane; vary in length from 36 to 55 cm; have one, two, or three lumens; and range in diameter from 7 to 16 French. These catheters are designed to be placed in a central vein, with their tip in the distal superior vena cava (SVC) or proximal right atrium (RA). Most catheters have an open-ended tip, although some, like a Groshong, have a valve at their tip to prevent reflux of blood into the catheter lumen. Some commonly used catheters are listed in Table 6–1.

Several centimeters of catheter are tunneled beneath the dermis. The catheters usually have a Dacron cuff and often an antimicrobial cuff. The Dacron cuff secures the catheter in place after 5 to 10 days by fibrosis. The antimicrobial cuff is impregnated with silver chloride. The cuff is positioned near the exit site to act as a barrier to organisms extending centrally to the subcutaneous tunnel or vein. The catheters all have luer lock-type connections for use with syringes and intravenous tubing.

Ports

Ports have reservoirs of different materials attached to silicone or polyurethane catheters (Fig. 6–1). Similar to the tunneled catheters, the tip is placed in the distal SVC or proximal RA. Ports support single- or dual-lumen catheters. Most cath-

Table 6–1 Tunneled Catheters

Name	Company	Material	Comments
Broviac	Bard	Silicone	S
Hickman	Bard	Silicone	S,D,T
Leonard	Bard	Silicone	D
Groshong	Bard	Silicone	S,D
Infus-a-Cath	Strato	Silicone, polyurethane	S,D
Raaf	Quinton	Silicone	S,D,T
Hemed	Gish	Silicone	S,D
Chemo Cath	HDC	Silicone	S,D

S, single; D, double; T, triple lumen catheters.
From Mauro MA, Jaques PF. Radiologic placement of long-term central venous catheters: a review. *J Vasc Interv Radiol.* 1993;4:127–137, with permission.

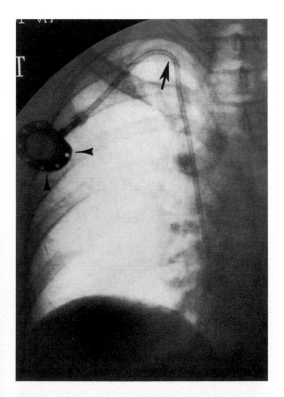

Figure 6–1 Port-A-Cath. The reservoir (*arrowheads*) is attached to a silicone catheter, which is tunneled subcutaneously and enters the vein (*arrow*). The port is implanted beneath the skin and can be accessed with a special noncoring needle.

eters have a single lumen with an open end hole, although a valve-tip Groshong-type catheter is available. The subcutaneous reservoirs are made of plastic or metal (usually titanium). The upper surface is silicone that can be punctured repeatedly without significant loss of integrity. The ports are generally round with a flat bottom that can be sutured to underling tissues. Table 6–2 lists some common ports, their features, and their manufacturers.

PLACEMENT TECHNIQUES

Placement of central venous access catheters can be broken into three basic steps: preprocedure imaging, obtaining vascular access, and catheter placement.

Preprocedure Imaging

To begin, it is important to review recent chest films for local chest-wall disease or possible mediastinal disease that could affect catheter placement. The patient is placed supine, flat on the angiography table. Trendelenberg may be the ideal position; however, most angiography tables do not tilt to provide this position. The veins

Table 6–2   Chest Ports

Name	Company	Material
A-Port	Therex	Ti
Chemo-Port	HDC	SS, silicone
Hickman	Bard	Plastic, Ti, silicone
Infuse-A-Port	Strato	Plastic
Life Port	Strato	Ti, silicone, polyurethane
Medtronic	Medtronic	Ti, silicone
Norport	Norfolk	SS, silicone
Port-A-Cath	Pharmacia Deltec	Ti, silicone
Q-Port	Quinton	
SEA Port	Harbor Medical	Silicone
Vasport	Gish	Ti

SS, stainless steel; Ti, titanium.

typically targeted for access are the sub-clavian, internal jugular, and cephalic. Ultrasound, with 7- or 5-MHz linear array transducer, of the infraclavicular fossa and neck is performed to evaluate the target vein, looking for altered anatomy or thrombosis. Venography can be useful to define the anatomy further when the ultrasound is abnormal, but it is rarely necessary. Translumbar and transhepatic access to the inferior vena cava is an option in cases where upper-extremity access and femoral access are not possible.[24]

Vascular Access

Patient Preparation

Prophylactic antibiotics (1 g of IV cefazolin) were given routinely during the procedure early in our experience, but this practice has been found to be unnecessary.[19,25] Midazolam and fentanyl are used for sedation and analgesia. Standard aseptic techniques used in the radiology suite include the wearing of caps, masks, gowns, and sterile gloves; a 5-minute hand scrub by the implanting radiologist; and preprocedure room cleaning with Vesphene IIse (Vestal Laboratories, Inc., St. Louis, MO).

To obtain suitable vascular access, it is important to study all the information available to choose an access site. A brief examination of the patient and a review of any available imaging studies (chest radiograph, chest computed tomography, or venography) should be done to look for potential problems that could be avoided. Some situations include mastectomy, mediastinal masses, and thrombosed veins; then the intended access vein should be evaluated directly using ultrasound or venography.

Once a patent access vein has been identified, the skin is widely prepared with Betadine, and the field is sterilely draped. The skin is anesthetized with 1% lidocaine (with or without epinephrine), and a small incision is made. Using real-time ultrasound or fluoroscopic guidance, a micropuncture needle is advanced into the vein. Ultrasound guidance is preferred because it does not require IV access or IV contrast material and is suitable for jugular, subclavian, and cephalic vein access.

Real-time ultrasound guidance of the access needle can be obtained in the longitudinal or transverse plane.[11,24,26] Using the longitudinal approach, the vein and needle path can be observed simultaneously and continually. Problems may arise from not keeping the needle in the plane of the transducer and the ultrasound beam. Using the transverse scanning approach, it is sometimes difficult to keep track of the depth of the needle tip. When scanning in the transverse plane, however, the artery and vein can be observed simultaneously to ensure a venous puncture. Many ultrasound units have a needle guide to control the needle path.

In axillary/subclavian vein access, longitudinal ultrasound guidance is the best choice for access. It is important to know the depth of the needle to prevent inadvertently entering the chest cavity and causing a pneumothorax. The upper chest lends itself to longitudinal positioning of the ultrasound transducer. In addition, longitudinal ultrasound guidance promotes a more lateral approach to the axillary/subclavian vein, which prevents the "pinch-off" syndrome (see later discussion).

When using the internal jugular and external jugular vein for tunneled catheters or ports, it is helpful to access the vein just cephalad to the clavicle for two reasons. First, it is difficult to create a tunnel from the chest to the midneck or vice versa. Second, access close to the clavicle results in a gentle curve of the catheter that prevents kinking (Figs. 6–1 and 6–2). Achieving access close to the clavicle with longitudinal ultrasound guidance is difficult because the length and, to a lesser extent, the width of most transducers puts the needle several centimeters above the clavicle. Whether using the longitudinal or transverse approach, it is often helpful to place the ultrasound transducer cephalad to the access site and needle so that the transducer does not push the needle above the clavicle. Fortunately, the jugular veins

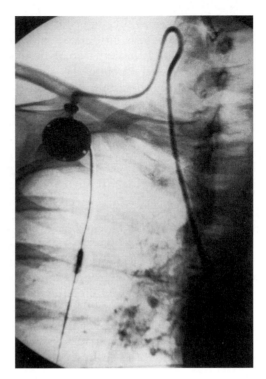

Figure 6–2 High jugular puncture. Puncture of the jugular vein too high in the neck can result in catheter kinking because of the acute angle necessary to enter the vein. Contrast this to the angle created by a low puncture (Fig. 6.1). Poor positioning of the port within the subcutaneous pocket, too close to the clavicle, could result in the device rubbing against the clavicle, causing irritation and pain.

are relatively superficial and easy to access with ultrasound guidance.

Catheter Placement

Tunneled Catheters

Venous access always is obtained first because this is the essential step in the process. The order of intravascular placement and subcutaneous tunneling depend on the catheter type. The Groshong catheter is placed through a peel-away sheath into the SVC and tunneled subcutaneously as previously described.[1,6] A similar approach is used for the Hickman catheter except this catheter is tunneled first and then it is placed intravascularly.

When making the subcutaneous tunnel, the tunneling device is introduced into the subcutaneous space through a small dermatotomy and passed through the subcutaneous fat, bluntly dissecting a tract to the access site. The catheter then is attached to the tunneler and pulled through the tunnel. Do not attach the catheter prior to tunneling because the force of gripping and pushing the tunneling device can damage the catheter tip at the attachment to the tunneling device.

HELPFUL HINTS

Blunt plastic tunneling devices usually are used to tunnel from the dermatotomy (skin exit site) to the venous puncture site. Stiff metal tunneling devices are intended to be used in the opposite direction, from venous puncture site to skin exit site, and a dermototomy need not be made in advance. The sharp point can be pushed through the skin at the desired exit site.

The access site is closed with absorbable suture (4-0 Vicryl), nonabsorbable material (3-0 Dermalon), or Steri-strips (Shur-strip, Shur Medical Corp., Beaverton, OR). We prefer to close the access site with absorbable suture because it involves less bleeding and follow-up care. The exit site is sterilely dressed using a small 2 × 2-inch gauze.

The external portion of the catheter can be secured in several ways. Most catheter kits come with anchoring devices that can be sutured to the skin. Patients often have difficulty cleaning around the anchoring devices that trap blood and debris beneath them. The catheters can be sutured directly to the skin using half-hitches. Another approach is to tape a safety loop to the chest until the Dacron cuff scars into place. A completion chest radiograph or fluoroscopic image is performed to document position and to evaluate for pneumothorax or other complications.

Pocket Creation and Port Placement

Once venous access is obtained, a subcutaneous pocket for placement of the port is created. The pocket for chest ports is planned over the anterior chest wall, in an area with bony support, away from breast tissue and radiation ports, and with adequate thickness of subcutaneous tissue to cover the port (at least 0.5 cm). Also, the port must be positioned far enough away from the clavicle that it does not rub against this bone (Fig. 6–2). Table 6–3 lists surgical instruments not commonly available in a radiology department that are useful in placing chest ports. A 3- to 5-cm incision is planned just above the proposed port site such that it bisects the perpendicular line from the access site to the center of the port site.

Table 6–3   Useful Instruments for Port Placement

Needle driver

Rat-tooth pickup

Army Navy retractor

Small rake

Metsembaum scissors

Suture cutting scissors

Good overhead light source

Battery powered cautery (Aaron Medical, St. Petersburg, FL)

Pacemaker drape

Lidocaine with epinephrine

HELPFUL HINT
When making the incision for the port, the incision should be made just large enough for the port to fit barely through. It is best to err on the side of making the incision too small; it can be extended if necessary.

The incision and port site are anesthetized with 1% lidocaine with epinephrine (up to 30 mL). The incision is made with a no. 10 or 15 blade scalpel.

HELPFUL HINTS
Make the incision with the rounded portion of the blade, not with the point. Make the incision in one continuous motion, not in multiple small-connected cuts, which can result in a wound with jagged edges. Cut through the skin and fascia. Part the underlying subcutaneous tissue using blunt dissection.

The pocket is formed by a combination of blunt and sharp dissection until adequate to house the intended port.

HELPFUL HINTS
Perform blunt dissection by pushing a clamp or needle driver into the subcutaneous tissues with the jaws closed and then spread the jaws apart. The finger also can be used to dissect bluntly any residual fibrous strands.

HELPFUL HINTS
Hemostasis can be obtained (if necessary) using electrocautery; however, in most instances, hemostasis can be obtained by tightly packing the pocket with a moist 4 × 4 gauze left in place for 2 to 3 minutes. If pulsatile bleeding is identified from a small skin artery, the site of bleeding must be localized and the bleeder clamped until no more bleeding is seen. A thin (4.0) nonabsorbable suture is tied around the clamp and slid off the tip of the clamp and tightened on the clamped tissue.

The port is sutured to the fascia or muscle with 3-0 Prolene on either side of the port pocket incision. Absorbable suture (3-0 Vicryl) also can be used because the port should be scarred into place before the suture absorbs. After the ends of the suture are lightly clamped, they can be pulled to the side so that they are ready for tying after placing the port in the pocket.

HELPFUL HINTS
Regardless of which suture material is used, the port should be anchored to the tissues to guarantee that the port does not flip within the pocket. The position of the sutures and which port holes the sutures are placed through must be carefully considered so that these sutures do not alter the intended position of the port. That is, a misplaced anchoring suture can cause the port to rotate or displace within the pocket.

The subcutaneous tissue from the venous access site to the midpoint of the pocket is anesthetized with lidocaine. The catheter is tunneled with a tunneling device from the access site to the pocket or vice versa. The tunneling of the catheter from the access site to the port pocket allows the port to be in an ideal location on the chest wall. Ports that are placed in a pocket created as an extension of the access incision often lead to catheter kinking and suboptimal positioning of the port. The catheter is attached to the port, flushed, and trimmed to ideal length. Trimming the catheter to the correct length is hard to estimate. The ideal position of the catheter tip is at the junction of the SVC and RA. The proper length can be measured fluoroscopically using a wire from the access incision. The alternative technique for determining the catheter length is to place the catheter tip at the junction of the SVC and RA. Then the catheter is cut to length and attached to the port. The latter technique is more likely to result in kinking of the catheter in the subcutaneous tissue and therefore is not recommended.

A retractor is useful for visualization of the pocket and for insertion of the port into the pocket. Once the port and catheter are in place, the system should be checked before closing the incisions. A Huber needle is inserted into the port through the skin, and the port is flushed and aspirated. Fluoroscopy can be used to check that the catheter tip is in good position and that there are no kinks. The port should be sutured into the pocket with two anchoring sutures. The catheter is placed in the SVC through a peel-away sheath under fluoroscopic guidance. The best way to avoid air embolism during catheter insertion is to have the patient suspend respiration or hum for the few seconds during catheter placement into the sheath.

After testing the port for flushing and blood aspiration, the pocket is closed in two layers using 2-0 or 4-0 absorbable suture for the deep layer, and 4-0 absorbable suture for the subcuticular layer. The pocket must close without tension being placed on the suture line or the skin over the port. A pocket that is too small or tight can result in pressure necrosis and erosion of the port through the skin. The access site is closed using a single Steri-strip or a subcuticular layer of 4-0 Vicryl. The Huber needle is left in place to use to avoid painful attempts at access into a freshly placed port. The incisions and Huber needle should be dressed sterilely. A completion chest radiography or fluoroscopic image is obtained to document position and to evaluate for pneumothorax. The port is immediately available for use.

COMMON PROBLEMS DURING CATHETER PLACEMENT

Additional problems encountered during placement not discussed in the preceding include catheter malposition, hematoma and bleeding, pneumothorax, and air embolism. It is important to be familiar with these potential complications and their correction.

Catheter Malposition

The ideal position for the catheter tip is in the proximal RA (Fig. 6–1). This position limits thrombosis at the catheter tip, catheter ensheathment with fibrin, and possibly central venous thrombosis. Significant shifts in

the catheter tip position occur in subclavian catheters, in obese patients (Fig. 6–3), in women, and when changing from supine to upright position (Fig. 6–4).[27] Catheters placed with their tip in the brachiocephalic vein or upper SVC have a 29% rate of thrombotic complications (Figs. 6–5 and 6–6).[28] These problems should be avoided when possible.

Occasionally, it will be difficult to advance the catheter through the peel-away sheath. This occurs commonly when using the right subclavian approach because of the short distance between the site of venous access and the acute angle between the right subclavian vein and SVC. There are solutions to this problem. The first is to pull the sheath back proximal to where it is kinked and then advance the catheter. The second is to insert a hydrophilic glidewire through the peel away and advance the catheter over the wire.

Hematomas and Bleeding

Hematomas during catheter placement usually result from inadvertent arterial puncture or from a skin vessel disrupted during tunneling. Manual pressure over the site of bleeding is usually adequate treatment as long as the bleeding is not into the chest cavity. When the axillary, subclavian artery or branch is punctured in the midclavicular line or more lateral, it is easy to apply adequate pressure to the puncture site to achieve homeostasis. This is another advantage of the lateral approach for subclavian access mentioned in the preceding section. In patients with continued bleeding at the access site, exit site, or port pocket, using a cautery device or sutures should be used to achieve hemostasis.

HELPFUL HINTS
When bleeding persists from the skin exit site, it is important to determine whether the bleeding is from the venous puncture or from a vessel in the subcutaneous tunnel. To make this determination, apply

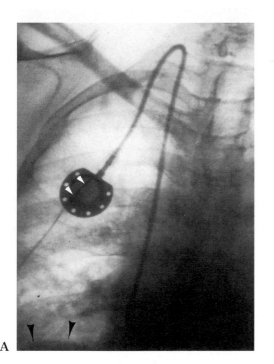 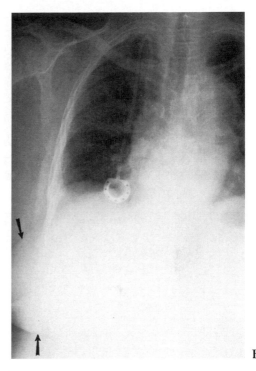

A   B

Figure 6–3   Catheter shift in an obese woman. **(A)** A completion image with the patient in the supine position shows adequate position of the port and catheter with the catheter tip in the right atrium. The Huber needle is in place (*white arrowheads*). Diaphragm (*black arrowheads*). **(B)** A chest radiograph obtained with the patient in the upright position shows that the abundant soft tissues of the chest wall (*black arrows*) have dropped, pulling the port caudally and pulling the attached catheter back. The catheter tip now lies in the superior vena cava. Note the distance that the port has migrated away from the clavicle.

pressure to the venous entry site, which should stop bleeding from the internal jugular vein. If bleeding persists, the bleeding is likely from the subcutaneous tunnel, and pressure should be held over the tract.

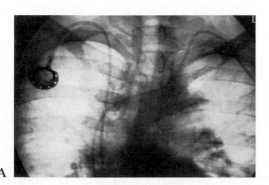 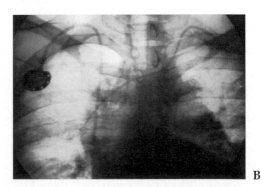

A   B

Figure 6–4   Catheter migration in the upright position. **(A)** Following placement, with the patient in the supine position, the right internal jugular Port-A-Cath and the left internal jugular 9 French Hickman catheter are in good position with catheter tips well into the right atrium. **(B)** After obtaining the upright position, both catheters have significantly migrated.

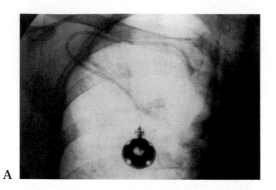

A

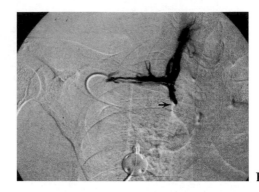

B

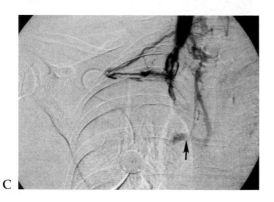

C

Figure 6–5 Catheter tip in the innominate vein. **(A)** A Port-A-Cath was placed via the axillary/subclavian vein approach, but the catheter was too short, with the catheter tip in the innominate vein. **(B)** Infusion of hyperosmolar, sclerosing materials resulted in venous thrombosis of the innominate vein (*arrow*) with reflux into the jugular vein. **(C)** Later images show collateralization to the left innominate vein (*arrow*).

Pneumothorax

A pneumothorax following catheter placement should be treated similar to a post-biopsy pneumothorax. Patients with large pneumothorax, respiratory distress, or risk of tension pneumothorax can be treated with a small chest tube with a Heimlich valve. A midaxillary approach is needed because the access device usually precludes the midclavicular line/anterior third rib approach.

Air Embolism

Air embolism occurs when a peel-away sheath or large central catheter is open to air during inspiration. A gurgling sound may be heard. The patient must be quickly turned in the left lateral decubitus position. This situation most commonly occurs when placing a catheter through the peel-away sheath in an uncooperative or deeply sedated patient. In this event, a catheter should be inserted and the peel-away sheath removed; then the patient is turned quickly to the decubitus position. The air in the RA must be aspirated using the catheter that was just inserted. The patient is left in the decubitus position until the air embolus resolves. Progress can be monitored by checking the RA with fluoroscopy. The patient should be given 100% oxygen.

POSTCATHETER FOLLOW-UP

Outpatients recover for an hour after the procedure, during which time their vital signs are monitored and bleeding checked. The radiology or oncology nurse gives the initial catheter care instructions. Inpatients recover in their rooms, with care instructions given by the nurses. Postprocedure examinations are at 24 hours and at 5 days to check the incisions and remove Steri-strips or sutures.

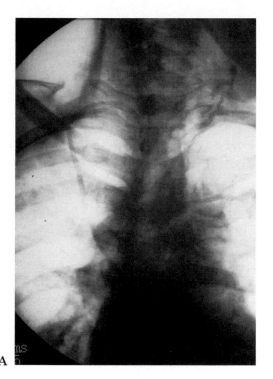
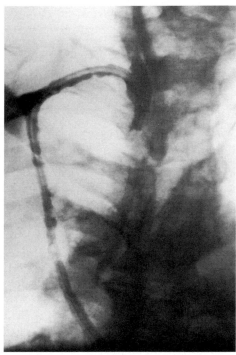

A   B

Figure 6–6 Catheter malposition causing vein thrombosis. **(A)** A Port-A-Cath was placed via the right internal jugular vein and tunneled to the sternum, where the port was implanted; however, the catheter is malpositioned, with the catheter tip in the right innominate vein or possibly the jugular vein. **(B)** After several days of use, blood could not be aspirated from the port and the patient complained of pain when the port was used for infusion of medications. Contrast injected through the Port-A-Cath showed occlusion of the jugular vein with reflux of contrast around the catheter into the subcutaneous tunnel.

Management of Problems

The most common complication after catheter placement is infection. Other significant problems include an inability to withdraw blood, extravasation of injected material, arm swelling, catheter rupture, and embolization (Table 6–4).

Infection

Catheter-related infections can be of three types: (1) exit-site infection (confined to 1 cm around the catheter), (2) tunnel infection, and (3) catheter-related bacteremia. The cutaneous infections (exit site, tunnel, and port-pocket infection) are usually clinically obvious with induration, redness, warmth, and exudate. Patients may be febrile and have an elevated white blood cell count. These infections are treated with antibiotics and local care. On the other hand, tunnel and port-pocket infections are more severe and may be harbingers of a subcutaneous abscess, which will require device removal and incision and drainage.

Catheter-related bacteremia (CRB) usually manifests with fever. Blood cultures through the catheter are positive. All patients with CRB should be treated with IV antibiotics for 10 days. *Staphylococcus epidermidis* is the most common organism, followed by *Staphylococcus aureus*. Patients who remain febrile and/or have a persistently elevated white blood cell count after 3 to 5 days of antibiotics should have their catheters removed, especially if their blood cultures have been positive. If no other infection source is found, these patients are presumed

Table 6–4 Common Problems and Their Treatment

Clinical Problem	Cause	Treatment
Arm swelling	Central vein thrombosis	Arm elevation, anticoagulation, leave catheter in place or Treat with urokinase and remove catheter
No blood return	Catheter thrombosis, valve malfunction in Groshong, possible ensheathment	Urokinase 5 K units × 2, then venogram to R/O ensheathment
Ensheathment found on venogram	Fibrin sheath formed around catheter so that injected fluid tracks back to venipuncture and extravasates extravascularly	In Groshong and Hickman pass wire to break fibrin sheath; strip catheter with snare; replace cath over wire, especially if catheter not at SVC/RA junction; replace dialysis catheter; prolonged infusion of a thrombolytic
Exit site infection (confined to 1 cm around catheter)	Most common form of infection often due to poor local care	Increase local care and treat with antibiotics (oral or IV)
Tunnel infection	More severe infection, possible abscess in tract	Will require IV antibiotics; catheter saved 60–80%
Catheter-related bacteremia	Colonization of catheter with pathogen	Blood culture from catheter and peripheral vein; treat with IV antibiotics for 3–5 days, remove cath if not better (fever and WBC) o/w continue Rx 10 days

RO, rule out; SVC, superior vena cava; RA, right atrium; WBC, while blood cell count; o/w, otherwise; Rx, treatment; IV, intravenous.

to have CRB and are treated with IV antibiotics.

Catheter removal is necessary in certain infections that are less likely to respond to antibiotic treatment, such as *Candida, Corynebacterium JK, Bacillus* species, *Mycobacterium fortuitum* (usually has accompanying exit site or tunnel infection), and in many patients with *S. aureus* and *Pseudomonas* infections. Catheter removal is necessary when a neutropenic, febrile patient develops hypotension or multiple organ failure to address the possible reservoir of infection.

Placement-Related Infection (Less Than 30 Days) The 30-day infection rate of external catheters is 10% as reported in the literature.[1–6] Most of these infections are minor exit-site infections occurring in immunocompromised patients and can be successfully treated with antibiotics. Reported infection rates for Hickman and Groshong catheters are variably reported to be 2.8 to 35.0% for sepsis[1,3–6] and 5 to 9.7% for local skin infection.[1,2,4] Often the early and late infectious complications are not reported separately, making analysis of the literature difficult.[1–6] Most infections occur after the first 7 days and probably are related to postplacement care.

Postplacement Infection (More than 30 Days) The infection rate after 30 days is 35% in chemotherapy patients with tunneled catheters.[29] This figure includes all unexplained febrile illnesses with positive blood culture. The high number of infections in the oncology group is partially due to the neutropenia and fever in these patients. All neutropenic and febrile patients are treated with antibiotics, and catheter-related infection is suspected if no other source is found. Using this treatment protocol, 68% of infected catheters can be salvaged in these patients. Patients who are not neutropenic usually have significantly lower infection rates.

Arm Swelling
Arm, neck, or face swelling on the side of a central venous catheter often is due to complete thrombosis of the central vein. The treatment is arm elevation and anticoagulation with heparin and then coumadin. Most patients treated conservatively do well with no appreciable sequelae. Thus, the catheter stays in place and spares the patient a lengthy thrombolysis procedure. Young patients who are active and have a long life expectancy may be candidates for thrombolysis and catheter removal, as they are more likely to have long-term sequelae if untreated.

Thrombosis of central veins after venous access is common but usually asymptomatic, occurring in 17% of patients in an autopsy series[30] and in 70% in a comparative, prospective study of Hickman and Groshong catheters,[31] with occlusive thrombus causing symptoms in 30% (3 of 10) of patients.[31] Most patients can be treated with arm elevation and anticoagulation without catheter removal. A recent study found a higher incidence of thrombosis in left subclavian catheters where the tip of the catheter is positioned in the high SVC.[19,32]

The thrombosis rate is similar regardless of the type of access device used.

Inability to Aspirate
A catheter that flushes but cannot aspirate is a common problem. Sometimes, changing the patient's position will allow the return of blood. Other causes are a clot in the catheter, venous thrombosis, and fibrin ensheathment of the catheter. The initial management is to treat with urokinase 5000 to 10,000 U or 1 to 2 mg of tissue plasminogen activator (TPA) into the catheter on the ward. In many cases, the clot will dissolve restoring catheter patency.

If this maneuver is unsuccessful, a venogram through the existing catheter may be required to ensure free flow into the central veins. Running a hydrophilic wire through the catheter may improve flow and allow blood return. When dealing with a Groshong catheter, a Rosen wire works better because it will pass reliably through the slit valves at the catheter tip. The venogram may show thrombosis near the catheter tip; however, catheter function may return after advancing a wire through the catheter to dislodge the clot. If there is arm swelling, anticoagulation may be necessary.

The success of restoring dialysis catheters to normal function by using thrombolytic agents or wire passage has been poor. Placement of a new catheter either at a new site or over a wire through the same tract is a better alternative. Occasionally, angioplasty is needed to clear residual thrombus on the SVC wall at the tip of the original catheter.

Ensheathment
The formation of a fibrin sheath around a central catheter causing injected fluid to track back along the catheter and extravasate is a common and serious problem, especially when cytotoxic drugs are being administered. When blood return cannot be obtained from a catheter, ensheathment is suspected (Fig. 6–7). To evaluate for possible catheter ensheathment when blood

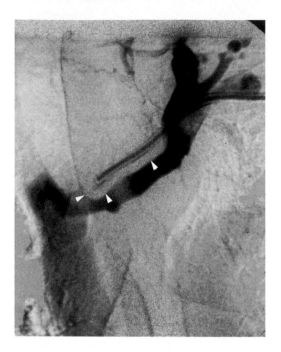

Figure 6–7 Fibrin sheath. A halo of fibrin sheath or clot (*arrowheads*) has formed around the catheter, resulting in an inability to aspirate blood through the Port-A-Cath. Infusion of tissue plasminogen activator resulted in complete lysis of the sheath; however, because of poor positioning of the catheter tip within the innominate vein, further fibrin sheath formation and venous thrombosis can be expected.

cannot be aspirated, a venogram through the existing catheter is required.

The venogram may show contrast returning along the catheter toward the venous site entry (Fig. 6–8). This represents fibrin ensheathment of the catheter. Passing a wire through the catheter often restores normal function. Alternatively, a Nitinol snare from a femoral access to strip the fibrin sheath can be done.[33] Infusion of thrombolytic agent through the catheter also may lyse the fibrin sheath. Placing a balloon catheter through a sheath and performing a fibrin sheath balloon disruption, followed by catheter placement, also has been used successfully. Ensheathment of a dialysis catheter requires replacement of the catheter. Venous stripping does not restore adequate flows for dialysis.[34]

Extravasation

Extravasation occurs most commonly with subcutaneous ports and is usually due to poor needle access (Fig. 6–9).[19,35] Poor placement can affect the ability to palpate adequately the port for access. Ports are accessed more easily if placed over muscle or bone and not too deep beneath fat and subcutaneous tissue. Extravasation occurs from catheter breaks or leaks, sometimes as a result of the device being vigorously flushed when obstructed or malfunctioning. In these cases, the catheter needs to be removed.

Catheter Rupture and Embolization

The pinch-off syndrome occurs when access to the subclavian vein is medial to the junction of the first rib and clavicle.[36–40] Catheters in this position can be compressed, fractured, and embolized.[36–40] Pinching of a catheter sometimes can be recognized on chest radiographs as a focal narrowing. Once pinching is recognized, these catheters should be removed. Embolized catheter fragments can be snared and removed. The pinch-off syndrome can be prevented by using the ultrasound-guided lateral approach; the subclavian or axillary vein is usually punctured in the midclavicular portion away from the junction of the first rib and clavicle.

Catheter Removal

Tunneled Catheters

The tunneled catheters can be removed by simply pulling the catheter out or by dissecting out the Dacron cuff, which holds the catheter firmly in the subcutaneous tissues. The catheter and the tunnel are sterilely prepped and draped. The skin at the exit site and at the Dacron cuff is anesthetized with lidocaine. With steady tension, the cuff may break free from the tissue and the catheter is easily removed with the cuff. Alternatively, the catheter can break free from the cuff and the catheter can be removed easily, but the cuff remains behind. Sometimes, an incision over the cuff parallel to the catheter is made, the incision is carried down until fibers

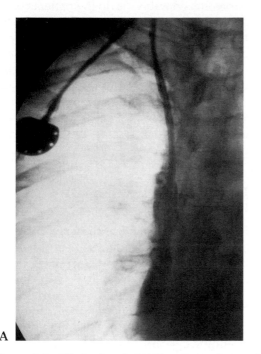
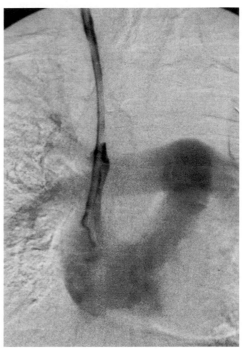

A B

Figure 6–8 Fibrin sheath. **(A)** Despite perfect positioning of the Port-A-Cath with the catheter tip in the proximal right atrium, a fibrin sheath formed around the catheter. **(B)** The digital subtraction images of the same study show reflux of contrast along the catheter within the fibrin sheath.

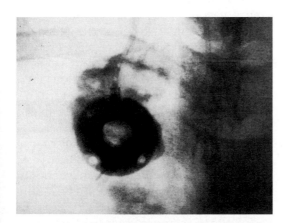

Figure 6–9 Poor needle access of a Port-A-Cath. The patient complained of pain when medication was infused into her Port-A-Cath. A small amount of contrast was injected through the indwelling Huber needle, showing extravasation of contrast. The needle did not adequately penetrate the diaphragm of the port. The port had been placed too deeply in the subcutaneous tissue and was not easily palpable, making needle access difficult.

of the cuff appear, the cuff then is sharply dissected away from the surrounding fibrous tissue, and the catheter with the cuff then is removed.

Ports

Removal of subcutaneous ports requires the same instruments as for placement (Table 6–3). The skin is sterilely prepped and draped. The skin along the old incision is anesthetized with lidocaine. An incision along the original scar is made. The port and catheter are exposed. Sutures holding the port in place, if present are identified, are removed. The port then is dissected free from the epithelialized surface of the subcutaneous pocket and tunnel. The port and catheter are removed. Pressure is held for 5 minutes over the venous entry site. The incision is closed in two layers as after catheter placement. A gauze dressing is applied to the incision and changed routinely.

111

RESULTS OF RADIOLOGIC ACCESS AND PLACEMENT OF PORTS AND CATHETERS

Successful access and port and catheter placement approach 100% in adults with radiologic placement (Table 6–5a). Complications have occurred with acceptable frequency. Longer-term results also have been favorable.

Venipuncture

Ultrasound-guidance has been shown to decrease the number of needle passes required for venipuncture and to decrease the rate of complications compared with other techniques.[3,7] Image guidance provides more confidence to the operator, especially in unusual or difficult cases. Ultrasound-guided subclavian venipuncture had no venipuncture-related complications, in the radiology suite in a report from Lameris and colleagues, compared with 10% puncture-related complications during blind placement in the operating room.[3] If ultrasound is not available, fluoroscopy, venography, and road mapping can be used for evaluation and access guidance.[9,41,42] A summary of the radiology literature is presented in Table 6–5.

The main problems during central venous access are arterial puncture and pneumothorax. Arterial puncture is the source of most bleeding complications in patients with normal coagulation. Bleeding complications (hematoma or hemothorax) are reported to occur in 3 to 7.5%.[24] Ultrasound-guided venipuncture decreases bleeding complications of venipuncture by decreasing threefold the number of needle passes and the number of inadvertent arterial punctures.[7]

Infection, catheter obstruction, central vein thrombosis, catheter fracture, or displacement limits long-term catheter function. Long-term (more than 30 days) infection is dependent on the patient and the catheter care. In radiologic series, the infection rates are reported to be 2.5 to 22.5% (Table 6–5). The definition of infection varies considerably, as do the patients being studied. Malpositioning of catheters leads to higher rates of catheter dysfunction and central venous thrombosis.[28] Good catheter position in the lower SVC or RA approaches 100% in radiologic series (Table 6–5). Clinically evident thrombosis occurs in 0.5 and 4.9% of patients (Table 6–5). Catheter fracture or pinch-off is rare with radiologic placement.[43]

Radiologic Versus Surgical Placement

Radiologic placement of tunneled catheters and ports has results similar to those reported in surgical series. A review of the literature (Tables 6–5 and 6–6) shows comparable results in most categories.

The literature suggests that radiologic placements have a higher success rate for obtaining access, lower access complications, and fewer catheter malpositions. The long-term complications of thrombosis and infection appear similar (Table 6–6).

A radiologist's ability to find and access a vein allows that radiologist to build a central venous access service. Patients and clinicians frustrated by multiple failed attempts at central venous access are grateful for the radiologist's ability to gain access in these problem patients. Successful imaging-guided central venous access is 99 to 100%. In addition, the radiologist is usually able to deliver these services on demand.

Lower access complications for central venous access with radiologic guidance was first reported by Lameris and colleagues in 1990.[3] In this landmark article, a statistically significant absence of access complications was reported, compared with 10% complication during blind surgical placement. As many subsequent articles have shown, however, this does not guarantee an absence of complications in all radiologists' hands. Pneumothorax rates during central venous access in radiology continue to be reported in the 0 to 2.5% range (Table 6–5). The high numbers of pneumothoraces, which occurred in several series, are due

Table 6–5a Radiology Access Literature

Authors (ref)	Year	No.	Type	Tech Fail	PNTX	Art Punc	Air Embo	Mal position	Pinch-Off	Infection	Thrombosis
Funaki et al.[48]	1997	80	Ports	0	0	0	NA	0	NA	2 (2.5)	1 (1.3)
Hull et al.[24]	1992	50	Groshong	0	1 (2.0)	2 (4.0)	0	0	0	6 (12)	0
Konen et al.[43]	1997	203	Hickman	1 (0.5)	1 (0.5)	NA	NA	NA	2 (1.0)	11 (5.4)	1 (0.5)
Lund et al.[44]	1996	237	Hickman	NA	6 (2.5)	NA	2 (0.8)	0	NA	32 (14)	2 (0.8)
Morris et al.[25]	1992	103	Ports	1 (1)	1 (1)	1 (1)	1 (1)	3 (2.9)	NA	5 (4.9)	4 (3.9)
Robertson et al.[4]	1989	60	Hickman	1 (1.7)	1 (1.7)	1 (1.7)	1 (1.7)	1 (1.7)	NA	7 (11.7)	1 (1.7)
Shetty et al.[42]	1997	350	Ports	0	7 (2.0)	0	0	4 (1.1)	0	4 (1.1)	10 (2.9)
Simpson et al.[49]	1997	161	Ports	0	2 (1.2)	NA	2 (1.2)	1 (1.06)	NA	9 (5.6)	8 (5.0)
Struk	1994	41	Ports	0	1 (2.4)	0	0	0	0	9 (22)	2 (4.8)

Techfail, technical failure; PNTX, pneumothorax; Embo, embolism; NA, not available.

Table 6-5b Surgery Access Literature

Authors (ref)	Year	No.	Type	Tech Failure	PNTX	Art Punc	Air Embolism	Malposition	Pinch-Off	Infection	Thrombosis
Biffi et al.[50]	1997	178	Port	NA	6 (3.3)	3 (1.7)	NA	2 (1.1)	3 (1.7)	5 (2.8)	2 (1.1)
Brothers et al.[19]	1988	329	Port	3 (0.9)	8 (2.4)	5 (1.5)	2 (0.6)	8 (2.4)	0	54 (16.4)	16 (4.9)
Delmore et al.[1]	1989	72	Groshong	NA	0	NA	NA	1 (1.4)	NA	6 (8.3)	1 (1.4)
Freytes et al.[35]	1990	134	Port	NA	1 (0.7)	NA	NA	3 (2.2)	NA	4 (2.5)	1 (1.07)
Malviya et al.[5]	1989	41	Groshong	NA	2 (4.8)	NA	NA	2 (4.8)	0	3 (7.3)	0
Ray et al.[51]	1996	560	Hickman	NA	9 (1.6)	21 (3.8)	NA				
Schwarz et al.[52]	1997	707	Port	6 (0.8)	0	NA	NA	18 (2.5)	11 (1.6)	62 (8.8)	0

PNTX, pneumothorax; NA, not available; Art Punc, arterial puncture.

Table 6-5c Comparative Studies

Author	Year	No.	Type	Tech Failure	PNTX	Art Punc	Air Embolism	Mal Position	Pinch Off	Infection	Thrombosis
Lameris et al.[3]	1990	40	Rad Hickman	0	0	0	NA	0	NA	10	3 (7.5)
		40	Surg Hickman	2 (5)	3 (7.5)	1 (2.5)	NA	1 (2.5)	NA	14	2 (5.0)
McBride et al.[53]	1997	120	Rad Hickman	0	4 (3.3)	NA	NA	0	NA	27 (22.5)	4 (3.3)
		133	Surg Hickman	6 (4.5)	1 (0.8)	NA	NA	5 (3.7)	NA	50 (37.6)	5 (3.7)

PNTX, pneumothorax; Art Punc, arterial puncture; NA, not available.

Table 6–6   Placement Complications

Placement	Radiology	Surgery
Access failure	0–1%	0.8–5%
Pneumothorax	0–2.5%	0–7.5%
Arterial puncture	0–4%	1.5–2.5%
Pinch-off	0–1%	0–1.7%
Malpositioning	0–2.9%	1.1–4.8%
Postplacement Complications		
Infection	1.1–22.5%	2.5–37.6%
Thrombosis	0–7.5%	0–5%

to the use of fluoroscopy and venography instead of ultrasound.[42,44]

Proper positioning of catheters by radiologists is very good, indeed (Table 6–5 and 6–6). Exact placement of catheters has been at the heart of angiography since its inception. Radiologists have had a great advantage with high-quality fluoroscopy and ultrasound.

Once a catheter has been inserted properly, whether by surgery or radiology, the long-term results should be similar. There has been concern that the infection rates might be higher in catheters and ports placed in the radiology suite compared with those placed in the operating room, but the reported infection rates have been similar (Tables 6–5 and 6–6).

The technical results of radiologic placement of central venous catheters reported in the literature do not explain the tremendous shift from the surgery to the radiology department for placement of these devices. Radiology has provided routine access with results similar to those of our surgical colleagues; however, radiologists have been able to provide reliable access in problem patients when others have failed. This success, combined with convenient service, is [likely] the source of growth in the central access for radiology.

SUMMARY

Radiologic placement of long-term central venous access devices is very successful.[3,4,6,11,24–26,45] There is no single device that will accommodate all patients. A variety of devices is available, and each has unique features.[11,46] In selected patients, ports have advantages over other devices. A port usually takes less than an hour to place, whereas an external catheter typically takes less than 30 minutes as reported by other researchers.[11,47] The radiologist should provide the best access device for an individual patient.

REFERENCES

1. Delmore JE, Horbelt DV, Jack BL, Roberts DK. Experience with the Groshong long-term central venous catheter. *Gynecol Oncol.* 1989;34:216–218.
2. Takasugi JK, O'Connell TX. Prevention of complications in permanent central venous catheters. *Surg Gynecol Obstet.* 1988;167:6–11.
3. Lameris JS, Post PJ, Zonderland HM, Gerritsen PG, Kappers-Klunne MC, Schutte HE. Percutaneous placement of Hickman catheters: comparison of sonographically guided and blind techniques. *AJR Am J Roentgenol.* 1990;155:1097–1099.

4. Robertson LJ, Mauro MA, Jaques PF. Radiologic placement of Hickman catheters. *Radiology.* 1989;170:1007–1009.

5. Malviya VK, Deppe G, Gove N, Malone JM Jr. Vascular access in gynecologic cancer using the Groshong right atrial catheter. *Gynecol Oncol.* 1989;33:313–316.

6. Dick L, Mauro MA, Jaques PF, Buckingham P. Radiologic insertion of Hickman catheters in HIV-positive patients: infectious complications. *J Vasc Interv Radiol.* 1991;2: 327–329.

7. Denys BG, Uretsky BF, Reddy PS, Ruffner RJ, Sandhu JS, Breishlatt WM. An ultrasound method for safe and rapid central venous access [letter to the editor]. *N Engl J Med.* 1991;324:566.

8. Knudson GJ, Wiedmeyer DA, Erickson SJ, et al. Color Doppler sonographic imaging in the assessment of upper-extremity deep venous thrombosis. *AJR Am J Roentgenol* 1990;154:399–403.

9. Surratt RS, Picus D, Hicks ME, Darcy MD, Kleinhoffer M, Jendrisak M. The importance of preoperative evaluation of the subclavian vein in dialysis access planning. *AJR Am J Roentgenol.* 1991;156:623–625.

10. Borst CG, de Kruif AT, van Dam FS, de Graaf PW. Totally implantable venous access ports—the patients' point of view: a quality control study. *Cancer Nurs.* 1992;15: 378–381.

11. Mauro MA, Jaques PF. Radiologic placement of long-term central venous catheters: a review. *J Vasc Interv Radiol.* 1993;4:127–137.

12. Alastrue A, Rull M, Escudero LE, et al. Experience with 150 subcutaneous venous reservoirs for venous access and infusion for the treatment of adult patients with oncologic and hematologic disorders and acquired immunodeficiency syndrome [in Spanish]. *Med Clin Barc.* 1992;99:444–449.

13. Ingram J, Weitzman S, Greenberg ML, Parkin P, Filler R. Complications of indwelling venous access lines in the pediatric hematology patient: a prospective comparison of external venous catheters and subcutaneous ports. *Am J Pediatr Hematol Oncol.* 1991;13:130-136.

14. Mirro JJ, Rao BN, Kumar M, et al. A comparison of placement techniques and complications of externalized catheters and implantable port use in children with cancer. *J Pediatr Surg.* 1990;25:120–124.

15. Ross MN, Haase GM, Poole MA, Burrington JD, Odom LF. Comparison of totally implanted reservoirs with external catheters as venous access devices in pediatric oncologic patients. *Surg Gynecol Obstet.* 1988;167: 141–144.

16. Mirro JJ, Rao BN, Stokes DC, et al. A prospective study of Hickman/Broviac catheters and implantable ports in pediatric oncology patients. *J Clin Oncol.* 1989;7: 214–222.

17. Pegues D, Axelrod P, McClarren C, et al. Comparison of infections in Hickman and implanted port catheters in adult solid tumor patients. *J Surg Oncol.* 1992;49:156–162.

18. Schrder M, Pedersen IR, Rasmussen RB. Permanent central venous catheters in oncologic patients. *Ugeskr Laeger.* 1991;153: 2491–2494.

19. Brothers TE, Von Moll LK, Niederhuber JE, Roberts JA, Walker AS, Ensminger WD. Experience with subcutaneous infusion ports in three hundred patients. *Surg Gynecol Obstet.* 1988;166:295–301.

20. Skoutelis AT, Murphy RL, MacDonell KB, VonRoenn JH, Sterkel CD, Phair JP. Indwelling central venous catheter infections in patients with acquired immune deficiency syndrome. *J Acquir Immune Defic Syndr Hum Retrovirol.* 1990;3:335–342.

21. Mueller BU, Skelton J, Callender DP, et al. A prospective randomized trial comparing the infectious and noninfectious complications of an externalized catheter versus a subcutaneously implanted device in cancer patients. *J Clin Oncol.* 1992;10:1943–1948.

22. McCready D, Broadwater R, Ross M, Pollock R, Ota D, Balch C. A case-control comparison of durability and cost between implanted reservoir and percutaneous catheters in cancer patients. *J Surg Res.* 1991;51:377–381.

23. Biagi E, Arrigo C, Dell'Orto MG, et al. Mechanical and infective central venous catheter-related complications: a prospective non-randomized study using Hickman and Groshong catheters in children with hematological malignancies. *Support Care Cancer.* 1997;5:228–233.

24. Hull JE, Hunter CS, Luiken GA. The Groshong catheter: initial experience and early results of imaging-guided placement [comments]. *Radiology.* 1992;185:803–807.

25. Morris SL, Jaques PF, Mauro MA. Radiology-assisted placement of implantable

subcutaneous infusion ports for long-term venous access. *Radiology.* 1992;184:149–151.

26. Jaques PF, Mauro MA, Keefe B. US guidance for vascular access [technical note]. *J Vasc Interv Radiol.* 1992;3:427–430.

27. Nazarian GK, Bjarnason H, Dietz CA Jr, Bernadas CA, Hunter DW. Changes in tunneled catheter tip position when a patient is upright. *J Vasc Interv Radiol.* 1997;8: 437–441.

28. Puel V, Caudry M, Le Metayer P, et al. Superior vena cava thrombosis related to catheter malposition in cancer chemotherapy given through implanted ports. *Cancer.* 1993;72:2248–2252.

29. Hunter CS, Hull JE, LaFleur B. Infectious complications of vascular access devices placed in the radiology suite. *Proc ASCO.* 1993:448.

30. Anderson AJ, Krasnow SH, Boyer MW, et al. Thrombosis: the major Hickman catheter complication in patients with solid tumor. *Chest.* 1989;95:71–75.

31. Haire WD, Lieberman RP, Lund GB, Edney JA, Kessinger A, Armitage JO. Thrombotic complications of silicone rubber catheters during autologous marrow and peripheral stem cell transplantation: prospective comparison of Hickman and Groshong catheters. *Bone Marrow Transplant.* 1991;7:57–59.

32. Hayward SR, Ledgerwood AM, Lucas CE. The fate of 100 prolonged venous access devices. *Am Surg.* 1990;56:515–519.

33. Crain MR, Mewissen MW, Ostrowski GJ, Paz-Fumagalli R, Beres RA, Wertz RA. Fibrin sleeve stripping for salvage of failing hemodialysis catheters: technique and initial results. *Radiology.* 1996;198:41–44.

34. Haskal ZJ, Leen VH, Thomas-Hawkins C, Shlansky-Goldberg RD, Baum RA, Soulen MC. Transvenous removal of fibrin sheaths from tunneled hemodialysis catheters. *J Vasc Interv Radiol.* 1996;7:513–517.

35. Freytes CO, Reid P, Smith KL. Long-term experience with a totally implanted catheter system in cancer patients. *J Surg Oncol.* 1990; 45:99–102.

36. Aitken DR, Minton JP. The "pinch-off sign": a warning of impending problems with permanent subclavian catheters. *Am J Surg.* 1984;148:633–636.

37. Hinke DH, Zandt-Stastny DA, Goodman LR, Quebbeman EJ, Krzywda EA, Andris DA. Pinch-off syndrome: a complication of implantable subclavian venous access devices. *Radiology.* 1990;177:353–356.

38. Franey T, DeMarco LC, Geiss AC, Ward RJ. Catheter fracture and embolization in a totally implanted venous access catheter. *JPEN J Parenter Enteral Nutr.* 1988;12: 528–530.

39. Noyen J, Hoorntje J, de Langen Z, Leemslag JW, Sleijfer D. Spontaneous fracture of the catheter of a totally implantable venous access port: case report of a rare complication. *J Clin Oncol.* 1987;5:1295–1299.

40. Rubenstein RB, Alberty RE, Michels LG, Pederson RW, Rosenthal D. Hickman catheter separation. *JPEN J Parenter Enteral Nutr.* 1985;9:754–757.

41. Selby JB, Tegtmeyer CJ, Amodeo C, Bittner L, Atuk NO. Insertion of subclavian hemodialysis catheters in difficult cases: value of fluoroscopy and angiographic techniques. *AJR Am J Roentgenol.* 1989;152: 641–643.

42. Shetty PC, Mody MK, Kastan DJ, et al. Outcome of 350 implanted chest ports placed by interventional radiologists. *J Vasc Interv Radiol.* 1997;8:991–995.

43. Konen E, Garniak A, Morag B, Hardan I, Rubinstein Z. Insertion of Hickman catheters in an interventional radiology suite. *Harefuah.* 1997;132:454–457,527,528.

44. Lund GB, Trerotola SO, Scheel PF Jr, et al. Outcome of tunneled hemodialysis catheters placed by radiologists. *Radiology.* 1996;198: 467–472.

45. Cockburn JF, Eynon CA, Virji N, Jackson JE. Insertion of Hickman central venous catheters using angiographic techniques in patients with hematologic disorders. *AJR Am J Roentgenol.* 1992;159:121–124.

46. Moran BJ, Sutton GL, Karran SJ. Clinical evaluation of percutaneous insertion and long-term usage of a new cuffed polyurethane catheter for central venous access. *Ann R Coll Surg Engl.* 1992;74:426–429.

47. Page AC, Evans RA, Kaczmarski R, Mufti GJ, Gishen P. The insertion of chronic indwelling central venous catheters (Hickman lines) in interventional radiology suites. *Clin Radiol.* 1990;42:105–109.

48. Funaki B, Szymski GX, Hackworth CA, et al. Radiologic placement of subcutaneous infusion chest ports for long-term central venous access. *AJR Am J Roentgenol.* 1997;169: 1431–1434.

49. Simpson KR, Hovsepian DM, Picus D. Interventional radiologic placement of chest wall ports: results and complications in 161 consecutive placements. *J Vasc Interv Radiol.* 1997;8:189–195.

50. Biffi R, Corrado F, de Braud F, et al. Long-term, totally implantable central venous access ports connected to a Groshong catheter for chemotherapy of solid tumours: experience from 178 cases using a single type of device. *Eur J Cancer.* 1997;33: 1190–1194.

51. Ray S, Stacey R, Imrie M, Filshie J. A review of 560 Hickman catheter insertions. *Anaesthesia.* 1996;51:981–985.

52. Schwarz RE, Groeger JS, Coit DG. Subcutaneously implanted central venous access devices in cancer patients: a prospective analysis. *Cancer.* 1997;79:1635–1640.

53. McBride KD, Fisher R, Warnock N, Winfield DA, Reed MW, Gaines PA. A comparative analysis of radiological and surgical placement of central venous catheters. *Cardiovasc Interv Radiol.* 1997;20:17–22.

Chapter 7

Access for Hemodialysis

Melvin Rosenblatt

How frail is man, for despite his wisdom and strength, it is a mere few drops of water that spare his life. More so, how frail is the hemodialysis-dependent patient for whom the basic essentials of life are not enough. For this patient, vascular access is as important for survival as water. As physicians caring for these patients, the onus to provide and maintain this type of access has fallen squarely on our shoulders. Since the 1940s, we have acknowledged our responsibility toward these patients and have explored various vascular access methods.[1–11]

Today, more than half a century later, despite all our efforts, a method for obtaining reliable and completely trouble-free, high-flow vascular access still eludes us. This does not mean that progress has not been made over the past 60 years. To the contrary, modern vascular access methods, such as surgically created native and prosthetic arteriovenous fistulas (AVFs), are a vast improvement over earlier solutions and have gained universal acceptance in the dialysis community. Unfortunately, although these methods are close to ideal, they have many failings.

Native AVFs take a long time to mature or, in many patients, never mature.[12–15] Prosthetic AVFs mature rapidly but fail frequently.[16,17] Additionally, neither method provides immediate access for hemodialysis. Only intravenous catheters can offer this attribute.

Intravenous catheters are readily available, can be inserted easily, and can be used immediately. As such, these catheters have gained remarkable popularity. In 1993, 37% of newly diagnosed end-stage renal disease (ESRD) patients were receiving hemodialysis using a central venous catheter 1 month after initiation of their treatment.[18] Additionally, it is estimated that 30% of hemodialysis-dependent patients have central venous catheters as their permanent type of vascular access.[19] Unfortunately, the "ideal" features of central venous catheters are offset by the high morbidity associated with these devices relative to that of other types of access.[20] Malfunction, infection, and central venous stenoses are frequent occurrences.[21–27] For these reasons, the National Kidney Foundation Dialysis Outcomes Quality Initiative (NKF-DOQI) Work Group recommends that fewer than 10% of chronic dialysis patients be maintained on long-term catheter-based hemodialysis.[28]

As meritorious as the DOQI recommendation is, widespread attainment of this goal in the United States is unlikely to occur in the near future. The dialysis population is aging, and more of these patients have severe cardiac and peripheral vascular disease limiting their access options. Additionally, the current well-entrenched practice pattern of delaying the establishment of vascular access until the last possible moment continues to increase the clinician's dependence on central venous catheters for both short- and long-term access solutions. Given this state of affairs, it is essential that clinicians placing these catheters must understand how to maximize the function of these devices while minimizing adverse consequences, which not only cause immediate patient morbidity but also often destroy central veins and ultimately prevent establishing durable arteriovenous (AV) accesses. Thus, this chapter discusses the different types of dialysis catheters and the indication for their use, and it highlights the techniques for proper implantation. Additionally, immediate and long-term outcomes as well as the cost-effectiveness of image-guided placement are reviewed.

HEMODIALYSIS CATHETERS

Catheter Design

To accomplish hemodialysis, blood must be removed from the body and passed through a system containing a semipermeable membrane to remove toxic metabolites and unwanted fluid. Once cleansed, the flowing blood is returned to the systemic circulation. Thus, for continuous hemodialysis, a circuit must be established with two separate access channels moving blood in opposite directions. To avoid recirculating the same treated blood, each of these channels must be located away from the other. This concept of separated dual-channel circulatory access is the basis of every hemodialysis catheter design. The challenge has been to translate this concept into a device that maximizes dual-channel flow rates and minimizes recirculation.

Recirculation has been the easiest challenge to overcome. Catheter channels do not need to be separated by great distances to reduce recirculation to an acceptably low level. If the draw channel is upstream to the return channel, a separation of only 2 to 3 cm is all that is needed.[29,30] Unfortunately, establishing and maintaining high flow rates have presented a much greater challenge. On average, 120 L of blood must be processed at each hemodialysis session. For this to occur in a reasonable time frame, blood flow rates of 350 to 500 mL per minute are required. Attaining flow rates of this magnitude through a central venous catheter requires that the channels possess a suitably large diameter. Additionally, the wall of at least one of the channels must be rigid enough to withstand a draw pressure of 150 to 250 mm Hg without collapsing. Because flow rates are predominantly dependent on the inner diameter of each channel (*Poiseuille law*), an increase in this diameter is the primary way to achieve higher flow rates. The most direct manner in which this can be accomplished is to increase the overall diameter of the catheter. Unfortunately, the morbidity associated with central venous catheters increases as the outer diameter is enlarged. Thus, in designing these devices, a balance between catheter diameter and optimal flow rates must be achieved to maximize the risk-to-benefit ratio.

Current adult hemodialysis catheters range in size from approximately 10 to 14.5 French (F).[31–33] Many of these catheters are designed as a single tube with two separate channels. Other designs rely on a two-catheter system, which consists of two separate single-channel catheters that are placed independently.[31] All these devices are constructed of polyurethane or silicone rubber. Polyurethane, in comparison to silicone rubber, possesses a high tensile strength.[34] This property allows for the construction of catheters with thinner walls that can withstand high flow rates. A thinner wall translates into a larger ratio of the inner diameter to the outer diameter, which in turn means higher sustainable flow rates for a given outer diameter. Unfortunately, polyurethane is susceptible to kinking with acute angulations. Additionally, polyurethane undergoes an enzymatic degradation process known as *environmental stress cracking*.[34,35] This process, albeit quite slow, can weaken the catheter and result in catheter fragmentation and embolization. Silicone rubber, in contrast to polyurethane, is extremely biostable. It is soft and very flexible, which reduces the likelihood of endothelial injury and catheter kinks. Silicone rubber, however, has a low tensile strength, necessitating a smaller ratio of the inner diameter to the outer diameter compared with polyurethane. In today's environment, this feature is problematic. Higher flow rates have been the focus of most new dialysis catheter designs, and manufacturers have all but abandoned the use of silicone rubber in favor of polyurethane materials.

Catheter Types

Central venous catheters for hemodialysis are designed for either short- or long-term use. Short-term, or acute, catheters, as opposed to long-term catheters, do not have a Dacron retention cuff and are not tunneled. They are designed specifically for rapid over-the-wire placement. For this type of placement to be possible, the catheter shaft must be rigid so that it can be advanced through the subcutaneous tissues. For the same reason, the catheter tip also must be tapered. Thus, once access is established into a central vein, the hemodialysis catheter can be advanced over the wire into position. The advantage of this type of catheter is in its ease of placement, which enables these catheters to be inserted at the patient's

bedside with minimal difficulty. Additionally, the rigid catheter can withstand high negative aspiration pressures, permitting adequate flow rates with a smaller catheter diameter. A smaller catheter diameter obviously contributes to the ease of implantation.

With implantation ease at the core of this catheter design, it is no surprise that a vast majority of these catheters are placed at the bedside, through the internal jugular, subclavian, or femoral vein without image guidance. These catheters are available in a straight or curved shaft configuration (Fig. 7–1). The straight shaft catheter is ideal for subclavian and femoral placement. The extension limbs of a straight shaft catheter, however, when placed in the internal jugular vein (IJV), often assume an awkward and uncomfortable position just below the patient's ear. The curved shaft design displaces the extension limbs of the catheter downward, away from the patient's neck onto the chest wall. This configuration is far more comfortable for the patient when the IJV is used for access. Another design modification involves curving the

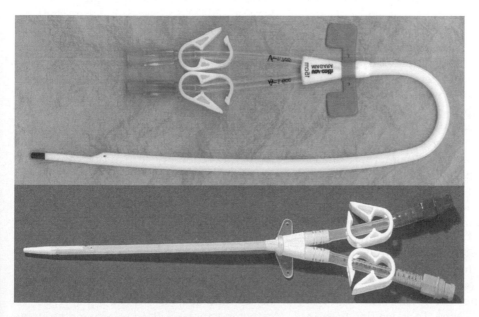

Figure 7–1 Straight (Mahurkar Catheter; Tyco Health Care, Kendall, Mansfield, MA, U.S.A.) and curved acute hemodialysis catheters (Niagra Bard Access Systems, Salt Lake City, UT, U.S.A.)

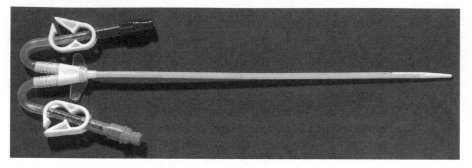

Figure 7–2 Mahurkar curved extension catheter (Tyco Health Care, Kendall, Mansfield, MA, U.S.A.).

extension limbs back on themselves instead of the catheter shaft (Fig. 7–2). This design, similar to the curved shaft design, displaces the extension limbs downward into a more comfortable position.

Chronic Catheters

Unfortunately, the characteristics of the acute hemodialysis catheter, which include a rigid catheter shaft and a tapered tip, do not make this type of catheter suitable for long-term use.[36] Conceptually, it is easy to see how a stiff, pointed catheter could cause significant injury to the superior vena cava (SVC) or right atrium (RA) if left in place a long time.[37] What constitutes a long period never has been precisely defined; however, it is generally accepted that this type of catheter should not remain implanted for more than 2 to 3 weeks when access is through the subclavian or IJV.[38] When the femoral vein is accessed, this type of catheter should not be left in place longer than 5 days.[39] Therefore, for long-term catheter access, a different catheter design is required.

Long-term or chronic catheters are designed to be soft so that endovascular trauma can be minimized. These catheters are constructed from soft polyurethane or silicone rubber and therefore have little column strength. Consequently, these catheters do not possess the rigidity necessary to permit over-the-wire placement through subcutaneous tissues. To place this type of catheter into the central venous system, a pathway must be created through which the soft catheter shaft can be advanced. This can be accomplished through the use of a peel-away sheath consisting of a rigid dilator supporting a thin, circular tube designed to split lengthwise into two. The sheath-dilator combination is rigid enough to be advanced through subcutaneous tissues over a wire. With the sheath in the central vein, the rigid dilator is removed, leaving only the thin-walled tube, which is of sufficient diameter to allow passage of the soft access catheter through it into the central venous system. Once the access catheter is placed, the sheath is split and torn away, leaving only the access catheter in place.

The flexibility and softness of the catheter shaft are not the only distinction between the acute and chronic hemodialysis access catheter. Chronic hemodialysis catheters are also tunneled and possess a polyester retention cuff. Tunneling helps to reduce the likelihood of infection and enables the catheter's exit site to be positioned away from the venotomy to a more convenient location.[40] The polyester cuff promotes tissue ingrowth, which prevents the catheter from dislodging and helps to create a barrier against infection.[41] These features enable this type of catheter to remain within the central venous system for a prolonged period.[42] Currently, there is no maximum implantation time recommendation for these catheters. If needed, this type of catheter can be left in place indefinitely; however, vascular injury and vessel occlusion are the inevitable consequences of

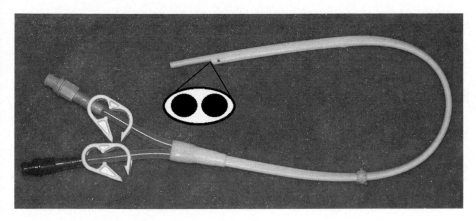

Figure 7–3 Quinton Permacath catheter (Tyco Health Care, Kendall, Mansfield, MA, U.S.A.).

having any type of catheter in the central venous circulation for a prolonged period. Therefore, a strenuous effort should be made to reduce the overall length of time a central venous dialysis catheter remains in place. In the hemodialysis-dependent patient, this can be accomplished by hastening the creation of more permanent arterial–venous access solutions. With this mindset, chronic hemodialysis catheters, as a bridge to more permanent access, should rarely remain in place for longer than 3 months.

Three months can be a very long time when a chronic access catheter fails to perform adequately. Ideally, this type of catheter should deliver a flow rate of at least 300 mL per minute.[43] Unfortunately, achieving and maintaining this goal have been problematic. In addressing this problem, many different chronic catheter configurations designed to improve function have been marketed to implanting physicians. These catheter designs can be divided into three broad groups: single-catheter design, dual-catheter design, and a composite design.

The single-catheter design consists of a single tube with two separate channels. The shape of the catheter and the configuration of channels within it are what individualize each of the access catheters in this group. An oval-shaped catheter with two round channels is one of the earliest catheter designs (Fig. 7–3). This design has a large outer diameter relative to the diameter of each channel. For this reason, catheters of this design are no longer popular. The most popular single-catheter configuration is the "double D." This design takes a round catheter and places a septum down the center. This septum divides the catheter into two D-shaped channels (Fig. 7–4). This configuration uses available space very efficiently, and the overall inner diameter of each of the channels is large in relation to outer diameter of the catheter. A similar catheter configuration to the "double D" is the Circle C (Horizon Medical Products, Manchester, GA, U.S.A.). This catheter is a circular tube that has an asymmetrically positioned smaller circular tube within it (Fig. 7–5). A configuration of this type has a draw channel that is larger than the infusion channel, permitting a higher flow rate through the more functionally vulnerable of the two channels.

The dual-catheter design involves placing two single-lumen catheters through independent venous access points. Typically, these two points of access are adjacent to each other in the same vein; however, this need not be the case. Each individual catheter can be placed through a different central vein with the distal ends positioned in the RA. Each of the catheter ends must be positioned so that recirculation is avoided. This is accomplished by positioning the aspiration cannula 3 to 5 cm upstream from

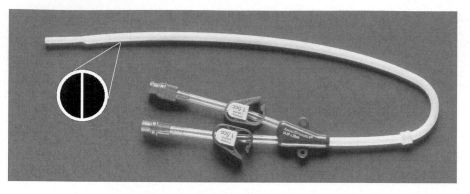

Figure 7–4 More-Flow catheter (AngioDynamics, Inc., Queens-bury, NY, U.S.A.).

the infusion cannula. The Tesio catheter (Medical Components, Inc., Harleysville, PA, U.S.A.) and the SchonCath (Angio-Dynamics, Queensbury, NY, U.S.A.) are two commercially available catheters that utilize this design.

The Tesio catheter consists of two 10-F single-lumen catheters that are inserted through a central vein and tunneled inde-pendently onto the chest wall (Fig. 7–6). Each of these catheters is held in place by a large polyester cuff. This design enables high flow rates with reduced diameter venotomies. Reducing the caliber of each venotomy may reduce implantation compli-cations. Additionally, two independent, free-floating cannulas may help to eliminate catheter occlusion. The extra time required

to implant this device and the overall presence of more catheter material in the central vein, potentially causing central vein occlusion, are clear disadvantages.

The SchonCath is two 9-F single-lumen catheters that are conjoined for a short segment at their midportion (Fig. 7–7). Just beyond this junction, each of the two catheter segments is inserted into a central vein. The attachment point then is buried in the subcutaneous tissue at the venous entry site, and the back ends of each catheter are tunneled to a site on the chest wall. Hence, the attachment point between the two cath-eters, referred to by the manufacturer as the Hemolock anchoring hub, holds the entire catheter in place without using polyester cuffs. This device possesses the same theo-

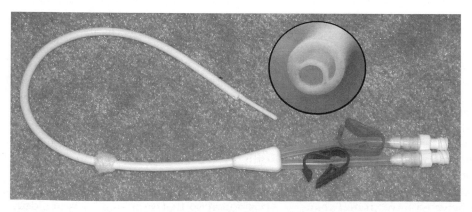

Figure 7–5 Circle C catheter (Horizon Medical Products, Man-chester, GA, U.S.A.).

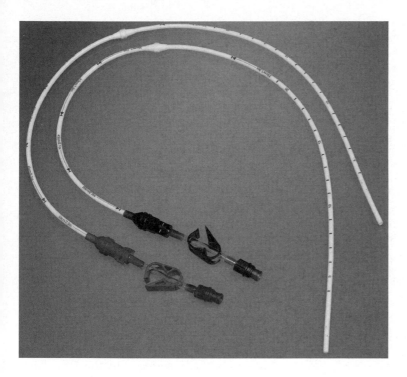

Figure 7–6 Tesio catheter (Medical Components, Inc., Harleys-ville, PA, U.S.A.).

retic advantages of the Tesio catheter, but it does not rely on tissue ingrowth into a cuff to prevent dislodgment. Disadvantages are analogous to the Tesio catheter, with the added difficulty of having to perform a more extensive dissection at the venotomy site to remove or replace the catheter.

A recent catheter design collages the advantages of the dual- and single-catheter systems. This composite design is easy to implant as a single-catheter device yet has two independent free-floating cannulas. This patented design, known as the Ash-Split Catheter (Medical Components, Inc.) has two D-shaped cannulas joined together to form a round catheter (Fig. 7–8). The joint holding these two cannulas together is designed to give way easily so that each of the two lumens can be split apart just before the device is placed in the central vein. Splitting the catheter gives rise to two separate free-floating lumens in the same vessel, which, similar to the dual catheter design, theoretically improves flow and increases long-term patency. Unfortunately, no data are currently available to support or refute this contention.

HEMODIALYSIS PORTS

Externalized catheters, such as those previously described, are easy to place and provide immediate high-flow access for hemodialysis. Unfortunately, these devices malfunction frequently and are susceptible to infection. In an effort to reduce the complications associated with these catheters, manufacturers have explored the idea of attaching these catheters to a subcutaneous reservoir. The concept of totally implanted venous access devices is not new. Totally implanted infusion devices have been available since the early 1980s; however, the high flow requirement of hemodialysis and the need of repetitive access present significant technical challenges.

The most significant challenge for these devices is that of repetitive transcutane-

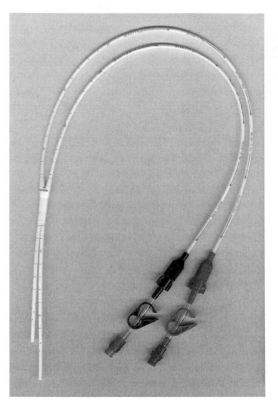

Figure 7–7 SchonCath (AngioDynamics, Queensbury, NY, U.S.A.).

ous, large-bore cannula access. The device, which is a gateway to the central circulation, must open wide once a cannula is inserted and then rapidly close tightly when it is removed. Additionally, with frequent access, the device must be extremely resistant to bacterial contamination and the tissue and skin around the device must remain intact. Other important issues that must be addressed are ease of device access, functional longevity, and ease of repair. Currently, two devices address these issues in different ways: the Dialock Port, manufactured by Biolink Corp. (Middleboro, MA, U.S.A.) and the LifeSite, manufactured by Vasca, Inc. (Tewksbury, MA, U.S.A.).

The Dialock Port is a single titanium rectangular container that has two needle-accessible passageways (Fig. 7–9). Each passageway incorporates a normally closed valve assembly. The valves are opened only by insertion of the specifically designed Dialock needles. The device is accessed along its side in such a way that the cannulas are in line with the access catheters. The access catheters themselves are designed of thin-walled silicone reinforced with a metal braid. The catheters normally are implanted into the IVJ by separate IJV punctures. The device then is placed subcutaneously on the chest wall. Currently, this device is available overseas but is not yet approved by the U.S. Food and Drug Administration (FDA) for sale in the United States.

The LifeSite device is a stainless steel port containing a single valve. The valve is connected to a 12 F silicone catheter, which is inserted into the central venous circulation (Fig. 7–10). For hemodialysis, the standard approach involves two valves implanted adjacent to one another, with both cannulas inserted into the IJV. Alternatively, the valves could be implanted at separate locations, with each cannula entering a different central vein. The device is accessed with standard 14-gauge fistula needles inserted perpendicularly into the device. When the needle enters the device channel, the valve is opened, allowing direct communication with the venous cannula (Fig. 7–11).

In the initial clinical trial, the valve entry channel was cleansed with Chlorpactin, a mild bleach solution, to prevent device contamination and infection. Subsequent investigation demonstrated 70% isopropyl alcohol to be a better cleansing solution that substantially reduces the infection rate for this device.[44] Cleansing is accomplished by insertion of a 25-gauge needle into the valve channel and the injection of 1 mL of the alcohol solution. The 25-gauge needle does not actuate the valve mechanism, and no communication with the central venous system is established during the alcohol wash. This device had been under clinical investigation in the United States since June 1997 and was approved for sale in the United States by the FDA in August 2000.

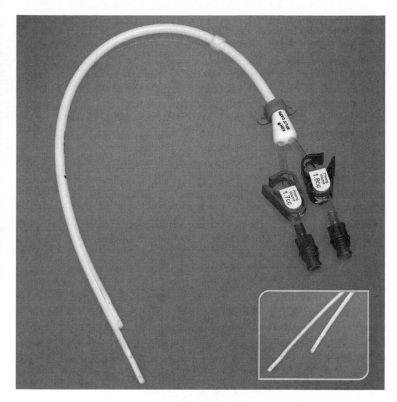

Figure 7–8 Ash-Split catheter (Medical Components, Inc., Harleysville, PA, U.S.A.).

Catheter Selection

In the past, hemodialysis access catheter diversity was limited, and as a consequence catheter selection was simple. With one or two less-than-ideal catheters of each type, acute or chronic, the implanting physician chose the one with which he or she was most comfortable. For the better, in the past decade, the number of available access catheters has increased dramatically. Currently, several manufacturers produce hemodialysis access catheters, each unique and yet similar in design. In many instances, only subtle differences, such as the number of side holes at the catheter tip, distinguish one catheter from another. In this era of abundance, it has become increasingly difficult to determine which catheter is best. Given these difficulties, it is important to keep in mind the criteria used to select a hemodialysis catheter. These criteria, in order of priority, include: function, risk,

ease of insertion, maintenance ease, patient comfort, and cost.

Catheter function is without question the most important criterion to consider when selecting a suitable catheter. Adequate function, defined by the DOQI as a sustained blood flow rate of greater than 300 mL per minute, was difficult to achieve with many of the older, small-diameter catheters. Recently, larger-diameter (i.e., more than 14.0 F) polyurethane devices have been introduced that can sustain flow rates greater than 400 mL per minute.[33] In most adults, these newer catheters should be chosen over smaller-diameter, lower-flow devices. Not every hemodialysis patient requires catheters with very high flow rates, however. Some patients cannot tolerate high-flux hemodialysis and are dialyzed at a rate that is well below the capacity of these large-bore devices. Additionally, the recommended hemodialysis flow rate for

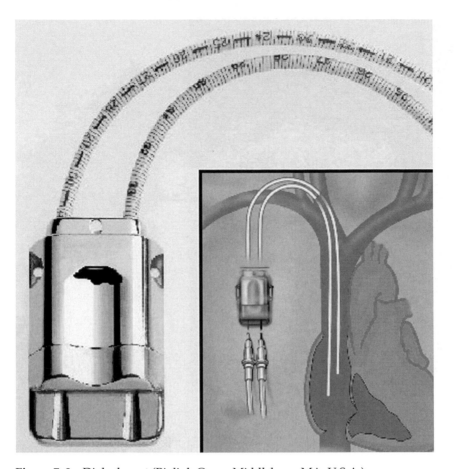

Figure 7–9   Dialock port (Biolink Corp., Middleboro, MA, U.S.A.).

pediatric patients is only 5 mL per kilogram per minute, and catheter flow capacities above 250 mL per minute are unnecessary. In this small group of patients, the potential risks associated with larger-diameter, high-flow catheters can be avoided by using smaller-diameter 8 F and 13.5 F catheters.

Effort always should be made to minimize the risks of placing a chronic hemodialysis catheter. It is therefore imperative that the device selected for implantation help in this goal. For most devices, the overall risk is similar. Some devices, however, by virtue of their design, are inherently more risky than others. Large-bore devices inserted through large-bore peel-away sheaths are intuitively more likely than smaller-diameter catheters to result in an air embolus. Additionally, the large-bore Ash-Split catheter, because of the separation

between the two lumens, is likely at greater risk for air embolus. Other devices possess different risks, some of which include excessive thrombogenicity and material instability. Material instability, usually the consequence of a manufacturing flaw, can result in device fracture and embolization (Fig. 7–12). The implanting physicians must be familiar with the unique risks of each device and weigh these risks against any potential benefits when selecting a suitable hemodialysis access catheter.

Ease of insertion and maintenance are other factors that should be considered when selecting a hemodialysis access device. Single-catheter, dual-lumen devices are easier to insert than dual-catheter devices, which require the vein to be accessed twice, the placement of two peel-away sheaths, and the creation of two separate subcutaneous tunnels. Additionally, dual-catheter systems are more difficult to maintain. When a dual-catheter system malfunctions, often both catheters need to be exchanged. This requires the placement of two guidewires, the dissection of two retention cuffs, and, if appropriate, disruption of two fibrin sleeves. Even removing dual-catheter systems is more time consuming than single-catheter systems simply because two retention cuffs, as opposed to one, must be dissected free.

Cost is always an important consideration when selecting a hemodialysis access device. In most instances, the cost difference between two devices is negligible, allowing outcome parameters to carry greater weight in the selection decision. The cost difference between a tunneled and a totally implanted device is dramatic, however, and therefore must be taken into consideration. The cost of a totally implanted hemodialysis device is approximately $3,600.00, which, on average, is more than 12 times that of a tunneled catheter. To justify this initial cost, the totally implanted device, over time, must reduce the overall

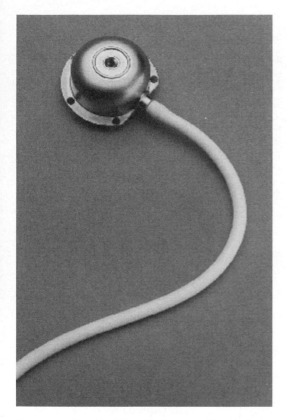

Figure 7–10 LifeSite (Vasca, Inc., Tewksbury, MA, U.S.A.).

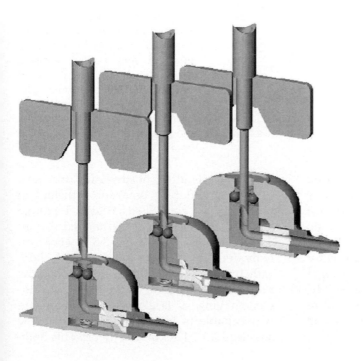

Figure 7–11 The 14-gauge needle displaces two ball bearings laterally as it passes through the opening of the device. These bearings force the access cup downward, releasing the pinch on the valve at the base, opening a channel to blood flow.

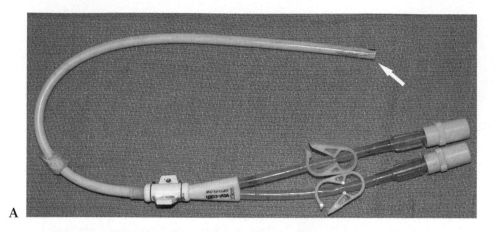

A

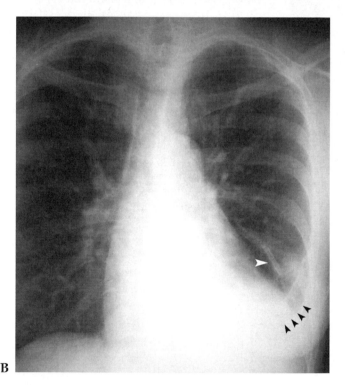

B

Figure 7–12 A chronic hemodialysis access catheter was placed in this patient 3 months earlier. Removal of the catheter was required for persistent fever. **(A)** When the catheter was removed, it was noted that the tip had separated from the catheter (*arrow*). **(B)** The tip embolized to the lung and lodged in a pulmonary artery branch (*white arrowhead*) resulting in a chronic infection and pleural effusion (*black arrowheads*). The tip could not be removed percutaneously, and the patient eventually required a lobectomy to resolve the infection.

cost of catheter maintenance by minimizing risk and maximizing function and device longevity. Whereas early data suggest that this is true, this cost-to-benefit ratio can be obtained in a patient who will require veno–venous hemodialysis for several months or years. Thus, proper patient selection is critical. Ultimately, further studies will be required to confirm the cost savings that these devices can afford.

Only a handful of investigators have compared different types of catheters in randomized, controlled trials. Trerotola and colleagues compared the 14.5 F Ash-Split catheter with the 13.5 F Hickman hemodialysis catheter and found both catheters able to provide acceptable flow rates.[33] Not surprisingly, the Ash-Split catheter, having a larger luminal diameter, was capable of higher flow rates than the smaller 13.5 F Hickman catheter. This higher flow capability can enhance dialysis efficiency and reduce the incidence of catheter failure. The tradeoff, as noted in this study, is a slightly longer insertion time and higher complication rate. More recently, Richard and co-workers evaluated hemodialysis catheters of similar luminal diameter.[45] The 14.5 F Ash-Split catheter (Medcomp, Harleysville, PA, U.S.A.), the 14.5 F Opti-flow catheter (Bard Access Systems, Salt Lake City, UT, U.S.A.), and the 10 F Tesio catheter (Medcomp) were investigated in this comparative trial. The investigators concluded that the Opti-flow and Ash-Split catheters were faster and easier to place than the Tesio catheter; however, no significant difference in function or catheter longevity was found. The risk of catheter placement was minimally higher for the Tesio catheter, but this difference was not statistically significant.

Few, if any, additional studies exist that prospectively compare the functionality of hemodialysis catheters. Furthermore, new hemodialysis catheters, which have never been evaluated, are constantly being introduced into the marketplace. The manufacturers promote each of these devices as being superior to all others. Unfortunately, in most instances, there is no evidence to support these claims. Given the dearth of data on this topic, it is nearly impossible to make recommendations on which specific catheter to select.

HEMODIALYSIS CATHETER IMPLANTATION

Site Selection

The most important aspect of placing a central venous catheter for hemodialysis is access site selection. Commonly, the subclavian and the jugular veins are used to introduce these large-bore catheters into the central circulation. Traditionally, the subclavian veins have been the most frequently used point of access because of their convenient chest wall location and the clinician's broad familiarity with subclavian access techniques.[41,46–51] Unfor-

tunately, for many reasons, the incidence of complications associated with subclavian vein access is high.[52,53] Complications such as pneumothorax and central venous thrombosis are more likely to occur with subclavian vein access, even when imaging techniques are used.[54,55] These complications, which are infrequent, are almost always symptomatic. However, subclavian vein stenosis, which is normally asymptomatic, is a significant problem for the hemodialysis-dependent patient because of its devastating effect on future long-term access options and the frequency with which it occurs. Barrett and colleagues reported a 50% incidence of subclavian vein stenosis in patients with acute subclavian access catheters.[26] They also noted that the incidence of stenosis was related to the duration of catheterization. Others reported similar findings.[53,56–61] In our practice, we also found this to be true, and we believe that the incidence of subclavian vein stenosis approaches 100% if the access catheter is left in place for a long enough period. Therefore, every effort should be made to avoid subclavian vein cannulation in any patient who is a candidate for upper-extremity AV access.[51] So critical is this point that this practice restriction should not be limited to large-bore dialysis catheters; rather, it should be applied to any type of infusion catheter in this patient population. Additionally, the patient population subjected to this restriction should include not only patients with chronic renal failure but also those with borderline renal function who someday might develop renal insufficiency.

HELPFUL HINT

The only scenario in which subclavian vein access would be considered appropriate is for the patient who has exhausted all surgical access options in the extremity ipsilateral to the desired site of access. In all other situations, the jugular vein is the preferred point of access.

Internal jugular vein access should be considered the access site of choice when

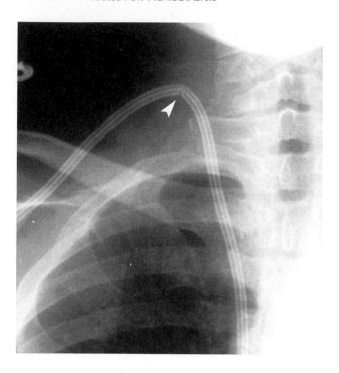

Figure 7–13 The anterior or middle approach to the jugular vein forces the soft-access catheter to assume an acute angle as it is tunneled into the chest wall (*arrowhead*).

placing hemodialysis access catheters. This access, over the short term, reduces the risk of pneumothorax and over the long term is less likely to cause problematic central vein stenoses.[58–61] Yet IJV access is still avoided occasionally when placing central venous access devices for hemodialysis. The explanation for this practice is likely attributable to the acute angulation that the catheter sometimes must make as it comes down the neck to its exit site on the chest wall. This angulation often results in a catheter kink that compromises luminal diameter and hence reduces blood flow rates (Fig. 7–13). In our early experience, this was a significant problem. Our initial solution was to modify the course of our subcutaneous tunnel tract. This, unfortunately, resulted in odd catheter exit sites that were poorly tolerated by patients. So uncomfortable was this solution that patients would obstinately refuse jugular vein access. In searching for an alternative solution to this problem, we developed the low posterior approach to the IJV. This technique, described in detail later in this chapter, permits the catheter to assume a gentle, kink-free curve as it courses through its subcutaneous tunnel

to a comfortable, unobtrusive exit site on the chest wall (Fig. 7–14). As a consequence of this new approach, catheter function improved, and patient satisfaction increased. The disadvantages once commonly associated with IJV access were eliminated, allowing us to completely abandon subclavian vein access with just one caveat: The jugular veins had to be traversable with a guidewire.

When the IJVs are occluded, alternate approaches are necessary. Before considering an alternate access site, aggressive attempts at securing access through a neck vein should be made. Sometimes the IJV, even though it is occluded, can be accessed and used as a passageway to the RA. If this fails, the external jugular veins should be considered for catheter access. If they, too, are occluded, a careful search for large neck vein collaterals should be undertaken. Often these collateral vessels can be used as passageways to the central venous circulation. If, after a careful search, all access in the neck has been exhausted, an alternate site must be chosen. The subclavian vein would be the next catheter access site choice if, as mentioned earlier, peripheral AV

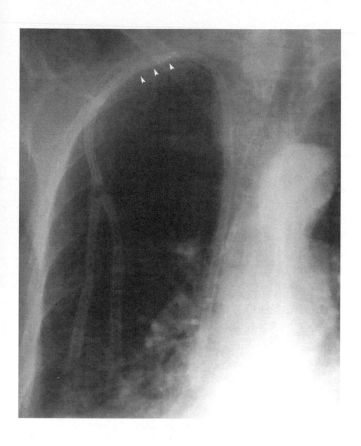

Figure 7–14 The low posterior approach to the jugular vein permits the access catheter to assume a broad gentle course as it travels away from the neck to the chest wall (*arrowheads*).

options in the ipsilateral arm have been completely exhausted. If the upper extremities are still able to support an AV access option, our next preferred access site choice is the inferior vena cava (IVC) through a translumbar approach. With good radiologic guidance, this approach is not difficult, and the short- and long-term complication rates are acceptable.[62–65] Femoral access is an option; however, this approach is associated with a high incidence of lower extremity deep venous thrombosis, and the infection risk is greater.[66] Additionally, as with the subclavian vein, lower-extremity AV access options can be obliterated through the use of femoral catheters. Our access site of last resort is the IVC through a trans-hepatic approach.[67–71] This approach, because it traverses liver parenchyma, poses a greater risk to the patient. Moreover, in our experience, there is a high likelihood of catheter tip migration resulting in catheter malfunction.

Site Preparation

Ultrasound Survey

Before preparing the skin for catheter implantation, it is important to know whether the intended access vein is patent. It is a waste of time and effort and exposes the patient to unnecessary risk if it is discovered that the intended access vein is occluded after the site has been prepared and attempts at access have been made. Knowledge of the patient's prior access history and a quick physical examination can help to determine the patency of central veins. Occasionally, the patient may know which veins are patent and which veins are occluded. If not, physical findings, such as large venous collaterals on the chest wall and shoulder, can suggest the presence of an occluded vein. Whereas these techniques are helpful, the best way to determine whether the vein is patent is to perform a quick ultrasound examination. The IJV can be imaged easily using ultra-

133

sound. If it is found to be easily compressible and can be followed down into the brachiocephalic vein in the chest, access difficulties are unlikely.

Skin Preparation

It is impossible to sterilize the skin completely. Therefore, the goal in preparing a surgical site is to remove the transient and pathogenic bacteria and to decrease the resident flora to the lowest possible level. This can be accomplished best through the combined effects of a mechanical scrub and an effective antiseptic agent.[72] Before preparing the skin, it might be necessary to remove hair; however, shaving with a razor can traumatize the skin surface and enhance bacterial growth. This only occurs if shaving is performed several hours before the procedure.[73,74] If hair removal is absolutely necessary because it interferes with the surgery, mechanical clipping is preferable to shaving.[72] If mechanical clippers are unavailable, shaving should be done just before surgery, using an antiseptic scrub as a lubricant.

The antiseptic preparation of the skin should be a two-step process. The first step is a mechanical scrub with Betadine soap. The second step involves painting an antiseptic solution over the skin. Usually, iodophor compounds, such as povidone–iodine, are used to accomplish this. These compounds are effective against a wide range of bacteria.[75] Once applied, the iodophor compound can be allowed to air-dry on the skin, but several studies have shown that this step is not essential.[76,77] If patients are sensitive to iodine-based compounds, other agents, such as isopropyl alcohol and chlorhexidine (Hibiclens, Stuart Pharmaceuticals, Wilmington, DE, U.S.A.) can be used. Chlorhexidine is effective against a wide range of gram-positive and gram-negative bacteria. Many studies have shown chlorhexidine to be superior to iodophors and alcohol as an antiseptic agent.[78–80] Chlorhexidine, once applied, leaves an antiseptic film behind. If other antiseptics are subsequently applied, this film can be washed away, negating the antibacterial effects of this agent. Thus, this agent, when it is used, should be applied in a one-step scrub. Newer scrub solutions have recently become available. These products combine two different antiseptics agents to be used effectively as a single-step skin preparation. Duraprep (3M Corp.) combines an iodophor compound with isopropyl alcohol. This combined agent is effective against many organisms, including methicillin-resistant *Staphylococcus aureus*, methicillin-resistant *Staphylococcus epidermidis*, vancomycin-resistant enterococcus, and gentamicin-resistant bacteria. It can be applied rapidly and leaves behind an antibacterial film that lasts for 12 hours.[81,82]

Prophylactic Antibiotics

Whenever an inert object is implanted in a body cavity, the risk of infection is of some concern. The question of whether to use intravenous antibiotics before placing a device has been asked and addressed by several investigators. Two published studies, one randomized and done to evaluate acute access catheters, the other nonrandomized and done to evaluate tunneled catheters, suggest that prophylactic intravenous antibiotics can reduce the incidence of catheter-related sepsis.[83,84] Another prospective study evaluating patients undergoing bone marrow transplantation demonstrated a significant reduction in catheter-related sepsis with perioperatively administered vancomycin.[85] Several other randomized prospective studies have arrived at completely opposite conclusions, showing no benefit from prophylactic therapy.[86–88]

Internal Jugular Vein Access

There are several approaches to the IJV. The middle and the anterior approaches are the most common. The anterior approach involves accessing the internal jugular vein 4

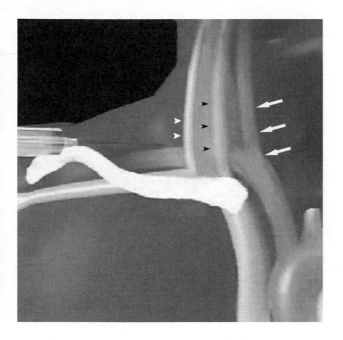

Figure 7–15 With the low posterior approach, the access needle is inserted posterior to the sternocleidomastoid muscle, above the external jugular vein (*white arrowheads*), and directed parallel to the procedure table or clavicle and perpendicular to the neck. The carotid artery (*arrows*) is almost always posterior and medial to the jugular vein (*black arrowheads*), making inadvertent puncture of this vessel unlikely from this approach.

to 5 cm above the clavicle from a point medial to the anterior belly of the sternocleidomastoid muscle. From this point, the access needle is directed caudally and laterally to enter the IJV. The middle approach is similar to the anterior approach, except the access point is between the two heads of the sternocleidomastoid muscle. With each of these approaches, the IJV is accessed from medial to lateral; thus, the access catheter must curve more than 180 degrees to track down along the neck to the chest wall. With such an acute angle, there is a likelihood that the catheter will kink and subsequently occlude. This is particularly true of double-lumen catheters.

The low posterior approach to the IJV avoids this predicament. With this approach, the needle is inserted posterior to the posterior belly of the sternocleidomastoid muscle just above the clavicle. From this location, the needle is directed from lateral to medial across the neck parallel to the operating table (Fig. 7–15). When the vein is accessed in this fashion, the catheter need curve only 90 degrees or less to track down to the chest wall, hence significantly reducing the likelihood of catheter kink-

ing. This, however, is only one of several advantages of this particular technique. Other advantages include the reduced risk of pneumothorax because the needle is being directed across the neck away from the lung and the ability to stand on the side of the procedure table when obtaining venous access. When accessing the IJV, a 21-gauge needle is used for entry. Ultrasound guidance is helpful in directing the needle into the vein. The ultrasound probe can be placed on the anterior aspect of the neck so that the needle can be visualized longitudinally as it traverses the subcutaneous tissues and enters the internal jugular vein (Fig. 7–16). Once the needle accesses the vein, the hub must be retracted cranially so that the 0.018-inch mandrill guidewire of the Micropuncture Systems (Cook, Inc., Bloomington, IN, U.S.A.) will advance caudally into the SVC (Fig. 7–17). Fluoroscopy is used to confirm that the wire is in the proper location. Once confirmed, the 3 F/5 F transitional catheter is inserted over this guidewire into the vein (Fig. 7–18). Inner elements of this coaxial system are removed to allow placement of a 0.035- or 0.038-inch guidewire.

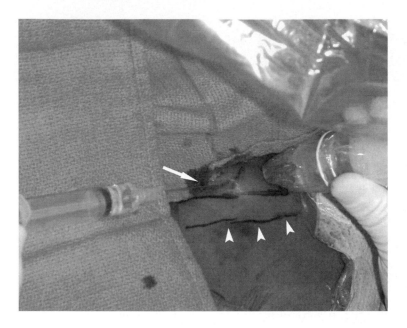

Figure 7–16 The ultrasound probe can be positioned perpendicular to the access needle as it is inserted underneath the sternocleidomastoid muscle (*arrow*) and directed parallel to the clavicle (*arrowheads*) to enter the internal jugular vein. Scanning longitudinally permits visualization of the needle throughout its course.

Subclavian Vein Access

The subclavian vein is best never used as an access point for the placement of temporary or permanent hemodialysis catheters. With this said, little time will be spent describing this access technique. If, however, access into this vessel is the only option, it should be done under direct image guidance. Ultrasound or contrast venography, using iodinated contrast or CO_2, can be used to visualize the vein as the needle is directed into it.[89,90] The medial aspect of the subclavian vein should be avoided because the needle might inadvertently traverse the costoclavicular ligament. Placing a hemodialysis catheter through this ligament can lead to catheter compression, malfunction, and fracture.[91–94]

Exit-Site Selection

For acute hemodialysis catheters, the venotomy is also the catheter exit site. Once access is established, the distance between the venotomy and the desired catheter tip location is measured and a catheter of appropriate length selected. The venotomy then is dilated to accommodate the access catheter, and the catheter is placed and sutured to the skin.

HELPFUL HINT
Some temporary dialysis catheters are inserted with a stiffener in place to give the catheter more "pushability" over the wire. Occasionally, it can be a challenge to load the wire through the stiffener. The wire instead will go between the stiffener and the catheter lumen. As a result, the wire will not exit through the end hole of the stiffener. If this occurs repeatedly, detach and remove the stiffener from the catheter, advance the wire out of the catheter hub, place the stiffener over the wire, and reattach the stiffener to the catheter.

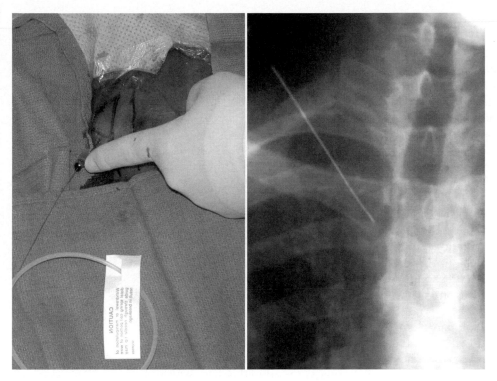

Figure 7–17 The hub of the access needle is pushed cranially to direct the 0.018-inch guidewire into the right atrium.

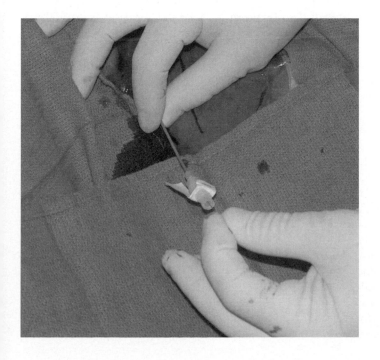

Figure 7–18 A coaxial catheter system, tapered to the 0.018-inch guidewire, is inserted into the vein. When the wire and inner catheter are removed, the outer catheter will allow a 0.038-inch guide to pass.

For tunneled catheters, an appropriate site away from the venotomy must be chosen for the catheter to exit. If access is gained through central neck veins, the catheter exit site typically is located on the chest wall, either medially or laterally, several centimeters below the clavicle. Exactly where the catheter will exit depends on the type of catheter being implanted. For cuffed catheters, it is the distance between the cuff and the catheter tip that determines the catheter exit site. Ideally, the hemodialysis catheter tip, which is specialized and cannot be trimmed, should be positioned in the upper to midportion of the RA to maximize function. Additionally, the polyester retention cuff should be no more than 2 to 3 cm away from the catheter exit site. Cuff placement too far into the subcutaneous tunnel can complicate eventual catheter removal. Thus, the position of the catheter exit site can be chosen only after the catheter tip position has been determined. The first step in determining a catheter exit site is to measure the distance between the venotomy and the desired catheter tip location. The measurement obtained is then used to select a catheter with a cuff-to-tip length that is greater than this measurement. The next step is to create a template of the cuff-to-tip length of the chosen catheter. This is accomplished by inserting a wire into the lumen of the selected catheter and positioning its end at the catheter tip. The catheter wire combination then is bent 2 cm proximal to the cuff (Fig. 7–19). The wire template is removed from the hemodialysis catheter and inserted into the previously placed 5 F Micropuncture catheter (Cook, Inc.). The tip of the wire is positioned fluoroscopically in the RA, where the hemodialysis catheter tip should be. The bend in the back of the wire indicates where the catheter exit site should be, and the curve simulates the course of the catheter (Fig. 7–20). The wire bend can be positioned laterally or more medially on the chest wall. A lateral exit site just below the deltopectoral groove helps to conceal the catheter because in this location it is

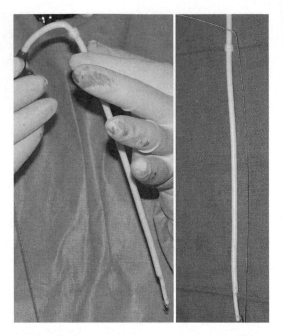

Figure 7–19 The short 0.035-inch wire that is often included with the catheter insertion kit is inserted into the hemodialysis catheter, and the catheter and wire are bent together just beyond the catheter cuff. This bent wire now can serve as a template for determining the catheter exit site.

almost always covered by the patient's shirt. In women, a lateral location is sometimes uncomfortable if the catheter exit site is just underneath the bra strap. Therefore, it is important to tailor the precise catheter exit point to meet the needs of each patient.

After choosing a suitable catheter exit site, the area and tract leading to the venotomy is anesthetized with lidocaine. A small stab wound is made at the catheter exit site, and a tunneling tool is used to pull the catheter through the tract to the venotomy (Fig. 7–21). When tunneling to the IJV, one should make an effort initially to tunnel laterally and then direct medially so that the catheter will take a broad gentle curve as it traverses over the clavicle to the venotomy.

HELPFUL HINT
When pulling the catheter through the subcutaneous tunnel, it is best to pull it as far as possible, even though the catheter

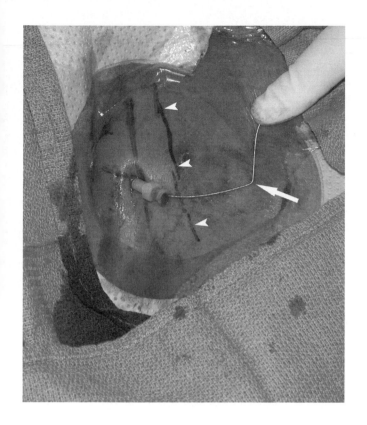

Figure 7–20 The wire template is inserted into the 5 French catheter, and its tip is positioned in the proximal right atrium with fluoroscopy. Once this is done, the bend in the rear of the wire template indicates the proper hemodialysis catheter exit site (*arrow*) on the chest wall below the clavicle (*arrowheads*).

will be too long in this position. After advancing the catheter through the pull-away sheath and removing the sheath, the catheter can be pulled back until the tip is in an ideal position. The act of pulling the catheter back will remove any

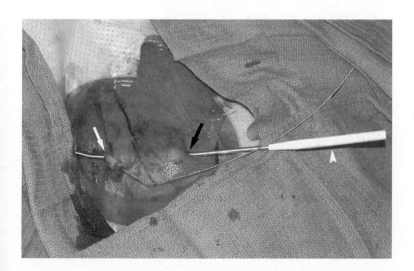

Figure 7–21 A tunneling tool (*arrowhead*) is used to create a subcutaneous path from the catheter exit site (*black arrow*) to the venotomy (*white arrow*).

kink that might have formed while stuffing it through the sheath. Remember, the final catheter tip position is more important than the final position of the cuff—as long as the cuff is within the tunnel.

Access Catheter Insertion

Chronic hemodialysis catheters are soft and have no intrinsic stiffness. Therefore, these devices must be inserted through peel-away sheaths. Once the template wire is removed, a stiff 0.035- or 0.038-inch guidewire is placed. The tip of this guidewire can be left in the SVC, or it can be negotiated into the IVC to avoid inadvertent dislodgment. Care should be taken not to allow the wire to migrate into the right ventricle and cause an arrhythmia.

Over the indwelling guidewire, a peel-away sheath of the appropriate diameter is advanced only as far as needed (Fig. 7–22). One must take great care not to over-advance these stiff peel-away sheaths to avoid inadvertent injury to the brachioce-

phalic vein. After placing the peel-away sheath, the dilator and guidewire must be removed so that the venous access catheter can be advanced to its final position. When removing the dilator and guidewire, it is critically important to avoid inadvertent introduction of air through the peel-away sheath into the venous system.[95,96] To prevent this occurrence, the wire should be removed first and the peel-away sheath pinched tightly while the dilator is being removed (Fig. 7–23). The patient is also instructed to hold his or her breath, hum, or preferably perform the Valsalva maneuver as the access catheter is rapidly introduced into the peel-away sheath and advanced into the central venous system.[97]

HELPFUL HINT
Have a towel near the venous entry site ready to absorb the surge of blood.

The tip of the access catheter must be positioned appropriately. Typically, the tip should be positioned in the upper to middle portion of the RA at full inspiration. High catheter tip positioning should be avoided

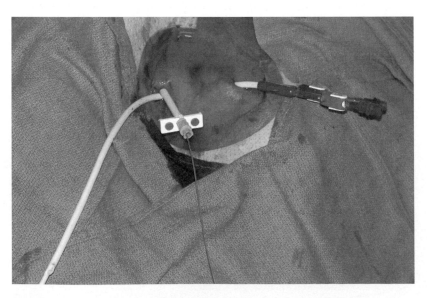

Figure 7–22 The large-diameter peel-away sheath is inserted over a sturdy guidewire. The peel-away sheath should be advanced only as far as needed to allow the hemodialysis catheter to be inserted into the vein.

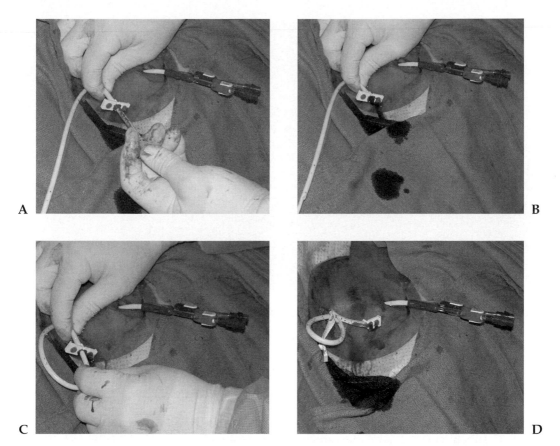

Figure 7–23 **(A)** *Upper left:* The dilator is removed from peel-away sheath, and the sheath is pinched before it is completely removed. **(B)** *Upper right:* With the dilator removed, the peel-away is pinched tight to prevent the introduction of air. **(C)** *Lower left:* The soft access catheter is rapidly inserted into the sheath. **(D)** *Lower right:* The sheath is split and torn away as the access catheter is advanced into the central venous system.

in anticipation of "device drop" to prevent retraction of the catheter tip into the brachiocephalic or subclavian vein when the patient assumes an upright position.[98] This phenomenon is more likely to occur with long tunnel tracts, lateral catheter exit sites, and in patients with an abundance of subcutaneous tissue on the chest wall. If this does occur, there is an increased risk of catheter malfunction and central vein thrombosis.[99] It is also important to avoid very low right atrial catheter tip placement. In this situation, the catheter, by being in contact with the right atrial wall, over time can cause an injury that can result in the formation of right atrial thrombus.[100] If right atrial thrombus occurs, catheter func-

tion is often severely hampered. Indeed, if a hemodialysis access catheter malfunctions frequently without apparent cause, one should consider the possibility that right atrial thrombus may be present. Interestingly, significant right atrial mural-based thrombus is often missed on venography. Transthoracic or transesophageal ultrasounds are the best modalities to confirm this diagnosis.

Implantation Completion

Once the access catheter tip is positioned appropriately, the peel-away sheath is split and removed. The entire course of the catheter should then be evaluated with

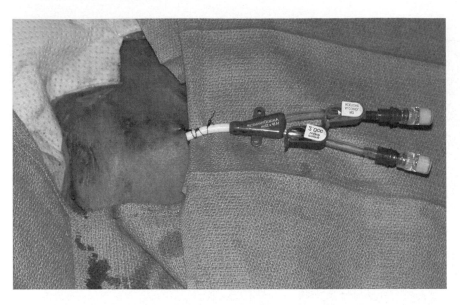

Figure 7–24 The venotomy is sutured closed, and the catheter is fixed in place with stitching.

fluoroscopy to ensure that no kinks are present that could limit flow in the catheter. If the catheter course is smooth and kink-free, then the venotomy is sutured closed. Wound closure is accomplished by placing a buried subcuticular absorbable stitch. Once this wound is closed, the catheter is sutured in place at the exit site to prevent early dislodgement (Fig. 7–24). Care should be taken to avoid applying this stitch too tightly to the catheter because this can cause a flow obstruction. This stitch is no longer needed once significant tissue ingrowth into the polyester cuff has occurred. This process usually takes 2 to 3 weeks, after which the retaining stitch can be removed. With the catheter fixed in position, a dressing is applied. Preferably, an absorbable gauze pad covered by a semipermeable adhesive dressing should be placed over the catheter's exit site. This type of dressing, as opposed to an impermeable dressing, helps to reduce the incidence of catheter infections.[101–104]

DIALYSIS PORT IMPLANTATION

The implantation of a dialysis port is similar to the implantation of an external hemodia-

lysis catheter, with the exception of the need to create a subcutaneous pocket for the needle entry port.

HELPFUL HINT
Become proficient at placement of infusion chest ports before attempting placement of dialysis ports, which are more complex to place.

The LifeSite device, which is currently the only FDA-approved hemodialysis port, consists of two separate valves with two separate catheters. Each of these catheters is inserted into the IJV through separate punctures. As with any access catheter, the first step is to obtain central venous access. Once access is achieved, two incisions are made on the chest wall, and a subcutaneous pocket is created to house the valve bodies (Fig. 7–25).

HELPFUL HINT
Create a pocket that is generous in size so that the port fits easily, not snugly, in the pocket. Because of the large size of these devices, if the skin is pulled tightly over the port (i.e., the pocket is too tight), the overlying skin can develop necrosis, presumably because of ischemia result-

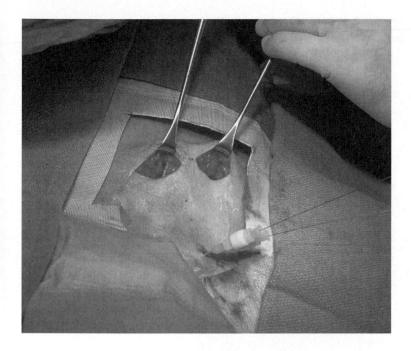

Figure 7–25   After access is gained twice into the jugular vein, two incisions are made on the chest wall to accommodate the valve bodies.

ing from the constant pressure of being pulled tightly over the port.

After the pockets are fashioned and hemostasis is achieved, the two 12-F access catheters are tunneled to the venotomy sites in the neck. The single-lumen access catheters are introduced one at a time through peel-away sheaths. The tips of each of the catheters are positioned in the RA in a staggered fashion to prevent recirculation. By convention, the medial valve catheter tip is positioned superior to the lateral valve catheter tip because this will be the draw port. After positioning the catheter tips, the rear of each catheter is cut to length and attached to the valve body (Fig. 7–26). The valves then are placed into the subcutaneous pockets and fixed to the chest wall with nonabsorbable suture (Fig. 7–27). The pocket opening then is closed in two layers with absorbable polyglactin sutures. Once device implantation is complete, the device is accessed transcutaneously with a 14-gauge hemodialysis access needle to

assess function and instill a heparin lock (Fig. 7–28). The access needle then is removed and the valve opening is cleansed with 70% isopropyl alcohol delivered through a 25-gauge needle.

The Dialock Port, which was described already, is inserted in a similar fashion. Access into the central vein must be obtained twice to insert the two large-bore catheters, which are tunneled from the subcutaneous pocket. Unlike the LifeSite device, only one larger incision and pocket are made to accommodate the valve body that houses both access channels. To prevent device contamination and infection, a new trial is being established to evaluate a locking solution of citrate, an anticoagulant, and taurolidine, an antimicrobial.

Clinical trials comparing these devices to external catheters have demonstrated equal or superior efficacy. Additionally, early data suggest that these devices have an overall reduced complication rate compared with tunneled catheters.[44,105–107] Controlled trials

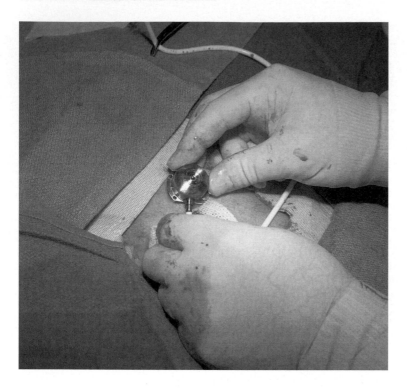

Figure 7–26 After the access catheters are tunneled and inserted into the jugular vein, the rear of each of these catheters is cut to the proper length and connected to the valve.

involving the LifeSite device demonstrated superior device function compared with the Tesio catheter as well as an overall reduction in device-related infections.[108] In the comparative trial, the Tesio catheter had 2.6 device-related infections per 1000 days of access compared with 1.3 for the LifeSite device. Additionally, device malfunction was three times less likely, and adverse events were nearly half as common for the LifeSite device. In our experience, these devices are susceptible to device malfunction and infection. The incidence of these complications appears less frequent, however, compared with that of tunneled catheters. Our concern about the breakdown of skin around the access point was ill-founded. Patients developed an area of thickened skin at the puncture site, which tolerated repeated large-bore needle punctures. Another concern was how to treat a malfunctioning device. For tunneled catheters, it has been our practice to exchange

these catheters over a guidewire and disrupt the fibrin sleeve with a balloon angioplasty catheter. With totally implanted devices, it would be moderately traumatic, time consuming, and expensive to replace the entire device. Fortunately, the LifeSite device has a catheter exchange kit, which allows the catheter to be exchanged without manipulation of the valve. This is accomplished through a small incision made over the subcutaneous portion of the catheter. Through this incision, the catheter is dissected free, transected, and a guidewire then is passed into the venous circulation. The venous portion of the catheter then can be removed, and if a fibrin sleeve is present, it can be disrupted. Once this is accomplished, a new catheter can be placed into the venous system and reconnected to the remaining portion of the catheter emanating from the valve body. This technique, although minimally more laborious than exchanging a tunnel catheter, was not difficult and was

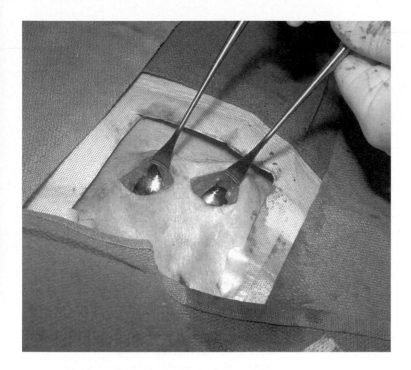

Figure 7–27 The valves are placed in the pockets and sutured down to the chest wall. The skin wounds then are closed.

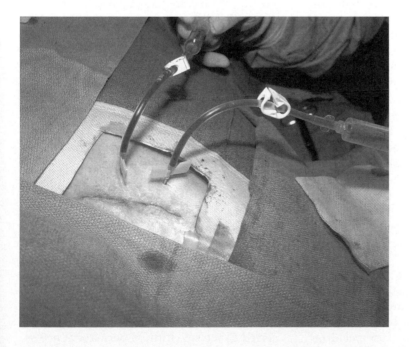

Figure 7–28 Inserted transcutaneously, 14-gauge dialysis needles open the valves and allow them to be flushed with saline and locked with heparin.

certainly less laborious and costly than exchanging the entire device.

IMPLANTATION SUCCESS RATE

It is not unreasonable to expect implantation success rates to approach 100% with image-guided techniques, particularly when ultrasound is used to assess the patency of the desired access vein before attempting catheter placement.[109–112] Additionally, proper placement techniques usually ensure adequate catheter function. The DOQI Work Group believes that 95% of initial catheter placements should achieve a blood flow rate greater than 300 mL per minute during the first attempted hemodialysis.[43]

COMPLICATIONS AND CATHETER SURVIVAL

Procedure-related complications are similar for all tunneled catheters and are reviewed in other chapters. There are, however, certain procedure-related complications that are more likely to occur with large-diameter hemodialysis catheters. Air embolus, which can occur during the placement of any tunneled catheter, is more likely to occur and more likely to be clinically significant when large-diameter peel-away sheaths are used. Severe hemothorax or hemomediastinum is also more likely to occur with the stiff inner dilators that accompany the large-diameter peel-away sheaths. Great care must be taken to avoid these potentially life-threatening complications. Meticulous adherence to appropriate image-guided implantation techniques should substantially reduce, if not eliminate, the likelihood of these complications.[109,113–115] Studies detailing the outcomes of surgically or non–image-guided hemodialysis catheter placements noted acute complication rates of about 2 to 5% and, as a consequence, a death rate between 0 and 1.25 per 1000 catheter placements.[46,116–118] Studies evaluating image-guided hemodialysis catheter insertions report an acute complication rate of 0 to 3%.[111,115,119] In light of these data, it is the opinion of the NKF-DOQI Vascular Access Work Group that acute complication rates associated with the insertion of hemodialysis catheters should be less than 2%.[120]

Late catheter malfunction is usually a consequence of fibrin deposition around the catheter tip end holes. This process is unpredictable and occurs more frequently in some and less frequently in others. Overall, this process is reported to occur in nearly half of implanted catheters.[41,116] Fibrin sleeve formation is likely to be inevitable, if the catheter is left in place long enough. Restoration of catheter function can be accomplished through a variety of techniques. These techniques are discussed in detail in other chapters.

Catheter infection is another vexing problem with a widely varying reported incidence that appears to be dependent on the duration of use.[47,121] Suhocki and colleagues reported a 50% cuffed catheter removal rate, secondary to infection, at 1 year.[122] With catheters in place for less than 3 months, infection rates lower than 10% have been reported.[122,123] It should be noted that the reported catheter infection rate for devices placed in interventional radiology (IR) has been quite low. Infection rates of 0.08 and 0.20 per 100 days of access after IR placement have been reported in separate studies.[47,115] Higher infection rates for surgically placed hemodialysis catheters have been noted in several studies.[124–126]

All the aforementioned complications contribute to the overall longevity of a hemodialysis access catheter. Unfortunately, accurate data on catheter longevity are difficult to obtain because most central venous catheters for hemodialysis are used as an interim solution and are removed once other access is established. Shaffer and colleagues reported on 51 patients in whom central venous access catheters were inserted as the sole form of permanent access. In this group, the primary survival rate was 53% at 6 months and 35% at 1 year. With revisions, the primary assisted survival rate was improved to 61 and 43% at 6 months and 1 year, respectively, with thrombosis and infection cited as the major limiting factors for device survival.[127] Other studies have reported widely variable device survival rates, with 1-year patency rates as high as 93% and as low as 35%.[31,41,116,127–130] Much of this variability reflects variations in the type of device used and the inconstancies of device placement and management. With such wide variability in the literature, it is difficult, if not impossible, to estimate an overall expected device survival rate.

COST-EFFECTIVENESS

In the era of cost containment, the cost of providing a medical service has become an important issue. In the hemodialysis-dependent patient, who is likely to undergo multiple costly procedures, this issue is of particular importance. Hemodialysis access catheter placement and its consequences can be costly. Costs can vary dramatically, depending on where and how these catheters are placed. Unfortunately, assessing the actual cost of a service within a particular environment is difficult to do in a complex health care system. Often procedural and hospital charges are used to gauge expenses because charge, as opposed to cost, data are usually more readily available for review. Charges bear little relation, if any, to the actual cost of performing a procedure, however.

To gain insight on how the implantation location can impact the cost of hemodialysis access catheter placement, Noh and colleagues reviewed the costs associated with the placement of 47 hemodialysis access catheters in the radiology department and compared them with 25 surgical placements.[131] This review revealed a 50% cost savings with radiologic placement, which averaged $926 per catheter placement compared with $1849 for surgical placement. At our institution, we performed a similar review but continued the analysis until a functional catheter was obtained to assess how outcomes could affect overall cost. In this study, we compared 132 primary chronic dialysis catheter implantations with 48 surgically implanted chronic dialysis catheters for the year 1996. The mean implantation time for surgically implanted catheters was 133 minutes (range, 65–360 minutes). For radiologically inserted catheters, the mean was 52 minutes (range, 30–130 minutes). A cost-accounting approach then was used to calculate the cost of implantation. For IR, the overall direct and indirect cost per hour totaled $327.45 per hour. The cost of equipment exclusive of the access device cost was $140.78, and the access device cost was $193.00. Thus, the average cost from the hospital perspective for implanting a dialysis catheter in the IR suite was $617.57 for the average 52-minute implantation. The cost for implantation in the surgical suite was assessed in a similar fashion. The average cost of insertion for an insertion time of 133 minutes was $1,386.77. Thus, from the hospital's perspective, the cost of implanting a dialysis catheter in the surgical suite was more than twice more costly than implanting it in the radiology suite.

Once the initial cost of implantation was assessed, we evaluated clinical outcome and its impact on overall cost. With dialysis catheters, more so than any other catheter, good function is mandatory. If the catheter malfunctions, the patient cannot receive adequate hemodialysis and must return for some intervention to restore the function. For this study, we define *acute functional failure* as a flow rate of less than 200 mL per minute from the catheter in two consecutive postimplantation dialysis sessions. Additionally, the function of the catheter was judged as poor by the nephrologist, who then referred the patient back to the implanting physician for repair or replacement. Using these criteria, 13 of the 48 catheters inserted in the surgical suite were classified as acute failures. Among the 132 catheters implanted in radiology, only three were classified as acute failures. To restore adequate catheter function in the surgical group, 21 additional procedures were performed on the 13 patients. Eleven were performed in the operating room (OR) suite, and 10 were performed in the IR suite. A total of 1.6 additional procedures per patient were required for this group. In the radiology group, each of the three failures was remedied with one additional procedure performed in the IR suite. The total additional procedure time required to obtain catheter function in the surgical group was 18.7 hours of OR time and 6.3 hours of IR time. In the radiology group, 2.3 hours of IR time was required to repair the malfunctioning catheter. Using the same cost-accounting approach, the cumulative cost of technical failure for the surgical group was $19,800.96. This cost, averaged out over all 48 cases, added an additional $412.52 per case. For the radiology group, the additional costs amounted to $1,754.06 and added a total of $13.29 per case. When these additional costs are added to the average cost of implantation, surgical implantation is three times more costly from the hospital's perspective than placement in the IR suite.

SUMMARY

Survival for the hemodialysis-dependent patient hinges on circulatory access. Central venous catheters can provide rapid circulatory access for these patients; therefore, they are an integral part of patient care. Unfortunately, these devices malfunction frequently, and placement can be associated with significant complications. For these reasons, it is critical that the implanting physicians be able to select the most appropriate access device and be thoroughly familiar with appropriate implantation technique and device management. With this knowledge, physicians can spare the already inflicted patient from the superimposition of unneeded iatrogenic morbidity.

REFERENCES

1. Clark PB, Parsons FM. Routine use of the Scribner shunt for haemodialysis. *BMJ.* 1966;5497:1200–1202.

2. Brescia MJ, Cimino JE, Appel K, Hurwich BJ. Chronic hemodialysis using venipuncture and a surgically created arteriovenous fistula. *N Engl J Med.* 1966;275:1089–1092.

3. Rohl L, Franz HE, Mohring K, et al. Direct arteriovenous fistula for hemodialysis. *Scand J Urol Nephrol.* 1968;2:191–195.

4. Zincke H, Aguilo JJ. Basilic vein swing-over for creation of arteriovenous fistula of forearm for hemodialysis. *Urology.* 1976;7:319–320.

5. Gorski TF, Nguyen HQ, Gorski YC, Chung HJ, Jamal A, Muney J. Lower-extremity saphenous vein transposition arteriovenous fistula: an alternative for hemodialysis access in AIDS patients. *Am Surg.* 1998;64:338–340.

6. Koontz PG Jr, Helling TS. Subcutaneous brachial vein arteriovenous fistula for chronic hemodialysis. *World J Surg.* 1983;7:672–674.

7. Pasternak BM, Paruk S, Kogan S, Levitt S. A synthetic vascular conduit (expanded PTFE) for hemodialysis access—a preliminary report. *Vasc Surg.* 1977;11:99–102.

8. Baker LD, Johnson JM, Goldfarb D. Expanded polytetrafluoroethylene (PTFE) subcutaneous arteriovenous conduit: an improved vascular access for chronic hemodialysis. *Trans Am Soc Artif Intern Organs.* 1976;22:382–387.

9. Payne JE, Chatterjee SN, Barbour BH, Berne TV. Vascular access for chronic hemodialysis using modified bovine arterial graft arteriovenous fistula. *Am J Surg.* 1974;128:54–57.

10. VanderWerf BA. Bovine graft arteriovenous fistulas for hemodialysis. *Proc Clin Dial Transplant Forum.* 1973;3:12–14.

11. Haimov M, Burrows L, Baez A, Neff M, Slifkin R. Alternatives for vascular access for hemodialysis: experience with autogenous saphenous vein autografts and bovine heterografts. *Surgery.* 1974;75:447–452.

12. Kinnaert P, Vereerstraeten P, Toussaint C, Van Geertruyden J. Nine years' experience with internal arteriovenous fistulas for haemodialysis: a study of some factors influencing the results. *Br J Surg.* 1977;64:242–246.

13. Winsett OE, Wolma FJ. Complications of vascular access for hemodialysis. *South Med J.* 1985;78:513–517.

14. Hodges TC, Fillinger MF, Zwolak RM, Walsh DB, Bech F, Cronenwett JL. Longitudinal comparison of dialysis access methods: risk factors for failure. *J Vasc Surg.* 1997;26:1009–1019.

15. Hakaim AG, Nalbandian M, Scott T. Superior maturation and patency of primary brachiocephalic and transposed basilic vein arteriovenous fistulae in patients with diabetes. *J Vasc Surg.* 1998;27: 154–157.

16. Palder SB, Kirkman RL, Whittemore AD, Hakim RM, Lazarus JM, Tilney NL. Vascular access for hemodialysis: patency rates and results of revision. *Ann Surg.* 1985;202: 235–239.

17. Raju S. PTFE grafts for hemodialysis access: techniques for insertion and management of complications. *Ann Surg.* 1987; 206:666–673.

18. Systems USRD. United States Renal Data System. 1994 Annual Data Report. Bethesda, MD: National Institutes of Health, National Institute of Diabetes and Digestive and Kidney Diseases, 1994.

19. Kapoian T, Sherman RA. A brief history of vascular access for hemodialysis: an unfinished story. *Semin Nephrol.* 1997;17: 239–245.

20. Butterly DW, Schwab SJ. Dialysis access infections. *Curr Opin Nephrol Hypertens.* 2000; 9:631–635.

21. Bolz KD, Fjermeros G, Wideroe TE, Hatlinghus S. Catheter malfunction and thrombus formation on double-lumen hemodialysis catheters: an intravascular ultrasonographic study. *Am J Kidney Dis.* 1995;25:597–602.

22. Marr KA, Sexton DJ, Conlon PJ, Corey GR, Schwab SJ, Kirkland KB. Catheter-related bacteremia and outcome of attempted catheter salvage in patients undergoing hemodialysis. *Ann Intern Med.* 1997;127: 275–280.

23. Taylor GD, McKenzie M, Buchanan-Chell M, Caballo L, Chui L, Kowalewska-Grochowska K. Central venous catheters as a source of hemodialysis-related bacteremia. *Infect Control Hosp Epidemiol.* 1998; 19:643–646.

24. Stalter KA, Stevens GF, Sterling WA Jr. Late stenosis of the subclavian vein after hemodialysis catheter injury. *Surgery.* 1986; 100:924–927.

25. Vanherweghem JL, Yassine T, Goldman M, et al. Subclavian vein thrombosis: a frequent complication of subclavian vein cannulation for hemodialysis. *Clin Nephrol.* 1986;26:235–238.

26. Barrett N, Spencer S, McIvor J, Brown EA. Subclavian stenosis: a major complication of subclavian dialysis catheters. *Nephrol Dial Transplant.* 1988;3:423–425.

27. Fant GF, Dennis VW, Quarles LD. Late vascular complications of the subclavian dialysis catheter. *Am J Kidney Dis.* 1986;7: 225–228.

28. Anonymous. III. NKF-K/DOQI Clinical practice guidelines for vascular access: update 2000. Guideline 30. *Am J Kidney Dis.* 2001;37:S137–S181.

29. Twardowski ZJ, Van Stone JC, Haynie JD. All currently used measurements of recirculation in blood access by chemical methods are flawed due to intradialytic disequilibrium or recirculation at low flow. *Am J Kidney Dis.* 1998;32:1046–1058.

30. Twardowski ZJ, Van Stone JC, Jones ME, Klusmeyer ME, Haynie JD. Blood recirculation in intravenous catheters for hemodialysis. *J Am Soc Nephrol.* 1993;3:1978–1981.

31. Tesio F, De Baz H, Panarello G, et al. Double catheterization of the internal jugular vein for hemodialysis: indications, techniques, and clinical results. *Artif Organs.* 1994;18:301–304.

32. Mankus RA, Ash SR, Sutton JM. Comparison of blood flow rates and hydraulic resistance between the Mahurkar catheter, the Tesio twin catheter, and the Ash split cath. *ASAIO J.* 1998;44:M532–M534.

33. Trerotola SO, Shah H, Johnson M, et al. Randomized comparison of high-flow versus conventional hemodialysis catheters. *J Vasc Interv Radiol.* 1999;10:1032–1038.

34. Szycher M, Siciliano A, Reed A. *Polyurethanes in Medical Devices.* Medical Design and Material 1991.

35. Phillips RE, Smith MC, Thoma RJ. Biomedical applications of polyurethanes: implications of failure mechanisms. *J Biomater Appl.* 1988;3:207–227.

36. Curelaru I, Gustavsson B, Hansson AH, Linder LE, Stenqvist O, Wojciechowski J. Material thrombogenicity in central venous catheterization. II. A comparison between plain silicone elastomer, and plain poly-

ethylene, long, antebrachial catheters. *Acta Anaesthesiol Scand.* 1983;27:158–164.

37. el-Shahawy A, Gadallah F. Acute hemodialysis catheters: how safe are they? [review]. *Int J Artif Organs.* 1996;19:571–573.

38. Anonymous. III. NKF-K/DOQI Clinical practice guidelines for vascular access: update 2000. Guideline 6a. *Am J Kidney Dis.* 2001;37:S137–S181.

39. Anonymous. III. NKF-K/DOQI Clinical practice guidelines for vascular access: update 2000. Guideline 6g. *Am J Kidney Dis.* 2001;37:S137–S181.

40. JJ OD, Clague MB, Dudrick SJ. Percutaneous insertion of a cuffed catheter with a long subcutaneous tunnel for intravenous hyperalimentation. *South Med J.* 1983;76: 1344–1348.

41. McDowell DE, Moss AH, Vasilakis C, Bell R, Pillai L. Percutaneously placed dual-lumen silicone catheters for long-term hemodialysis. *Am Surg.* 1993;59:569–573.

42. Schwab SJ, Buller GL, McCann RL, Bollinger RR, Stickel DL. Prospective evaluation of a Dacron cuffed hemodialysis catheter for prolonged use. *Am J Kidney Dis.* 1988; 11:166–169.

43. Anonymous. III. NKF-K/DOQI Clinical practice guidelines for vascular access: update 2000. Guideline 23. *Am J Kidney Dis.* 2001;37:S137–S181.

44. Beathard GA, Posen GA. Initial clinical results with the LifeSite Hemodialysis Access System. *Kidney Int.* 2000;58:2221–2227.

45. Richard HM III, Hastings GS, Boyd-Kranis RL, et al. A randomized, prospective evaluation of the Tesio, Ash split, and Opti-flow hemodialysis catheters. *J Vasc Interv Radiol.* 2001;12:431–435.

46. Swartz RD, Messana JM, Boyer CJ, Lunde NM, Weitzel WF, Hartman TL. Successful use of cuffed central venous hemodialysis catheters inserted percutaneously. *J Am Soc Nephrol.* 1994;4:1719–1725.

47. Lund GB, Trerotola SO, Scheel PF Jr, et al. Outcome of tunneled hemodialysis catheters placed by radiologists. *Radiology.* 1996;198:467–472.

48. Burdick JF, Maley WR. Update on vascular access for hemodialysis. *Adv Surg.* 1996;30: 223–232.

49. Queiros J, Cabrita A, Maximino J, Lobato L, Silva M, Xavier E. Central catheters for hemodialysis: a six-month experience of 103 catheters. *Nephrologie.* 1994;15: 113–115.

50. Dahlberg PJ, Agger WA, Singer JR, et al. Subclavian hemodialysis catheter infections: a prospective, randomized trial of an attachable silver-impregnated cuff for prevention of catheter-related infections. *Infect Control Hosp Epidemiol.* 1995;16: 506–511.

51. De Moor B, Vanholder R, Ringoir S. Subclavian vein hemodialysis catheters: advantages and disadvantages. *Artif Organs.* 1994;18:293–297.

52. Aggarwal S, Hari P, Bagga A, Mehta SN. Phrenic nerve palsy: a rare complication of indwelling subclavian vein catheter. *Pediatr Nephrol.* 2000;14:203–204.

53. Hernandez D, Diaz F, Rufino M, et al. Subclavian vascular access stenosis in dialysis patients: natural history and risk factors. *J Am Soc Nephrol.* 1998;9:1507–1510.

54. Hayashi N, Sakai T, Kitagawa M, Kimoto T, Ishii Y. Percutaneous long-term arterial access with implantable ports: direct subclavian approach with US. *Eur J Radiol.* 1998;26:304–308.

55. Gualtieri E, Deppe SA, Sipperly ME, Thompson DR. Subclavian venous catheterization: greater success rate for less experienced operators using ultrasound guidance. *Crit Care Med.* 1995;23:692–697.

56. Cavatorta F, Campisi S, Zollo A. Subclavian vein stenosis in hemodialysis patients. *Minerva Urol Nefrol.* 1998;50: 55–59.

57. Criado E, Marston WA, Jaques PF, Mauro MA, Keagy BA. Proximal venous outflow obstruction in patients with upper extremity arteriovenous dialysis access. *Ann Vasc Surg.* 1994;8:530–535.

58. Schillinger F, Schillinger D, Montagnac R, Milcent T. Central venous stenosis in hemodialysis: comparative angiographic study of subclavian and internal jugular access. *Nephrologie.* 1994;15:129–131.

59. Vanherweghem JL. Thrombosis and stenosis of central venous access in hemodialysis. *Nephrologie.* 1994;15:117–121.

60. Schillinger F, Schillinger D, Montagnac R, Milcent T. Post-catheterization venous stenosis in hemodialysis: comparative angiographic study of 50 subclavian and 50 internal jugular accesses. *Nephrologie.* 1992; 13:127–133.

61. Cimochowski GE, Worley E, Rutherford WE, Sartain J, Blondin J, Harter H. Superiority of the internal jugular over the subclavian access for temporary dialysis. *Nephron.* 1990;54:154–161.

62. Biswal R, Nosher JL, Siegel RL, Bodner LJ. Translumbar placement of paired hemodialysis catheters (Tesio catheters) and follow-up in 10 patients. *Cardiovasc Intervent Radiol.* 2000;23:75–78.

63. Rajan DK, Croteau DL, Sturza SG, Harvill ML, Mehall CJ. Translumbar placement of inferior vena caval catheters: a solution for challenging hemodialysis access. *Radiographics.* 1998;18:1155–1170.

64. Lund GB, Trerotola SO, Scheel PJ Jr. Percutaneous translumbar inferior vena cava cannulation for hemodialysis. *Am J Kidney Dis.* 1995;25:732–737.

65. Apsner R, Sunder-Plassmann G, Muhm M, Druml W. Alternative puncture site for implantable permanent haemodialysis catheters. *Nephrol Dial Transplant.* 1996;11: 2293–2295.

66. Trottier SJ, Veremakis C, J OB, Auer AI. Femoral deep vein thrombosis associated with central venous catheterization: results from a prospective, randomized trial. *Crit Care Med.* 1995;23:52–59.

67. Denny DF Jr. Placement and management of long-term central venous access catheters and ports. *AJR Am J Roentgenol.* 1993; 161:385–393.

68. Bergey EA, Kaye RD, Reyes J, Towbin RB. Transhepatic insertion of vascular dialysis catheters in children: a safe, life-prolonging procedure. *Pediatr Radiol.* 1999;29:42–45.

69. Mauro MA, Lacey SR. Percutaneous translumbar and transhepatic inferior vena caval catheters for prolonged vascular access in children. *J Pediatr Surg.* 1992;27:165–169.

70. Azizkhan RG, Taylor LA, Jaques PF, Mauro MA, Lacey SR. Percutaneous translumbar and transhepatic inferior vena caval catheters for prolonged vascular access in children. *J Pediatr Surg.* 1992;27:165–169.

71. Kaufman JA, Greenfield AJ, Fitzpatrick GF. Transhepatic cannulation of the inferior vena cava. *J Vasc Interv Radiol.* 1991;2: 331–334.

72. Sebben JE. Sterile technique and the prevention of wound infection in office surgery—Part II. *J Dermatol Surg Oncol.* 1989;15:38–48.

73. Cruse PJ, Foord R. The epidemiology of wound infection: a 10-year prospective study of 62,939 wounds. *Surg Clin North Am.* 1980;60:27–40.

74. Seropian R, Reynolds BM. Wound infections after preoperative depilatory versus razor preparation. *Am J Surg.* 1971;121:251–254.

75. Lowbury EJ, Lilly HA. Use of 4 per cent chlorhexidine detergent solution (Hibiscrub) and other methods of skin disinfection. *BMJ.* 1973;1:510–515.

76. Kutarski PW, Grundy HC. To dry or not to dry? An assessment of the possible degradation in efficiency of preoperative skin preparation caused by wiping skin dry. *Ann R Coll Surg Engl.* 1993;75:181–185.

77. Workman ML. Comparison of blot-drying versus air-drying of povidone-iodine-cleansed skin. *Appl Nurs Res.* 1995;8:15–17.

78. Smylie HG, Logie JR, Smith G. From Phisohex to Hibiscrub. *BMJ.* 1973;4:586–589.

79. Anonymous. Chlorhexidine and other antiseptics. *Med Lett Drugs Ther.* 1976;18: 85–86.

80. Peterson AF, Rosenberg A, Alatary SD. Comparative evaluation of surgical scrub preparations. *Surg Gynecol Obstet.* 1978;146: 63–65.

81. Larson E. Guideline for use of topical antimicrobial agents. *Am J Infect Control.* 1988;16:253–266.

82. Anonymous. Recommended practices: skin preparation of patients. Association of Operating Room Nurses. *AORN J.* 1992; 56:937–941.

83. Al-Sibai MB, Harder EJ, Faskin RW, Johnson GW, Padmos MA. The value of prophylactic antibiotics during the insertion of long-term indwelling silastic right atrial catheters in cancer patients. *Cancer.* 1987;60:1891–1895.

84. Bock SN, Lee RE, Fisher B, et al. A prospective randomized trial evaluating prophylactic antibiotics to prevent triple-lumen catheter-related sepsis in patients treated with immunotherapy. *J Clin Oncol.* 1990;8:161–169.

85. Vassilomanolakis M, Plataniotis G, Koumakis G, et al. Central venous catheter-related infections after bone marrow transplantation in patients with malignancies: a prospective study with short-course vancomycin prophylaxis. *Bone Marrow Transplant.* 1995;15:77–80.

86. Harms K, Herting E, Kron M, Schiffmann H, Schulz-Ehlbeck H. Randomized, controlled trial of amoxicillin prophylaxis for prevention of catheter-related infections in newborn infants with central venous silicone elastomer catheters. *J Pediatr.* 1995; 127:615–619.

87. Ranson MR, Oppenheim BA, Jackson A, Kamthan AG, Scarffe JH. Double-blind placebo controlled study of vancomycin prophylaxis for central venous catheter insertion in cancer patients. *J Hosp Infect.* 1990;15:95–102.

88. McKee R, Dunsmuir R, Whitby M, Garden OJ. Does antibiotic prophylaxis at the time of catheter insertion reduce the incidence of catheter-related sepsis in intravenous nutrition? *J Hosp Infect.* 1985; 6:419–425.

89. Post PJ, Lameris JS, Zonderland HM, Gerritsen GP, Kappers-Klunne MC, Schutte HE. Placing of Hickman catheters under ultrasonic guidance. *Ned Tijdschr Geneeskd.* 1992;136:747–749.

90. Higano ST, Hayes DL, Spittell PC. Facilitation of the subclavian-introducer technique with contrast venography. *Pacing Clin Electrophysiol.* 1990;13:681–684.

91. Magney JE, Staplin DH, Flynn DM, Hunter DW. A new approach to percutaneous subclavian venipuncture to avoid lead fracture or central venous catheter occlusion. *Pacing Clin Electrophysiol.* 1993; 16:2133–2142.

92. Magney JE, Flynn DM, Parsons JA, et al. Anatomical mechanisms explaining damage to pacemaker leads, defibrillator leads, and failure of central venous catheters adjacent to the sternoclavicular joint. *Pacing Clin Electrophysiol.* 1993;16:445–457.

93. Nace CS, Ingle RJ. Central venous catheter "pinch-off" and fracture: a review of two under-recognized complications. *Oncol Nurs Forum.* 1993;20:1227–1236.

94. Punt CJ, Strijk S, van der Hoeven JJ, van de Sluis R, Verhagen CA. Spontaneous fracture of implanted central venous catheters in cancer patients: report of two cases and retrospective analysis of the 'pinch-off sign' as a risk factor. *Anticancer Drugs.* 1995;6: 594–598.

95. Lucas CE, Irani F. Air embolus via subclavian catheter. *N Engl J Med.* 1969;281: 966–967.

96. Flanagan JP, Gradisar IA, Gross RJ, Kelly TR. Air embolus—a lethal complication of subclavian venipuncture. *N Engl J Med.* 1969;281:488–489.

97. Wysoki MG, Covey A, Pollak J, Rosenblatt M, Aruny J, Denbow N. Evaluation of various maneuvers for prevention of air embolism during central venous catheter placement. *J Vasc Interv Radiol.* 2001;12: 764–766.

98. Kowalski CM, Kaufman JA, Rivitz SM, Geller SC, Waltman AC. Migration of central venous catheters: implications for initial catheter tip positioning. *J Vasc Interv Radiol.* 1997;8:443–447.

99. Brown-Smith JK, Stoner MH, Barley ZA. Tunneled catheter thrombosis: factors related to incidence. *Oncol Nurs Forum.* 1990; 17:543–549.

100. Fincher ME, Caruana RJ, Humphries A, Gross CM, Rubin JW, Bowen PA. Right atrial thrombus formation following central venous dialysis catheter placement. *Am Surg.* 1988;54:652–654.

101. Hoffmann KK, Weber DJ, Samsa GP, Rutala WA. Transparent polyurethane film as an intravenous catheter dressing: a meta-analysis of the infection risks. *JAMA.* 1992;267:2072–2076.

102. Raad, II. The pathogenesis and prevention of central venous catheter-related infections. *Middle East J Anesthesiol.* 1994;12: 381–403.

103. Ouwendyk M, Helferty M. Central venous catheter management: how to prevent complications. *Anna J.* 1996;23:572–579.

104. Nielsen J, Kolmos HJ, Espersen F. Infections related to central venous catheters. *Ugeskr Laeger.* 1996;158:764–768.

105. Megerman J, Levin NW, Ing TS, Dubrow AJ, Prosl FR. Development of a new approach to vascular access. *Artif Organs.* 1999;23:10–14.

106. Levin NW, Yang PM, Hatch DA, et al. New access device for hemodialysis. *ASAIO J.* 1998;44:M529–M531.

107. Levin NW, Yang PM, Hatch DA, et al. Initial results of a new access device for hemodialysis technical note. *Kidney Int.* 1998;54:1739–1745.

108. Rosenblatt M, Stainken B, Weiss M, Caridi JG. LifeSite totally implanted HD system versus Tesio cath; results of a comparative trial. *J Vasc Interv Radiol.* 2002;(suppl).

109. Farrell J, Gellens M. Ultrasound-guided cannulation versus the landmark-guided technique for acute haemodialysis access. *Nephrol Dial Transplant.* 1997;12:1234–1237.

110. Nadig C, Leidig M, Schmiedeke T, Hoffken B. The use of ultrasound for the placement of dialysis catheters. *Nephrol Dial Transplant.* 1998;13:978–981.

111. Lin BS, Huang TP, Tang GJ, Tarng DC, Kong CW. Ultrasound-guided cannulation of the internal jugular vein for dialysis vascular access in uremic patients. *Nephron.* 1998;78:423–428.

112. Forauer AR, Glockner JF. Importance of US findings in access planning during jugular vein hemodialysis catheter placements. *J Vasc Interv Radiol.* 2000;11:233–238.

113. Page B, Souissi M, Legendre C, Moreau JF. Positioning of hemodialysis catheters after locating the internal jugular vein by echo-Doppler. *Nephrologie.* 1994;15:111–112.

114. Docktor BL, Sadler DJ, Gray RR, Saliken JC, So CB. Radiologic placement of tunneled central catheters: rates of success and of immediate complications in a large series. *AJR Am J Roentgenol.* 1999;173:457–460.

115. Trerotola SO, Johnson MS, Harris VJ, et al. Outcome of tunneled hemodialysis catheters placed via the right internal jugular vein by interventional radiologists. *Radiology.* 1997;203:489–495.

116. Moss AH, Vasilakis C, Holley JL, Foulks CJ, Pillai K, McDowell DE. Use of a silicone dual-lumen catheter with a Dacron cuff as a long-term vascular access for hemodialysis patients. *Am J Kidney Dis.* 1990;16:211–215.

117. Vanholder R, Lameire N, Verbanck J, van Rattinghe R, Kunnen M, Ringoir S. Complications of subclavian catheter hemodialysis: a 5-year prospective study in 257 consecutive patients. *Int J Artif Organs.* 1982;5:297–303.

118. Vanherweghem JL, Cabolet P, Dhaene M, et al. Complications related to subclavian catheters for hemodialysis: report and review. *Am J Nephrol.* 1986;6:339–345.

119. Prabhu PN, Kerns SR, Sabatelli FW, Hawkins IF, Ross EA. Long-term performance and complications of the Tesio twin catheter system for hemodialysis access. *Am J Kidney Dis.* 1997;30:213–218.

120. Anonymous. III. NKF-K/DOQI Clinical Practice Guidelines for Vascular Access: update 2000. Guideline 34. *Am J Kidney Dis.* 2001;37:S137–S181.

121. Levin A, Mason AJ, Jindal KK, Fong IW, Goldstein MB. Prevention of hemodialysis subclavian vein catheter infections by topical povidone-iodine. *Kidney Int.* 1991; 40:934–938.

122. Suhocki PV, Conlon PJ Jr, Knelson MH, Harland R, Schwab SJ. Silastic cuffed catheters for hemodialysis vascular access: thrombolytic and mechanical correction of malfunction. *Am J Kidney Dis.* 1996;28: 379–386.

123. Maki DG, Weise CE, Sarafin HW. A semiquantitative culture method for identifying intravenous-catheter-related infection. *N Engl J Med.* 1977;296:1305–1309.

124. Mosquera DA, Gibson SP, Goldman MD. Vascular access surgery: a 2-year study and comparison with the Permcath. *Nephrol Dial Transplant.* 1992;7:1111–1115.

125. Gibson SP, Mosquera D. Five years' experience with the Quinton Permcath for vascular access. *Nephrol Dial Transplant.* 1991;6: 269–274.

126. Uldall R, DeBruyne M, Besley M, McMillan J, Simons M, Francoeur R. A new vascular access catheter for hemodialysis. *Am J Kidney Dis* 1993;21:270–277.

127. Shaffer D, Madras PN, Williams ME, JA DE, Kaldany A, Monaco AP. Use of Dacron cuffed silicone catheters as long-term hemodialysis access. *ASAIO J.* 1992;38:55–58.

128. Kinnaert P, Hooghe L, De Pauw L, Dhaene M, Dratwa M, Vanherweghem JL. Use of the Hickman catheter as permanent vascular access for hemodialysis. *ASAIO Trans.* 1990;36:104–106.

129. Duszak R Jr, Haskal ZJ, Thomas-Hawkins C, et al. Replacement of failing tunneled hemodialysis catheters through pre-existing subcutaneous tunnels: a comparison of catheter function and infection rates for de novo placements and over-the-wire exchanges. *J Vasc Interv Radiol.* 1998;9: 321–327.

130. Sharma A, Zilleruelo G, Abitbol C, Montane B, Strauss J. Survival and complications of cuffed catheters in children on chronic hemodialysis. *Pediatr Nephrol.* 1999; 13:245–248.

131. Noh HM, Kaufman JA, Rhea JT, Kim SY, Geller SC, Waltman AC. Cost comparison of radiologic versus surgical placement of long-term hemodialysis catheters. *AJR Am J Roentgenol.* 1999;172:673–675.

Chapter 8

Catheter Placement in Pediatric Patients

Siobhan A. Dumbleton

The transition from surgical placement of venous access devices to their placement in the interventional radiology suite has occurred with the pediatric population in the same way that it has occurred in the adult population.

Typically, the placement of venous access devices in the pediatric population is performed by interventional radiologists or pediatric radiologists who have an interest and training in interventional radiology. Although the basic techniques for the insertion of venous access devices in children do not differ from those used in adults, some differences do exist. This chapter outlines the placement of venous access devices in pediatric patients and highlights the differences.

CATHETER TYPES AND SELECTION

Long-term catheters are made from polyurethane or silicone rubber. A Dacron cuff on tunneled catheters allows tissue ingrowth. Catheters and ports are available in the lower size ranges suitable for the pediatric population.

Catheters designed for the pediatric population include the Broviac catheter (Bard Access Systems, Salt Lake City, UT, U.S.A.), which was introduced in 1973.[1] This is a single-lumen tunneled catheter whose diameter ranges from 2.7 to 6.6 French (F). Although the diameter of the intravenous portion of this catheter is small, the tunneled and external portions are larger and therefore less likely to break. If a double-lumen tunneled catheter is required, the 7 F Hickman catheter (Bard Access Systems) is adequate for children.[2]

Regarding port catheters, the Cook Minivital port (Cook, Inc., Bloomington, IN, U.S.A.), which has a 5 F catheter, is suited for implantation in the chest in children, whereas the Braun Celsite port (Braun, Evanston, IL, U.S.A.) is suitable for placement in the arm. Double-lumen ports are not placed in children because of size considerations. Older teenagers receive single- or double-lumen ports, as in adults.

Peripherally inserted central catheters (PICCs) for children are the same as for adults. For small double-lumen PICC catheters, Luther Medical Systems (Luther Medical Products, Inc., Tustin, CA, U.S.A.) manufactures 2.6, 3.5, and 5 F double-lumen PICCs, the smaller sizes of which are suitable for neonates. Single-lumen Cook 3 or 4 F PICC catheters work well in children.

Dialysis or pheresis catheters are available in a variety of sizes. In older children, catheters used in the adult population can be placed. For smaller children and neonates, double-lumen catheters as small as 8 F are available from Medcomp (Medcomp, Harleysville, PA, U.S.A.). Varying lengths are available. A split-tip dialysis catheter is available from Medcomp (Ash-Split). This catheter is available in 10 F and 18 cm (13 cm cuff-to-tip) or 24 cm (19 cm cuff-to-tip) lengths. On occasion, despite the variety of catheters available, it is necessary to cut and tailor a dialysis catheter to suit the child. We avoid this whenever possible because it can be difficult to fashion the catheter enough to give adequate flow rates for dialysis or pheresis.

Close collaboration with the clinical service is required to determine the most suitable access device for children. Ideally, the catheter with the smallest diameter and the least number of lumens should be used because infectious and thrombotic complications are more common with increased diameter and greater number of lumens.[3,4] The access to be placed is determined by the treatment plan; however, consideration of cost, infection risks, supportive care needs, and the fears and phobias of patients and parents regarding needles should be considered.

Absolute contraindications for tunneled catheter and port placement include an active infection. A relative contraindication is thrombocytopenia or coagulopathy, and attempts should be made to correct coagulation abnormalities before placement. A platelet count greater than $50,000/mm^3$ is desired.

PATIENT PREPARATION AND SEDATION

Informed consent must be obtained from a parent or legal guardian. Occasionally, a child is a ward of the state, in which case consent is obtained by contacting the caseworker. Information can be obtained from the hospital social worker assigned to the child. Consent may be obtained from an older teenager if he or she is considered an emancipated minor.

In the younger patient, sedation is usually required even for PICC line placements or catheter exchange over a guidewire. Occasionally, in teenagers, a catheter can be placed using local anesthetic only. Frequently, even in the teenage population, sedation is required even for simple line procedures because many of these children have chronic illnesses and psychosocial issues.

Tunneled catheters, dialysis catheters, and ports always are placed at our institution with the patient under general anesthesia. Air embolism with serious complications can result from the patients being unable to hold their breath.[5,6]

Before conscious sedation, the risk factors as well as past and present medical history and past sedation history must be reviewed. Overall risks can be determined using the American Society of Anesthesia (ASA) classification system (Table 8–1).[7,8] Usually, patients sedated in the interventional radiology suite are class 1 or 2. For higher classes, either the department of anesthesia or critical care medicine provides assistance with sedation and control of the airway. For all cardiac patients, cardiac anesthesia provides sedation.

At the Children's Hospital of Philadelphia, most children who were allowed to drink clear fluids up to 2 hours before surgery had comparable gastric pH and residual gastric fluid values compared

Table 8–1 American Society of Anesthesiologists Physical Status Classification

Class	Patient
Class 1	Healthy patient
Class 2	Mild systemic disease
Class 3	Severe systemic disease
Class 4	Severe systemic disease that is a constant threat to life
Class 5	Moribund. Not expected to survive 24 hours with or without the surgery or procedure

Table 8–2   Fasting Requirements Prior to Procedure

	Fasting Guidelines	
Age	Clear Liquids	Semi-solids/Solids
0–up to 6 months	2 hours	4 hours
6–up to 36 months	2 hours	6 hours
Older than 36 months	2 hours	8 hours

Semi-solids includes breast milk.

with children who were fasted longer.[9] The guidelines for fasting, as recommended by the American Academy of Pediatrics Committee on Drugs (AAPCOD), are outlined in Table 8–2.[7] For conscious sedation, the same fasting guidelines are used because unconscious sedation can occur unexpectedly. It is important that parents clearly understand the fasting guidelines because failure to follow them can result in the procedure being delayed or canceled. For class 1 or 2 patients, the sedatives used will depend in part on personnel preference and expertise with any given agent as well as patient factors.

Faster onset of sedation occurs by using the intravenous route. Three classes of drugs represent the most commonly used sedative agents: barbiturates, benzodiazepines, and narcotics (Table 8–3). Ketamine hydrochloride also has been described as being useful in providing sedative and analgesia in young children.[10]

At the Children's Hospital of Philadelphia, toddlers and older children are given meperidine (Demerol) and pentobarbital (Nembutal) administered orally on call to radiology and receive intravenous sedation in the radiology department. Neonates receive intravenous sedation only, in the radiology department.

The JCAHO has adopted the AAPCOD's recommended minimum standards for monitoring children. The level of monitoring should reflect the depth of sedation required to complete the study. Baseline vital signs (blood pressure, heart rate, respiratory rate, oxygenation) should be obtained and documented at a minimum of 5-minute intervals. Oxygen should be administered as needed. It is important to monitor the level of consciousness and perfusion because the status of these can change rapidly in a child.[7,11]

Discharge criteria (based on the AAPCOD recommendations) include the following: cardiovascular and airway status is stable and satisfactory, the child can be aroused easily, protective reflexes are intact, and age-appropriate actions can be performed (e.g., talking, sitting up). In the very young child or handicapped child, the presedation level of responses should be present.[7,11] Hydration of the child must be adequate. Inpatients are transferred back to their clinical service; consequently, monitoring of the patient is also transferred.

Antagonist drugs for the sedatives given should be readily available in the radiology department (Table 8–4). In addition, full pediatric code facilities must be available, and it is helpful for personnel to be certified in Pediatric Advanced Life Support (PALS).

TECHNIQUES FOR CATHETER INSERTION

Tunneled Catheters

The placement of tunneled catheters and ports by the radiology department is well described.[5,12–16] We prefer internal jugular access rather than the subclavian route in all cases. This avoids the potential "pinch-off" syndrome, which can occur as the result of

Table 8–3   Sedative Agents

Drug	Class	Effect	Dose/Route
Morphine sulphate	Narcotic	Analgesic Sedative properties	*Neonates*: 0.05 mg/kg IV *Infants and Children* 0.05–0.1 mg/kg/dose up to 2 mgs IV. May repeat to total maximum dose of 15 mg *>12 years*: 3–4 mg IV. May repeat in 1–2 mg doses. Total dose of 15 mg
Chloral hydrate	NA	Sedative	*Neonates:* 25 mg/kg/dose PO *Children:* 50–75 mg/kg/dose PO. Maximum 1.5 gms 1 hour prior to procedure
Pentobarbital sodium	Barbiturate	Sedative	*>6 months:* 2 mg/kg/dose IV (PO). Maximum 100 mg; may repeat 1 mg/kg/dose up to maximum total dose of 8 mg/kg; do not exceed 200 mg
Meperidine	Narcotic	Analgesic Sedative properties	1–1.5 mg/kg/dose IV (PO), 100 mg is maximum initial dose. May repeat 1 mg/kg up to total maximum dose of 150 mg
Midazolam	Benzodiazepine	Sedative, anxiolytic Amnestic	0.02–0.05 mg/kg IV. Use half of original dose to titrate to effect 1 mg is maximum bolus dose
Fentanyl	Narcotic	Analgesic Sedative properties	1–2 mcg/kg IV. May repeat 1 mcg/kg every 5 minutes. Maximum dose of 5 mcg/kg or 100 mcgs
Lidocaine hydrochloride	Local anesthetic	Local anesthesia	Maximum 4.5 mg/kg/dose. May repeat after 2 hours
Lidocaine hydrochloride with epinephrine	Local anesthetic	Local anesthesia	Maximum 4.5 mg/kg/dose. May repeat after 2 hours

Dosing protocols will vary from institution to institution.
Parentheses indicate alternate routes of administration.

the catheter being caught between the first rib and clavicle. Ultimately, the catheter may fracture and embolize.[17] In addition, studies have shown a greater incidence of central venous thrombosis and stenosis when the subclavian vein is used compared with when the internal jugular vein is used.[18–20] This is important in the dialysis patient because arm grafts may be needed. Avoiding placement of catheters in the subclavian vein prevents subclavian vein stenoses. Also, the internal jugular vein is much more easily punctured than the subclavian vein, particularly in the very young child.

Sterile technique is used for all procedures. All personnel wear hat and mask. The

Table 8–4   Narcotic and Benzodiazepine Antagonists

	Sedative Antagonists	
Drug	Effect	Dose/Route
Naloxone hydrochloride	Narcotic antagonist	0.005–0.01 mg/kg/dose IV. May repeat in 2 to 3 minutes. Titrate to reversal. Maximum dose 2 mg
Flumazenil	Benzodiazepine antagonist	20 kg *initial*–0.01 mg/kg IV over 15 seconds. Maximum 0.2 mg *repeat*–0.005 mg/kg after 1 minute
		20–40 kg *initial*–0.2 mg over 15 seconds IV *repeat*–0.2 mg after 1 minute. Maximum cumulative dose 1 mg

operator performs a surgical scrub before putting on gown and gloves. The patient's skin is cleaned with povidone–iodine. The use of prophylactic antibiotics remains controversial, and several studies suggest that they are not of benefit.[21,22] At Children's Hospital, we do not use prophylactic antibiotics in the placement of tunneled catheters, dialysis catheters, or ports.

The right internal jugular vein is preferred because it provides a more direct route into the right atrium (RA) and therefore helps prevent sheath kinking. The vein should be accessed as low as possible to prevent an acute angle as the catheter turns toward the skin exit site. The vein should be accessed between the two heads of the sternocleidomastoid muscle because it is painful to bring a catheter through the muscle. Alternatively, a posterior approach into the vein can be used by commencing at a point just lateral to the lateral border of the lateral head of the sternocleidomastoid. The vein is localized using a small portable battery-powered ultrasound machine with a 3-inch screen (Siterite; Dymax, Pittsburgh, PA, U.S.A.).

Buffered lidocaine (9 mL of 1% lidocaine and 1 mL of sodium bicarbonate) is used to anesthetize the puncture site. Buffered lidocaine dramatically reduces the burning sensation associated with injecting lidocaine. This is of greater significance when dealing with patients in whom conscious sedation is being used. A no. 11 scalpel blade is used to make a dermatotomy.

A 21-gauge needle, 2 to 4 cm long, is used for entry into the vein (Micropuncture; Cook, Inc.). The needle is advanced under ultrasound guidance into the vein. Once the needle is seen resting on the vein, a short, sharp jab is used to enter the vein. A double-wall puncture is not performed, particularly if the carotid artery lies under the vein rather than at its lateral aspect. The vein wall can be resistant to entry, and the walls may coapt. Entry into the vein usually is felt as a "give" or "popping" sensation. A slip-lock syringe may be attached and blood aspirated to confirm intravascular placement. Alternatively, a short length of vena-tubing may be attached to the needle and the syringe attached to the vena-tubing. The syringe should not be attached directly to the needle while making the puncture because to do so is an awkward setup to control. If blood return is not obtained, the needle should be withdrawn slightly during aspiration.

The .018-inch mandril guidewire from the micropuncture set is advanced under fluoroscopic guidance into the inferior vena cava (IVC). The needle is removed and the dilator placed. The intravascular length of the catheter is measured by kinking the wire when the tip is in the RA (for dialysis catheters or catheters placed for chemotherapy) or at the superior vena cava (SVC)–RA junction (PICC lines). A forceps then is used to mark the skin exit site. Under fluoroscopic guidance, the wire is withdrawn to the level of the forceps. The wire then is clamped at this point. The distance between the clamp and the kink is the intravascular length for the catheter.

An 80-cm-long, .035-inch Rosen wire (Cook, Inc.) then is inserted and the tip placed in the IVC. Passage of any wire through the heart should be monitored fluoroscopically, and the anesthetist should be informed of such passage.

Following this, the exit site is chosen in the deltopectoral groove level. In older teenage girls, care should be taken to avoid breast tissue. The site is anesthetized with 1% lidocaine with epinephrine, a dermatotomy is made, and then the entire length of the tunnel is anesthetized through the dermatotomy with a 22-gauge Chiba needle (Cook, Inc.) or the micropuncture needle. The tunnel should not be punctured multiple times because to do so might increase the risk of infection. Initially, blunt dissection of the tunnel is made using a curved forceps, followed by the tunneling device with the lead end exiting the venotomy site in the neck. The catheter is brought through the tunnel, and its cuff is placed 1 to 2 cm into the tunnel. The catheter is cut as determined by the previously measured wire. The catheter then is pulled further into the tunnel because it is usually easier to pull back the catheter from the RA than to later advance it. The catheter should be flushed and the clamps closed.

The neck venotomy site may need to be progressively dilated, depending on the diameter of the catheter. The peel-away sheath then is inserted over the wire under fluoroscopic guidance to ensure that the sheath is following the line of the wire (i.e., advancing coaxially). When a left internal jugular vein approach is used, making a gentle curve in the sheath is useful to facilitate passage over curves.

At this point, respiration is suspended by the anesthetist, the wire and inner dilator of the peel-away sheath are removed, and the catheter is immediately inserted. Respiration is resumed as soon as the catheter is within the peel-away sheath. Intermittent fluoroscopy checks of the passage of the catheter should be made to ensure correct position. The sheath is removed in its entirety if the catheter is in adequate position. If the catheter is in farther than desired, it can be pulled back under fluoroscopic guidance until the tip is at the desired level.

HELPFUL HINTS
It is useful to hold gentle pressure over the neck entry site and to "jiggle" the catheter as it is pulled back to prevent pulling it back too far. The length of the catheter should be checked under fluoroscopy to ensure that no kinks are present. Each port of the catheter should be aspirated, flushed, and primed with heparin solution.

HELPFUL HINTS
Difficulty in passing the catheter through the peel-away sheath is usually due to the sheath being kinked. Peeling away some of the sheath will allow further catheter advancement. A hydrophilic guidewire can be inserted through the catheter and the catheter placed through the peel-away sheath over the hydrophilic guidewire.

The skin venotomy site is closed with an inverted 4-0 Vicryl subcuticular suture and Steri-strips. The catheter is secured at the skin exit site with a 2-0 or 3-0 nonresorbable suture (such as Prolene). A sterile nonocclusive dressing then is applied because infectious complications are greater with occlusive dressings. In teenagers, the suture may be removed in 10 to 14 days when the cuff has become incorporated. In younger children, the suture is left in place for extra stability.

Dialysis Catheters

Uncuffed or temporary dialysis catheters can be functional for up to 2 months in children.[23] Rigid short-term catheters should be placed with the tip in the SVC, not in the RA as usual because perforation and cardiac tamponade, although rare, have been reported.[24] For long-term dialysis, cuffed tunneled catheters are needed.

Access is obtained as described in the preceding section. The catheter length should be measured with the guidewire, and a subcutaneous tunnel is created; however, instead of trimming the catheter to length, the length is chosen before creation of the tunnel because dialysis catheters are designed with staggered tips and therefore should not be cut. For example, if the intravascular length of the catheter is measured to be 16 cm, the tunnel for a 13.5 F, 36-cm-long Bard dialysis catheter should be 5 cm long. This is calculated as follows: The cuff-to-tip length of the catheter is 19 cm. Therefore, 19 cm − 16 cm = 3 cm. Two centimeters is added for the cuff. The overall length of the tunnel is therefore 5 cm. To determine the tunnel length correctly, the catheter cuff-to-tip length must be known. Ideally, the subcutaneous tunnel should be 5 cm or longer.

On occasion, in infants, the dialysis catheter has to be trimmed. This involves staggering the ends and creating additional side holes so that adequate flow rates for dialysis can be achieved.

The remainder of the procedure is the same. The tip of the catheter must be placed in the proximal RA. The arterial port should be facing into the RA because, theoretically, if the arterial port faces the lateral right atrial wall, during aspiration it may "suck up" against the wall and therefore prevent adequate flow rates. This does not apply to newer-design catheters such as the "split-tip" or dual Tesio dialysis catheters.

Ports

Ports are placed in the arm or in the chest, depending on the age and size of the child, patient or guardian preference, and institutional bias. Children over the age of 10 are candidates for arm ports. Exceptions may occur; for example, a large 8-year-old may be a suitable candidate for an arm port, whereas a small 13-year-old may not be suitable. Judgment on the radiologist's part is required for determining the suitability of the child for arm port placement.

Ports are available with pre-attached catheters or where a catheter must be attached. The former are generally suitable for a left-sided approach, when tortuous vessels may lead to the catheter being too short.

For chest placement, access into the internal jugular vein and tunneling of the catheter are performed as described previously. For arm placement, access into the basilic vein is obtained with a micropuncture set. The port pocket is created over the medial aspect of the arm, above the elbow, and over the humerus.[12,16]

A subcutaneous pocket is created over the anterolateral chest wall, inferior to the clavicle but superior to breast tissue. It is important to ensure that the port hub is not resting on the clavicle. A no. 11 or no. 15 scalpel blade may be used to make an incision. An incision of only 2 to 3 cm is needed for pediatric ports. The incision should be made over a rib interspace for the port to rest on a rib to provide stability accessing the port. The incision, the port pocket, and the tunnel should be anesthetized with 1% lidocaine with epinephrine. Multiple punctures of the skin should be avoided. Blunt dissection with a sponge forceps, curved hemostats, or what is a very effective tool, the operator's little finger, is used to fashion the pocket. Residual fibrous bands can be cut with scissors. Retractors are used to allow better visualization of the pocket. Bleeding sites can be controlled with a Bovie or with suture ligation. Usually, packing the pocket with saline-soaked gauze for a few minutes will control minor bleeding or general ooze. Curved hemostats are used to start the tunnel. At this point, the port is placed in the pocket to ensure that an adequate fit and adjustments to the pocket can be made. When the pocket is completed, lavage with saline will ensure hemostasis.

To anchor the port in the pocket, either resorbable (e.g., 3-0 Vicryl) or nonresorbable (e.g., 3-0 Prolene) sutures can be used. A stitch is placed in each corner of the pocket to anchor the port later.

A tunneling device is brought through the tunnel, the catheter is attached to the device, and the catheter is brought through the tunnel. The catheter should be clamped to prevent blood loss during catheter insertion. A peel-away sheath is inserted and the catheter advanced under fluoroscopic guidance until the tip is in the proximal RA. The back end of the catheter is cut and attached to the port, and the locking mechanism is secured. The port is accessed, aspirated, and flushed to ensure integrity of the connection. The sutures to anchor the port should be brought through the openings on the port reservoir; then the port is placed in the pocket and the sutures tied.

The deep tissues of the pocket are closed with interrupted inverted 3-0 Vicryl sutures, and the subcuticular tissues are closed with a running 4-0 Vicryl suture. The deep sutures take the tension off the wound and should bring the wound together. Steri-strips and a sterile bandage then are applied. The skin neck puncture site is closed with a 4-0 deep Vicryl suture.

If the port is required for immediate use, it is accessed with a noncoring needle (Huber needle), flushed with heparin, and left accessed. If it is not required immediately, it is accessed and flushed with heparin, and then the needle is removed. Generally, because of soft-tissue swelling over the area, the port cannot be accessed for 7 to 10 days afterward.

The same technique is used to fashion a pocket for an arm port. The pocket should be made over bone, in this case the humerus. The basilic vein or alternatively the brachial vein is accessed. A tunnel is not needed for arm ports. The port should be placed in the patient's nondominant arm.

The placement of preattached ports is similar except the port must be placed in its pocket, the catheter portion brought through the tunnel, and the catheter trimmed to the appropriate length, determined by measuring with a wire. Port removal is done by anesthetizing along the scar, making the incision along the scar, and bluntly dissecting out the port. The pocket should be lavaged and hemostasis ensured. The pocket is closed with deep 3-0 Vicryl interrupted, inverted sutures and with a running 4-0 Vicryl subcuticular suture. Port removal in the younger child may need to be done with general anesthesia.

Peripherally Inserted Central Catheters

In the adult population, better results are achieved with placement of PICCs in the interventional radiology suite than at the bedside.[25] However, because it is more expensive to place PICCs in interventional radiology, placement at the bedside should continue for pediatric patients. If this fails, the PICC can be placed in interventional radiology. Success rates as high as 98% have been reported for placement of PICCs in pediatric patients by interventional radiologists.[26–28] Lower success rates are expected in children younger than 1 year and in children weighing less than 5 kg.[27,29]

In neonates, infants, and younger children, venographic guidance is used. About 5 mL of contrast per kilogram can be used. Sterile technique is necessary, but a full surgical scrub is not. Buffered lidocaine with sodium bicarbonate is preferred for local anesthesia. The arm is placed abducted and externally rotated. A tourniquet is applied on the arm. While the nonionic contrast is injected, a suitable vein is selected, preferably the basilic vein. If the brachial vein is used, care must be taken to avoid puncturing the brachial artery. The vein is cannulated with a 21-gauge needle under fluoroscopic guidance. When the needle is on the vein, contrast within the vein will be displaced. Once the needle has entered the vein, an .018-inch mandril guidewire is advanced centrally, the needle is removed, a dermatotomy is done, and the appropriately sized peel-away sheath is inserted. Measurements are made from the cavoatrial junction to the skin insertion site, and the PICC is trimmed to length. If the catheter has a transition portion from the hub that is a French size larger than the catheter, it can be buried within the subcutaneous tissues and vein to prevent bleeding. The PICC then is inserted through the peel-away sheath and advanced centrally. If a double-wall puncture rather than a single-wall puncture is made, the 0.018-inch wire is used to probe while slowly withdrawing the needle about 1 mm at a time under fluoroscopic guidance. Before withdrawing the needle, the wire must be pulled back into it. Remember that the wire can be advanced easily as far as the axilla and yet be in a perivascular location. The tourniquet is released as soon as the wire is in a central vein or if the wire appears to be hanging up at it.

If there is difficulty advancing the PICC, a hydrophilic guidewire (the diameter determined by the lumen size; for example, a 3.5 F double-lumen catheter takes a 0.014-inch wire) can be advanced and the PICC inserted over the wire, through the peel-away sheath. There is a tendency for venospasm to occur, most commonly in neonates and infants (Fig. 8–1). In these cases, it may be useful to attach a Tuohy–Borst adapter onto the PICC and inject saline as the catheter is advanced over the wire and through the peel-away sheath. Injection of nitroglycerin (3–5 µg/kg) via the catheter has been recommended in cases of persistent venospasm.[26] In addition, there can be a problem advancing catheters from the cephalic into the subclavian vein secondary to spasm or because of the right angle that can be present at this junction. Frequently, catheter placement via the cephalic vein must be done over a hydrophilic wire.

In older children, ultrasound guidance can be used to access the vein. The pro-

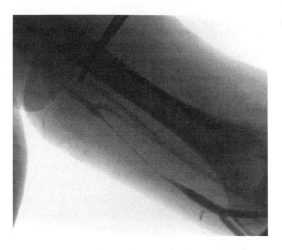

Figure 8–1 Follow-up venogram demonstrating venospasm, which occurred after one pass with a 21-gauge needle into the basilic vein in a 16-year-old boy.

cedure is performed as described. Note that usually it is not necessary to aspirate blood from the needle because, when the tourniquet is tied, blood will drip rapidly from the needle once it is in the vein. The advantage of placing PICCs in interventional radiology is that access is obtained higher in the arm than when placed on the floor, where access is usually at the elbow. This enables the child to bend his or her elbow. The PICC should be placed in the nondominant arm if possible. The PICC is secured with 2-0 or 3-0 Prolene, and a sterile dressing is applied. In neonates, infants, and younger children, a "no-no" is applied to prevent the arm bending and to protect the PICC.

HELPFUL HINT
If it is not possible to place a PICC in an arm vein, the saphenous vein can be used. A tourniquet is applied to the leg, and using venographic or ultrasound guidance, the saphenous vein is cannulated above the medial aspect of the knee. The procedure is the same as for placement in an arm vein, with the tip of the catheter placed in the proximal IVC.

On occasion, in premature infants or infants in whom placement in the arm or

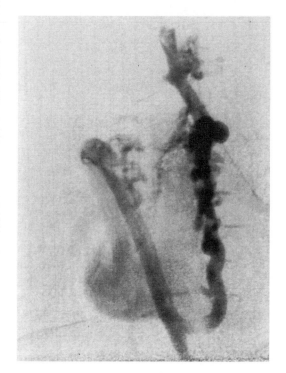

Figure 8–2 A 2-month-old female infant weighing 2.5 kg was a former 31-week prematurely delivered infant. A prior peripherally inserted central catheter (PICC) line was placed via the right internal jugular vein 1 month previously but had come out. A 16.5-cm, 3 French, single-lumen PICC catheter was placed via the left internal jugular vein. Note the venogram demonstrating left intercostals vein, accessory hemiazygos vein, azygos vein, and superior vena cava.

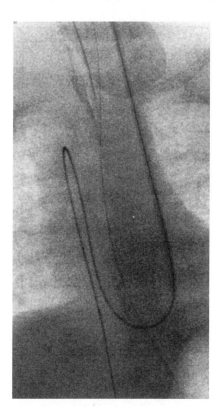

Figure 8–3 Guidewire tip in the inferior vena cava.

leg veins fail, a decision must be made whether to place the PICC via the internal jugular vein (Figs. 8–2, 8–3, and 8–4), or whether to place a Broviac catheter. If access is needed immediately, the internal jugular vein is an acceptable option for placing the PICC.

Alternative Sites

Rarely, a translumbar or trans-hepatic approach is needed. The techniques are similar to those used in adults.[30–32] In children, because of expected growth resulting in eventual shortening of the intravas-cular portion of the catheter, it may be preferable to use the trans-hepatic rather than the translumbar route.[30] It is also recommended that some slack be left in the catheter at its entry site into the liver.

CATHETER MAINTENANCE

Catheter maintenance includes instructions on flushing and dressing changes. For tunneled catheters and PICCs in children who weigh less than 10 kg, the catheters are flushed with 1 to 3 mL of heparin (10 U/mL) after each use or, if capped, every 24 hours. For children who weigh more than 10 kg, the catheters are flushed with 1 to 3 mL of heparin solution (100 U/mL) if capped, every 24 hours. For children who weigh more than 10 kg and require three to four flushes per day, a 10 U/mL heparin solution should be used. The max-

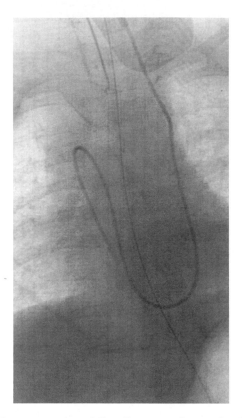

Figure 8–4 A peripherally inserted central catheter line in place.

imum daily heparin flush solution should not exceed 50 U/kg daily. For ports, 5 mL of 10 U/mL of heparin solution in children who weigh less than 10 kg and 5 mL of 100 U/mL of heparin solution in children greater than 10 kg are used. A Huber needle should be changed every 7 days. Ports should be flushed with heparin solution monthly or after completion of therapy, before the access needle is removed. Hemodialysis catheters are loaded with 1000 U/mL of heparin solution for inpatients, and the volume used should equal the exact volume of the catheter. For outpatients, 5000 U/mL of heparin solution is used, and the volume equals the exact volume of the catheter. Apheresis catheters are loaded with 1000 U/mL heparin solution, and the volume used equals the exact volume of the catheter. Home health nurses must do dressing changes at least

weekly for patients receiving therapy at home, and nursing staff do these changes for inpatients.

COMPLICATIONS

Complications occur during or after the procedure (periprocedural or postprocedural). Placement of central lines in the interventional suite compares favorably with surgical placement in the operating room.[33,34] The complications in children mirror those in adults. Management is also essentially the same. With careful technique, periprocedural complications can be minimized.

Air embolism is a potentially serious complication during tunneled catheter placement, with greater hemodynamic derangement occurring in a child than in an adult.[5,6] Heavily sedated and young children are unable to cooperate by holding their breath. The advantage of anesthesia is to provide positive pressure ventilation during insertion of the catheter through the peel-away sheath. Because of the seriousness of this complication in our experience, as well as in the experience of others, general anesthesia is preferred for the placement of all tunneled catheters, dialysis catheters, and ports.

In the pediatric age group, one of the greatest problems is the inadvertent removal of the catheter. To prevent this in the neonate, infant, or young child, a soft restraint may be fastened around the PICC line. Donaldson and colleagues[5] found that by suturing the line, using a K-lock and a soft bandage, inadvertent removal was reduced from 8 to 2%. For tunneled central catheters, it is helpful to have a suture secure the catheter at the skin exit site as well. In children (typically toddlers) in whom tunneled catheters are repeatedly, inadvertently removed, we find it helpful to tunnel the catheter over the shoulder, with the exit site over the back rather than over the chest.

Catheter-related thrombosis occurs in up to 10% of patients.[35,36] Urokinase, which will be re-released pending FDA approval of the package insert, may be used for the treat-

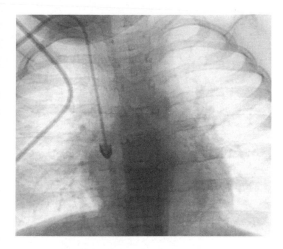

Figure 8–5 A 1-year-old child with a history of ability to flush a Broviac catheter but an inability to aspirate from the catheter. Contrast study revealed a fibrin sheath around the catheter.

ment of catheter thrombosis. The amount used is the catheter volume, with a concentration of 5000 u/ml. This may be repeated up to three times in 24 hours. tPA may also be used. The dose in children <10 kg is 0.5 mgs diluted in saline and in children >10 kg the dose is 1–2 mgs (1 mg/mL). Urokinase also can be used for management of a fibrin sheath around the tip of the catheter.[12] The typical history is the ability to flush the catheter but not aspirate from it. This results from the sheath forming a one-way valve at the catheter tip (Fig. 8–5).

Infection is a major cause of catheter failure in long-term use. There is an increased risk of infection with multiple lumens.[37] Ports have a decreased infection rate compared with tunneled catheters.[38,39]

Adherence to aseptic technique during implantation of the device is important. No advantage has been shown from using periprocedural antibiotics, although this practice is common.[21,22] Infection from contamination of the subcutaneous pocket or tract during placement of the device begins in the immediate postprocedural period.[12]

Delayed infection may be secondary to seeding of the device from a hematogenous source but frequently begins at the catheter hub or in a pocket that is entered by an

access needle. In 50 to 70% of cases, skin flora are responsible for catheter infection.[12] *Staphylococcus epidermidis* is found in 25 to 50% of cases.[12] To determine whether the infection is due to the device, Weightman and colleagues demonstrated that in cases of catheter sepsis there is at least a tenfold increase in colony counts in blood drawn from the catheter compared with peripheral blood.[40,41] This has an advantage over techniques in which removal of the catheter is required.[41,42] Recent work suggests that although sepsis is an indication for catheter removal, catheter exchange and antibiotics may suffice in the treatment of mildly symptomatic bacteremia.[43,44] Tunnel infections usually require catheter removal,

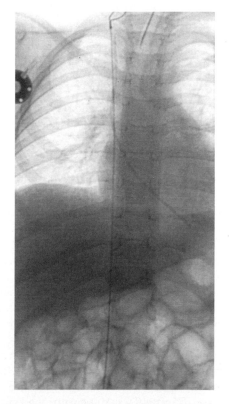

Figure 8–6 In this 2-year-old infant, it was not possible to aspirate from the port. Chest radiography revealed that port catheter was disconnected. The catheter fragment was retrieved using a partially deployed 10-mm loop snare. A right common femoral vein approach was used, and another port was placed.

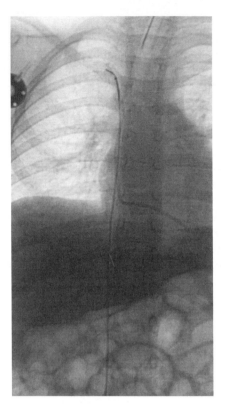

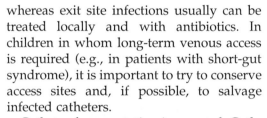

Figure 8–7 A right common femoral vein approach was used. Another port was placed.

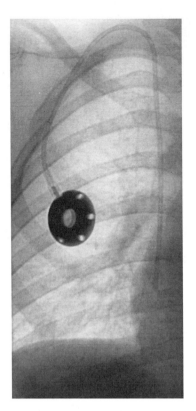

Figure 8–8 Cook Minivital port placed via the right internal jugular vein. A new port pocket was created.

whereas exit site infections usually can be treated locally and with antibiotics. In children in whom long-term venous access is required (e.g., in patients with short-gut syndrome), it is important to try to conserve access sites and, if possible, to salvage infected catheters.

Catheter fragmentation is unusual. Catheters placed via the subclavian route may fragment secondary to "pinch-off" phenomenon.[17] On occasion, catheters may be fragmented by inadvertent puncture with an access needle. Port catheters may detach from the port reservoir. Usually, these catheter fragments can be retrieved with the use of a loop snare (Microvena, White Bear Lake, MN, U.S.A.). In the younger patient, if a small snare is unavailable, a snare can be partially deployed and used to retrieve the catheter fragment (Figs. 8–6, 8–7, and 8–8).

SUMMARY

Pediatric interventional radiology is undergoing rapid change and expansion, with procedures ranging from central venous access to complex embolizations. Although the principles used in adults are applicable to children, differences do exist. When dealing with children, it must be remembered always that we are dealing with the patient as well as with the patient's parents and guardian. Sedation of children requires a thorough knowledge of drugs for adequate sedation to be achieved. General anesthesia is required in many children. We have tried to provide practical information for successful central venous access in children. With patience and flexibility, interventional radiologists can make the same positive impact on the placement of central venous catheters in children as has been done in adults.

References

1. Broviac JW, Cole JJ, Scribner BH. A silicone rubber atrial catheter for prolonged parenteral alimentation. *Surg Gynecol Obstet.* 1973;136: 602–606.
2. Hickman RO, Buckner CD, Clift RA, Sanders JE, Stewart P, Thomas ED. A modified right atrial catheter for access to the venous system in marrow transplant recipients. *Surg Gynecol Obstet.* 1979;148:871–875.
3. Early TF, Gregory RT, Wheeler JR, Snyder SO, Gayle RG. Increased infection rate in double-lumen versus single-lumen Hickman catheters in cancer patients. *South Med J.* 1990;83:34–36.
4. Openshaw KL, Picus D, Hicks ME, Darcy MD, Vesely TM, Picus J. Interventional radiologic placement of Hohn central venous catheters: results and complications in 100 consecutive patients. *J Vasc Interv Radiol.* 1994;5:111–115.
5. Donaldson JS, Jackson NT, Morello FP, Saker MC. Pediatric vascular access. *Semin Interv Radiol.* 1998;15:315–323.
6. Morello FP, Donaldson JS, Saker MC, Norman JT. Air embolism during tunneled central catheter placement performed without general anesthesia in children: a potentially serious complication. *J Vasc Interv Radiol.* 1999;10:781–784.
7. Committee on Drugs. Guidelines for monitoring and management of pediatric patients during and after sedation for diagnostic and therapeutic procedures. *Pediatrics.* 1992;89: 1110–1115.
8. Frush DP, Bissett GS III, Hall SC. Pediatric sedation in radiology: the practice of safe sleep. *AJR Am J Roentgenol.* 1996;167: 1381–1387.
9. Schreiner MS. Preoperative and postoperative fasting in children. *Pediatr Clin North Am.* 1994;41:111–120.
10. Cotesen MR, Donaldson JS, Uejima T, Morello FP. Efficacy of ketamine hydrochloride sedation in children for interventional radiologic procedures. *AJR Am J Roentgenol.* 1997;169:1019–1022.
11. American Society of Anesthesiologists Task Force. Practice guidelines for sedation and analgesia by non-anesthesiologist: a report by the American Society of Anesthesiologists Task Force on Sedation and Analgesia by Non-anesthesiologists. *Anesthesiology.* 1996; 84:459–471.
12. Denny DF. Placement and management of long-term central venous access catheters and ports. *AJR Am J Roentgenol.* 1993;161: 385–393.
13. Nosher JL, Shami MM, Siegal RL, DeCandia M, Bodner LJ. Tunneled central venous access catheter placement in the pediatric population: comparison of radiologic and surgical results. *Radiology.* 1994;192: 265–268.
14. Docktor BL, Sadler DJ, Gray RR, Saliken JC, So CB. Radiologic placement of tunneled central catheters: rates of success and of immediate complications in a large series. *AJR Am J Roentgenol.* 1999;173:457–460.
15. Crowley JJ, Pereira JK, Harris LS, Becker CJ. Radiologic placement of long-term subcutaneous venous access ports in children. *AJR Am J Roentgenol.* 1998;171:257–260.
16. Foley MJ. Radiologic placement of long-term central venous peripheral access system ports (PAS port): results in 150 patients. *J Vasc Interv Radiol.* 1995;6:255–262.
17. Hinke DH, Zandt-Stastny DA, Goodman LR, Quebbeman EJ, Krzywda EA, Andris DA. Pinch-off syndrome: a complication of implantable subclavian venous access devices. *Radiology.* 1990;177:353–356.
18. Cimochowski GE, Worley E, Rutherform WE, Sartain J, Blondin J, Harter H. Superiority of the internal jugular over the subclavian access for temporary dialysis. *Nephron.* 1990;54:154–161.
19. Schillinger F, Schillinger D, Montagnac R, Milcent T. Post catheterisation vein stenosis in haemodialysis: a comparative angiographic study of 50 subclavian and 50 internal jugular accesses. *Nephrol Dial Transplant.* 1991;6: 722–724.
20. Barrett N, Spencer S, McIvor J, Brown EA. Subclavian stenosis: a major complication of dialysis catheters. *Nephrol Dial Transplant.* 1988;3:423–425.
21. McKee R, Dunsmuir R, Whitby M, Garden OJ. Does antibiotic prophylaxis at the time of catheter insertion reduce the incidence of catheter-related sepsis in intravenous nutrition? *J Hosp Infect.* 1985;6:419–425.
22. Johnson A, Oppenheim BA. Vascular catheter-related sepsis: diagnosis and prevention. *J Hosp Infect.* 1992;20:67–78.

23. Goldstein SL, Macierowski CT, Jabs K. Hemodialysis catheter survival and complications in children and adolescents. *Pediatr Nephrol.* 1997;11:74–77.

24. Friedmann BA, Jurgelcit C. Perforation of the atrium by a polyethylene CV catheter. *JAMA.* 1968;203:1141–1142.

25. Cardella JF, Fox PS, Lawler JB. Interventional radiologic placement of peripherally inserted central catheters. *J Vasc Interv Radiol.* 1993;4:653–660.

26. Dubois J, Garel L, Tapiero B, Dube J, Laframboise S, David M. Peripherally inserted central catheters in infants and children. *Radiology.* 1997;204:622–626.

27. Crowley JJ, Pereira JK, Harris LS, Becker CJ. Peripherally inserted central catheters: experience in 523 children. *Radiology.* 1997; 204:617–621.

28. Donaldson JS, Morello FP, Junewick JJ, O'Donovan JC, Lim-Dunham J. Peripherally inserted central venous catheters: US-guided vascular access in pediatric patients. *Radiology.* 1995;197:542–544.

29. Chait PG, Ingram J, Phillips-Gordon C, Farrell H, Kuhn C. Peripherally inserted central catheters in children. *Radiology.* 1995; 197:775–778.

30. Azizkham RG, Taylor LA, Jaques PF, Mauro MA, Lacey SR. Percutaneous translumbar and transhepatic inferior vena caval catheters for prolonged venous access in children. *J Pediatr Surg.* 1992;27:165–169.

31. Robertson L, Jaques P, Mauro M, Azizkhan RG, Robards J. Percutaneous inferior vena cava placement of tunneled silastic catheters for prolonged vascular access in infants. *J Pediatr Surg.* 1990;25:596–598.

32. Denny DF Jr, Greenwood LH, Morse SS, Lee GK, Baquero J. Inferior vena cava: translumbar catheterization for central venous access. *Radiology.* 1989;170: 1013–1014.

33. McBride KD, Fisher R, Warnock N, Winfield DA, Reed MW, Gaines PA. A comparative analysis of radiological and surgical placement of central venous catheters. *Cardiovasc Interv Radiol.* 1997;20:17–22.

34. Davis SJ, Thompson JS, Edney JA. Insertion of Hickman catheters: a comparison of cutdown and percutaneous techniques. *Am J Surg.* 1984;50:673–676.

35. Gray WJ, Bell WR. Fibrinolytic agents in the treatment of thrombotic disorders. *Semin Oncol.* 1990;17:228–237.

36. Moss JF, Wagman LD, Riihimaki DU, Terz JJ. Central venous thrombosis related to the silastic Hickman-Broviac catheters in an oncologic population. *JPEN J Parenter Enteral Nutr.* 1989;13:397–400.

37. Early TF, Gregory RT, Wheeler JR, Synder SO, Gayle RG. Increased infection rate in double-lumen versus single-slumen Hickman catheters in cancer patients. *South Med J.* 1990;83:34–36.

38. Ross MN, Haase GM, Poole MA, Burrington JD, Odom LF. Comparison of totally implanted reservoirs with external catheters as venous access devices in pediatric oncologic patients. *Surg Gynecol Obstet.* 1988;167: 141–144.

39. Groeger JS, Lucas AB, Thaler HT, et al. Infectious morbidity associated with long-term use of venous access devices in patients with cancer. *Ann Intern Med.* 1993;119:1168–1174.

40. Weightman NC, Simpson EM, Speller DCE, Mott MG, Oakhill A. Bacteremia related to indwelling central venous catheters: prevention, diagnosis, and treatment. *Eur J Clin Microbiol Infect Dis.* 1988;7:125–129.

41. Maki DG, Weise CE, Sarafin HW. A semiquantitative culture method for identifying intravenous catheter related infection. *N Engl J Med.* 1977;296:1305–1309.

42. Cooper GL, Hopkins CC. Rapid diagnosis of intravascular associated infection by direct gram staining of catheter segments. *N Engl J Med.* 1985;312:1142–1147.

43. Robinson D, Suhocki P, Schwab SJ. Treatment of infected tunneled venous access hemodialysis catheters with guidewire exchange. *Kidney Int.* 1998;53:1792–1794.

44. Beathard GA. Management of bacteremia associated with tunneled cuffed hemodialysis catheters. *J Am Soc Nephrol.* 1999;10: 1045–1049.

Chapter 9

Placement of Central Catheters in Specific Circumstances

Philip C. Pieters
Jaime Tisnado

Several specific entities, some of which do not appear to be related to each other, are discussed in this chapter. These entities are of major concern because of abnormalities in hemostasis or immunity. Therefore, brief reviews of the hemostasis pathways and immunity/inflammation will be mentioned first, followed with a discussion of the entities.

BONE MARROW

The medullary cavity of certain flat bones (sternum, pelvis, ribs, and skull) contains red bone marrow/myeloid tissue. Components of myeloid tissue are: (1) a hetcro geneous population of developing blood cells; (2) vascular connective tissue stroma supported by a meshwork of collagenic and reticular fibers; (3) fat storage cells; and (4) sinusoids (thin-walled vascular channels consisting of simple squamous endothelium that allow newly formed blood cells to enter the bloodstream).

All types of blood cells are derived from a single type of ancestral stem cell called the *pleuripotential hemopoietic stem cell*. Stem cells remain poorly differentiated and uncommitted except that they will form blood cells of some kind. They are able to proliferate extensively and renew themselves. The myeloid tissue contains a mixture of stem cell offspring at various stages of differentiation.

The hemopoietic stem cell has the potential to differentiate into several different lines of specialized cells. Initially, the progeny of stem cells become restricted to undergo lymphoid (producing lymphocytes and plasma cells) or myeloid (producing other types of blood cells, such as megakaryocytes, erythrocytes, granulocytes, and monocytes) differentiation. The restricted orders of stem cells then give rise to progenitor cells committed to single lines of lymphoid or myeloid differentiation.

IMMUNE SYSTEM

The immune system consists of complex interactions between antibody production, cellular immunity, and components of the complement system and phagocyte function.

Lymphocytes

As previously discussed, the bone marrow stem cells may become restricted to the lymphoid line of differentiation and then differentiate further into two divergent and immunologic active populations: B lymphocytes and T lymphocytes and their subsets. The lymphocytes continuously interchange between blood and lymph (*recirculation*) to bring them into contact with any foreign antigen present in the body. The cells have the unique capacity to recognize antigen and respond to it. The production of circulating immunoglobulins in response to an antigen is termed the *humoral antibody response* and is mediated by B lymphocytes and their progeny (*plasma cells*), although helper T cells are required for this response. When a small lymphocyte responds to the antigen for which it is programmed, it develops intense cytoplasmic basophilia, enlarges rapidly, duplicates its DNA, and embarks in a series of divisions that generates a whole clone of identically programmed cells. This clone of cells then may respond to the antigen or the antigen-bearing cells. T lymphocytes mediate a wide range of immunologic activities. Individual T cells are programmed during differentiation to express only a limited range of functions (i.e., cytotoxic cells, helper T cells, or suppressor T cells). The T lymphocytes' importance in resistance to infection is through macrophage activation by lymphokines and cytotoxicity of virus-infected cells. T lymphocytes play a central role in resistance to infection by a variety of facultative intracellular microorganisms. Other functions of T lymphocytes include delayed hypersensitivity; immunologic memory; allograft rejection; destruction of neoplastic cells; and release of cytotoxic, chemotactic, and macrophage-reactive factors.

Inflammation

The acute phase of inflammation is of relatively short duration, lasting several hours, and is stereotypic, regardless of the nature of the injury. The main characteristics of acute inflammation are exudation of fluid and plasma proteins (*edema*) and the emigration of leukocytes from the bloodstream to inflamed tissues. Changes in vascular permeability and vasodilatation are responsible for the heat and redness associated with acute inflammation. The accumulation of leukocytes (predominantly neutrophils and monophils) is the most important feature of the inflammatory reaction. After 24 to 48 hours, the chronic inflammation response is less uniform and longer in duration. Lymphocytes and macrophages replace the short-lived neutrophils. Prolifer-

ation of blood vessels and connective tissue also takes place.

Neutrophils

Neutrophils have only one known function: to destroy microorganisms. The steps in neutrophils' response in host defense against invading microbes are mobilization, adherence, locomotion, chemotaxis, phagocytosis, and intracellular killing. Microbial invasion is followed by mobilization of both mature and round (*band*) forms of neutrophils from the bone marrow, resulting in the "left shift" present in many acute bacterial infections. The neutrophils adhere to the vascular endothelium and enter the tissue by locomoting between the endothelial cells (*diapedesis*). Once in the tissues, chemotaxis (*directed migration*) occurs as the neutrophils move in the direction of increasing concentrations of attractants (*chemotactic factors*). The most important chemotactic agents for the neutrophils (and also monocytes) are bacterial products, components of the complement system, and products of the lipooxygenase pathway of the arachidonic acid metabolism. As the neutrophils accumulate at the site of inflammation, contact with the microorganisms initiates phagocytosis. Many microorganisms resist ingestion by the neutrophils and can be engulfed only after being opsonized. *Opsonins* are antibodies or components of the complement system that coat the microbial surface and render it more ingestible. Opsonizing antibodies act as ligands between organisms and phagocytic cells. Neutrophils have specific membrane receptors for these opsonins, which enhances their initial attachment and ultimately ingestion. The microbes are engulfed by the neutrophils and destroyed by a variety of mechanisms, including a variety of oxygen-dependent and oxygen-independent microbicidal systems.

Complement System

Complement is a generic term for a group of distinct proteins that normally exist in plasma in inactive precursor forms but are activated during immunologically induced inflammation. This system functions by mediating a series of biologic reactions, all of which serve in the defense against microbial agents. The complement system is activated by antigen–antibody complexes or by such stimuli as bacterial endotoxins. When activated, these components have the ability to increase vascular permeability, attract leukocytes, opsonize microbial agents prior to phagocytosis, immobilize cells at the site of inflammation, and impair cell membrane function (which may lead to osmotic lysis of target organisms and cell death).

STATES OF IMMUNODEFICIENCY

As described, the immune system consists of multiple components, including antibody production, cellular immunity, and components of the complement system and phagocytic function. Immunodeficiency can result from disruption of any of these components in the complex chain of events. The following lists of causes of immunodeficiency are organized according to their functional deficiency.

Antibody-Deficiency Disorders

Considered as a whole, immunoglobulin deficiencies are not uncommon, occurring in about 1 in 600 in the general population. Several or only one of the immunoglobulin classes can be affected, and antibody production can be totally or partially disrupted (agammaglobulinemia versus hypogammaglobinemia). Clinically, infections in these patients frequently involve the sinopulmonary tract, ears, meninges, and skin. Bacteremia with metastatic spread of infection is not uncommon. Severe viral infections are uncommon. Recurrent infections with high-grade extracellular encapsulated pathogens (pneumococci, streptococci, and *Haemophilus* organisms) are typical entities in this category, which includes the following:

- Congenital X-linked hypogammaglobulinemia (Bruton type): This condition is marked by nearly complete absence of B cells in the circulation and becomes apparent at 5 to 6 months of age.
- Common variable immunodeficiency: This deficiency does not become apparent until age 15 or older. The presenting disease is often chronic progressive bronchiectasis. The B cells are either absent or unable to differentiate nto immunoglobulin-producing plasma cells.
- Transient hypogammaglobulinemia of infancy.
- Selective immunoglobulin A (IgA) deficiency: Most affected subjects are well clinically but may have sinopulmonary infections, atopy, gastrointestinal disorders, autoimmune disease, and malignancy.

Cellular Immunodeficiency Disorders

Acquired immunodeficiency syndrome (AIDS) is the most common acquired cellular immunodeficiency disorder; the human immunodeficiency virus (HIV) impairs normal T-cell function. Other causes of secondary immunodeficiency include chemotherapy, radiation therapy, and bone marrow transplantation (BMT). Congenital thymic hypoplasia (DiGeorge syndrome) is a rare condition that is a relatively pure form of T-cell immunodeficiency. Because of a hypoplastic thymus, these infants do not develop T cells and lack any form of cell-mediated immunity. The serum immunoglobulin concentrations are usually normal or elevated in these disorders, but B-cell function is compromised because of a deficiency of T-helper cells. Clinical characteristics of these conditions include recurrent infection with low-grade or opportunistic infectious agents (fungi, viruses, *Pneumocystis*), diarrhea, and a high incidence of malignancy.

Combined Immunodeficiency Disorders

Patients with combined immunodeficiency disorders suffer from antibody deficiency as well as cellular immunodeficiency. Entities in this category include the following:

- Severe combined immunodeficiency disorders, such as reticular dysgenesis and "Swiss-type" immunodeficiency, are due to a defect in relatively primitive hematopoetic precursor cells, resulting in profound deficit of both T cells and B cells. As a result, these infants have a marked susceptibility to infection and rarely live past infancy.
- Partial combined immunodeficiency disorders include ataxia telangiectasia and Wiskott–Aldrich syndrome. Ataxia telangiectasia patients initially present with ataxia during the first year of life and later in childhood suffer from recurrent susceptibility to infection. Telangiectasia of the conjunctiva and the skin may appear anytime from birth to several years of age. Increased susceptibility to sinopulmonary infections begins at about age 3 years. There is a selective IgA deficiency and variable degrees of T-cell deficiency. The cellular immunity becomes increasingly impaired with the passage of time, and patients are susceptible to viral and bacterial infections. Wiskott–Aldrich syndrome involves both cellular and humoral abnormalities. Patients display the triad of eczema, recurrent pyogenic infections, and thrombocytopenia. Children with this disorder commonly die within the first decade of life.

Complement Deficiencies

The complement system plays a critical role in the normal inflammatory reaction. Activation of the complement system (classic pathway or alternative pathway) involves a complex interaction between a variety of proteins. Deficiency of any component in this system can result in increased susceptibility to infection. Some patients with sickle cell anemia or patients who have had splenectomy have an unexplained defect in the alternative pathway of the complement system that may be linked to the susceptibility of these patients to infection by encapsulated organisms.

Phagocytic Dysfunction

The neutrophils, monocytes, and macrophages are the final link in the complex inflammatory reaction. Every event that has taken place during inflammation has occurred with the ultimate goal of bringing these phagocytes into contact with the offending microbial organisms such that these cells may kill the organisms. Again, the process of mobilization, adherence, locomotion, chemotaxis, phagocytosis, and intracellular killing is complex, and defects can occur at any point during the process from a variety of causes:

- Disorders of production result in a decrease in the number of circulating neutrophils. Neutropenia resulting from toxic depression of the bone marrow due to radiation or chemotherapy is common.
- Defects in adherence may be due to diabetes mellitus, acute alcohol intoxication, corticosteroids, and leukemia.
- Defects in chemotaxis may be due to complement deficiency, cell-derived agent deficiencies (e.g., lymphokines), or the production of inhibitors such as in patients with Hodgkin's disease or sarcoidosis. Chediak–Higashi syndrome and diabetes mellitus result in intracellular defects, which decrease chemotaxis.
- Defects in phagocytosis are most often due to opsonin defects, such as complement or immunoglobulin deficiencies.
- Defects of microbicidal activity involve abnormalities of either oxidative burst or granule function.
- Chronic granulomatous disease is a syndrome characterized by abnormal neutrophil oxidative metabolism, resulting in phagosomes lacking the microbicidal activity of superoxide and anion and hydrogen peroxide.

HEMOSTASIS

Hemostasis may be defined as the process by which the vascular system maintains its integrity as a closed system. Injury to soft tissues and to the endothelium of a blood vessel initiates a complex series of events that ultimately leads to formation of a clot. There are three basic phases in hemostasis: (1) vascular spasm, (2) formation of a platelet plug, and (3) blood coagulation. Vascular spasm occurs immediately after injury and results in decreased blood flow to the site of injury. Platelets play a critically important role in primary hemostasis and in initiating blood coagulation. The intact vascular endothelium is nonreactive to platelets; however, after an injury to the vessel wall, collagen fibrils of the vascular endothelium are exposed and platelets from the circulating blood adhere to the site of injury within seconds. The adherent platelets become activated and undergo the so-called platelet-release reaction. Released platelet factors, among other effects, activate the coagulation factor X to initiate the intrinsic coagulation sequence. Concomitantly, the release of tissue factors from injured cells participates in the activation of the extrinsic coagulation system.

Activation of platelets occurs by stimulation of receptors on the platelet surface by subendothelial collagen (other nonphysiologic surfaces, including glass, will also activate platelets). The discoid-shaped platelet responds by changing its shape to a more spheric form with filamentous cytoplasmic extensions and undergoes a release reaction. The release of storage granules, which contain adenosine diphosphate (ADP), serotonin, thromboxane A_2, biogenic amines, and potassium, serves to induce further platelet aggregation, secretion, and vasoconstriction. During the platelet-release reaction, glycoprotein Ib surface receptors on the platelet interact with Von Willebrand factor (vWF) and the exposed collagen, making the platelet "sticky."

The combination of platelet "stickiness" and the recruitment of additional platelets leads to the formation of an initial clot. The release of ADP modifies the surface of the platelet so that fibrinogen can attach to the heterodimer complex formed by glycoproteins IIb and IIIa on the platelet surface. This linkage of platelets creates a hemostatic plug; however, if not reinforced, the initial clot soon will begin to degenerate.

Secondary hemostasis occurs when internal and external coagulation pathways are initiated. As proteins present on the surface of the platelet come into contact with the damaged endothelial wall, factors VII and XII are activated. The intrinsic pathway is initiated by the activation of factor XII (*the Hageman factor*), which is converted into a proteolytic enzyme. The Hageman factor also activates the complement system. The cascade of the intrinsic pathway proceeds over a span of several minutes to the development of factor Xa.

The extrinsic pathway is triggered by the introduction of tissue factors containing thromboplastin into the blood. Tissue factor complexes with factor VII to activate it, and the resultant complex interacts with factor X to form factor Xa. Thereafter, with the facilitation of calcium ions and phospholipids, this prothrombin activator complex converts prothrombin to thrombin as the two pathways converge.

Thrombin is a serine protease that splits the fibrinogen molecule. The resulting fibrin molecules associate side by side to form a noncovalently linked fibrin polymer, which is highly susceptible to the proteolytic enzymes present in the plasma and is not sufficiently stable for normal hemostasis. Fibrin stabilization is achieved following activation of factor XIII by thrombin in the presence of calcium. The clot thus formed is significantly more effective in maintaining hemostasis. Incorporated into the clot are factors needed for later clot degeneration (*fibrinolysis*). The clotting system and the fibrinolytic system exist in a homeostatic balance.

Disorders of Primary Hemostasis (Platelet Dysfunction)

Platelet-associated bleeding disorders and hypercoagulable states can arise from several factors, either quantitative or qualitative. Platelets (thrombocytes) are fragments of megakaryocytes, the large cells in the bone marrow, which descended from pluripotent stem cells. The megakaryocytes shed platelets, which measure 2 to 6 μ in diameter and have a life span of 8 to 10 days. A normal platelet count is 150,000 to 400,000/mm^3 of blood.

Quantitative Platelet Disorders

Thrombocythemia results from an overproduction of platelets, and it occurs in patients with myeloproliferative disorders, usually as a result of abnormal stem cell reproduction, including polycythemia vera, chronic myelogenous leukemia, and idiopathic refractory sideroblastic anemia. Thrombocytosis is also an entity with overproduction of platelets, but it is not a primary disorder, such as thrombocythemia; rather, it is a reactive disorder secondary to an underlying malignancy or to a nonmalignant disease. Thrombocytosis may be due to production of plasma platelet-stimulating factor in response to a variety of factors, including malignancy, inflammation, and others. Splenectomy also can result in thrombocytosis as the spleen removes platelets from the blood; when the spleen is absent, the platelet count increases and may cause a hypercoagulable state. Both thrombocythemia and thrombocytosis exist when the platelet count is greater than 400,000/mm^3 and may present with diffuse thromboses, such as venous thrombosis, pulmonary embolism, transient ischemic attacks, or myocardial infarction. A severe condition exists if the count is greater than 800,000/mm^3. Therapy usually is directed at correcting the underlying disorder.

On the other hand, thrombocytopenia is defined as a platelet count of less than 150,000/mm^3 and is the most frequent platelet abnormality associated with malignancies. Patients with 40,000 to 60,000 platelets per mm^3 have an increased incidence of postsurgical and post-trauma bleeding, whereas patients with fewer than 20,000 platelets/mm^3 may have spontaneous bleeding. Thrombocytopenia may be caused by sequestration of platelets by the spleen (*hypersplenism*). Several drugs, including chemotherapeutic agents, and radiation therapy are common causes of thrombocytopenia in patients with malignancies. In fact, bone marrow suppression is a major dose-limiting effect of chemotherapy. Antimetabolites and antimitotic agents also cause generalized bone marrow hypoplasia or aplasia. Alcohol and estrogens may cause a decreased megakaryocyte production, and hence thrombocytopenia. Aspirin, furosemide, heparin, penicillin, and phenytoin also are associated with a decreased platelet survival time. Multiple blood transfusions also may result in thrombocytopenia. Although stored blood is viable for 21 days, the platelets lose their effectiveness after 24 hours of storage. Neoplasms such as multiple myeloma, lymphoma, leukemia, or any metastatic carcinoma involving the bone marrow displace the megakaryocytes with malignant cells, thus producing thrombocytopenia. Viral and bacterial infections decrease platelet production by releasing endotoxins, resulting in damaged platelets and decreased platelet survival time.

Idiopathic thrombocytopenic purpura (ITP) is a platelet dyscrasia. The mechanism of platelet destruction is unknown but is most likely due to binding of an immunoglobulin G (IgG) autoantibody to circulating platelets causing destruction of the platelets. ITP may be associated with pregnancy, malignant disease, HIV infection, and autoimmune diseases, such as systemic lupus erythematosus (SLE).

Qualitative Platelet Disorders

Several rare hereditary disorders can affect platelet adhesion or aggregation characteristics. Bernard–Soulier syndrome, Glanzmann thombasthenia, and storage pool disease are several such conditions.

An acquired platelet dysfunction may be associated with uremia, liver disease, anemia, autoimmune diseases, multiple myeloma, and myeloproliferative disorders. The mechanism of dysfunction varies but may include: (1) interference with the platelet membrane receptor, (2) inhibition of prostaglandin pathways, and (3) inhibition of platelet phosphodiesterase activity. Aspirin produces an acquired platelet dysfunction by irreversibly inactivating cyclo-oxygenase, an enzyme required for the synthesis of prostaglandins. The platelet abnormalities persist until the defective platelets are replaced by new, unaffected platelets. Nonsteroidal anti-inflammatory agents (NSAIAs) bind with the cyclo-oxygenase, but the defect is reversible, lasting approximately 24 hours.

Disorders of Secondary Hemostasis (Coagulation)

Abnormalities of coagulation can be congenital or acquired. Usually, congenital defects involve only a single factor, whereas acquired defects involve multiple factors.

Congenital disorders should be apparent from a history of bleeding problems and include hemophilia (a deficiency or abnormality of factor VIII procoagulant activity); Christmas disease (an abnormality of factor IX); von Willebrand disease (an abnormality of vWF); congenital deficiencies of factor II, factor V, factor VII, factor X, factor XII, and factor XIII (all rare); and afibrinogenemia.

The most common acquired disorders are associated with liver disease that results in decreased synthesis of vitamin K–dependent factors (II, VII, IX, and X) plus factor V, fibrinogen, and possibly other factors. Acquired disorders of hemostasis also may be secondary to the production of antibodies that bind to coagulation factors. Examples include inhibitors of factor VIII procoagulant activity and factor V. Most common acquired bleeding problems are complications of anticoagulation therapy with warfarin or heparin.

MALIGNANCIES

Central venous catheters are an essential device in the treatment of patients with malignancies; they provide reliable and long-lasting venous access for different purposes. Most of the chemotherapeutic agents and other drugs administered to these patients are toxic and sclerosing to the endothelium and result in thrombosis of peripheral veins. The prolonged contact with the endothelium in small, low-flow veins increases the risk of thrombosis. Peripheral veins are thus quickly depleted.

Central venous catheters allow infusion into high-flow veins such as the superior vena cava (SVC) and into the right atrium (RA); so the agents are diluted rapidly and therefore less likely to damage the endothelium with the resultant thrombosis. Furthermore, multiple blood transfusions require the placement of dependable high-flow catheters. Moreover, the development of new cocktails of agents and the success of BMT have allowed a more aggressive therapy, and an increased number of immunosuppressed and thrombocytopenic patients need reliable central venous accesses. Unfortunately, placement of central venous catheters in these immunocompromised patients is risky. An indwelling catheter breaking the epidermal barrier increases the risk of infection and sepsis. Data from the National Cancer Institute show that the risk of bacteremia in oncology patients who are not neutropenic is increased 40-fold by the sole presence of an indwelling catheter.

Cancer chemotherapy utilizes cytotoxic drugs to arrest or shrink tumor growth. Clinically useful anticancer agents have a greater toxicity for malignant cells than for normal cells (*selective toxicity*). In part, selective toxicity occurs because of differences between malignant and normal cells, such as the proliferative capacity of the cells, although the differences between normal and malignant tissues may be slight. Many normal tissues have a high proliferative capacity; therefore, bone marrow cells, gastrointestinal epithelium, and hair follicle cells are seriously affected by the toxic effects of anticancer agents.

The toxic effect of chemotherapeutic agents and radiation therapy on the bone marrow creates special problems for central catheter placement:

1. Neutropenia results in an increased risk of catheter-related infection.
2. Catheter infection may be difficult to diagnose because of the inability of immunocompromised host to mount a suppurative response.
3. Decreased bone marrow megakaryocytes result in thrombocytopenia and increased risk of bleeding. Furthermore, a hematoma can further increase the risk of catheter-related infections because blood products are an excellent culture medium.
4. Catheter placement in cancer patients who have hypercoagulability has an increased risk of venous thrombotic complications.

Catheter-Related Infections

Neutropenia from chemotherapy results in a high rate of morbidity attributable to complications of infection. BMT recipients are especially susceptible to fungal and bacterial nosocomial infections during and after "conditioning" therapy, which includes cytotoxic chemotherapeutic agents with or without adjuvant radiation, depending on the primary disease and the type of transplantation to be administered. The neutropenia may last 4 to 58 days until engraftment, when the absolute neutrophil count increased to greater than $500/mm^3$. In profound neutropenia, the patient remains susceptible to these infections throughout the transplant procedure until a successful engraftment has occurred. After engraftment, infections may be associated with complications of BMT, especially graft versus host disease and immunosuppressive therapy, both of which markedly suppress the immune system.

Neutropenia is the most important risk factor for development of catheter-related infections.[1] Neutropenia means an absolute count of fewer than $500/mm^3$. Severe neutropenia is fewer than $200/mm^3$. As previously described, the phagocytic action of neutrophils is essential in the complex inflammatory reaction and is the final link in the inflammatory reaction, with the offending microbial organisms being engulfed and destroyed by the neutrophils. The overall reported incidence of catheter-related infections is 0.7 to 3.3 per 1000 catheter days; however, an increased incidence has been reported in patients with neutropenia, especially in those who have undergone bone marrow transplantation.[2–12]

Morrison and colleagues[13] showed that 61% of septic episodes in patients with central venous catheters occurred during the time patients were neutropenic. Fever is the hallmark of infection in these patients. Other signs and symptoms of infection may be notoriously absent in immunocompromised patients. Empiric broad-spectrum antibiotic therapy in febrile neutropenic patients is begun while awaiting the results of cultures. On the other hand, febrile cancer patients who do not have central catheters and adequate neutrophil counts are observed until the clinical examination and laboratory tests are completed because of the low incidence of serious infection in these patients.[14–16] Other important considerations in cancer patients include suppression of lymphocyte function, compromise of mucosal barriers, poor nutrition, and altered bacterial colonization resulting from frequent hospitalizations and prolonged antibiotic therapy, even in the absence of neutropenia.

Neutropenia in cancer patients also may be due to bone marrow replacement by tumor cells and decreased production of neutrophils, most commonly seen in hematologic malignancies such as leukemia, lymphoma, myeloma, and other metastatic deposits.

Many infections in neutropenic patients will present as septicemia. It is critical to recognize the clinical signs and symptoms of hematogenous dissemination of infection and the diagnostic value of blood cultures. When one of these patients develops fever, as soon as cultures have been obtained,[17] an empiric, wide-spectrum antibiotic therapy such as the combination of mezlocillin, cefazolin, and gentamicin[18] must be instituted.

Most catheter-related infections can be controlled without removal of the catheter; however, if the patient's condition deteriorates and besides fever there is refractory hypotension, septic emboli, or persistent positive blood cultures, the catheter must be removed.[19,20] Riikonen and colleagues[20] showed that 78% of documented septicemias were curable without the need for removal of the catheter in children who were hematology–oncology patients with neutropenia. Others have reported similar success in the treatment of catheter-related bacteremia with the use of empiric wide-spectrum antibiotic therapy. Catheter removal rates were between 22 and 68% in these studies.[12,15,18,21–27]

Coagulase-negative staphylococci, once considered a nonpathogenic bacteria, living on the skin and mucous membranes as harmless commensals, have become increasingly significant clinically, causing considerable morbidity and even mortality. These bacteria are the most common cause of nosocomial bacteremia in BMT patients, both before and after the neutropenic period.[18,28–30] The worldwide emergence of methacillin-resistant coagulase-negative staphylococci has led to the inclusion of vancomycin in the initial empiric antimicrobial therapy in BMT patients, especially during the periods of febrile neutropenia.[18,23] Some are reluctant to include vancomycin because of the risk of development of vancomycin-resistant enterococci.

Patients with Hodgkin's disease, BMT recipients, and patients receiving remission maintenance therapy for acute lymphocytic leukemia also may have cellular immune dysfunction, which results in a different spectrum of infection than does neutropenia. Neutropenic patients receiving broad-spectrum antibiotics for a prolonged time develop fungal infections (*Candida* and *Aspergillus* organisms).

Bleeding Diathesis

Radiation and drug toxicity of the marrow-proliferating pool or marrow replacement by tumor also result in thrombocytopenia. Neoplasms involving the bone marrow displace the mature megakaryocytes with malignant cells. The toxic effects of chemotherapy deplete the radiosensitive stem cells. Bone marrow suppression is a major dose-limiting side effect of chemotherapy and affects the production of leukocytes and platelets most profoundly. Red blood cell production also is affected. Alkylating agents have the most prominent effect on the megakaryocyte line, and they cause severe hypoplasia and aplasia. Platelet counts typically fall 7 to 14 days after chemotherapy is begun and slowly recover 2 to 6 weeks later. Multiple myeloma and Waldenström macroglobulinemia, the monoclonal gamapathies, frequently are associated with bleeding diathesis. The monoclonal immunoglobulins interfere with platelet function, resulting in prolonged bleeding times and abnormal platelet aggregation tests.

Blood products often are given to patients with clotting abnormalities before central venous catheter placement because of the perceived increased risk of bleeding; however, the correction of coagulation abnormalities with transfusions of blood products has not been proven effective. Further, this practice has some disadvantages. An indicated procedure may be delayed while the abnormalities are corrected. Some operators may not place catheters because of the abnormalities of homeostasis, denying the patient needed access. In addition, blood products are costly and scarce. Furthermore, transfusion of blood products has risks of hepatitis, HIV, and cytomegalovirus transmission; fluid overload; and transfusion reactions.

Correcting abnormalities of homeostasis with blood-component transfusions is common; however, there are limited data on the efficacy of this practice. Recent literature suggests that the liberal use of blood products is not warranted and should be reserved only to correct severe hemostatic defects.[31] Overall rates of bleeding complications of central venous catheter placement range between 0.0 and 2.87%.[31–38] Deloughery and colleagues[31] had a significant complication rate (22%) only in patients with severe hemostatic defects, including low platelet count and elevated prothrombin time (PT) and partial thromboplastin time (PTT). Several other studies also showed that severe thrombocytopenia is the only risk factor statistically associated with minor bleeding.[31,33]

Therefore, we can make the following recommendations after reviewing the most recent literature:

- Mild to moderate hemostatic defects need not be corrected with blood components. The costs and risks to the patients are too significant for the benefits received.
- Severe hemostatic defects should be corrected before catheter placement. Patients with platelet counts lower than $20,000/mm^3$ should receive transfusion of platelets because thrombocytopenia is the greatest absolute risk for bleeding. Multiple defects (platelet count less than $20,000/mm^3$, PT more than 29 seconds, PTT more than 64 seconds, uremia) warrant efforts to correct abnormalities. Unless placement of the catheter is urgent, alternatives to blood products, such as vitamin K and protamine, should be considered.
- Most bleeding complications can be controlled with manual pressure; usually, it is necessary to spend considerable time compressing.

- Ultrasound-guided puncture of the veins decreases the risk of inadvertent arterial puncture.
- Experience of the operator placing the catheter is a major factor in bleeding complications.[31] Only operators with experience should place catheters in these high-risk patients.
- Bleeding time is not reliable for assessing the risk of perioperative bleeding and should not be used.[39]

Hypercoagulability

Patients with malignancies may have an apparent hypercoagulable state, which cannot be determined by routine laboratory tests of coagulation or platelet function. Occasionally, there is a thrombocytosis due to production of plasma platelet-stimulating factor in response to anemia, hemorrhage, malignancy, or inflammation. In most cases, however, hypercoagulable states of malignancy are not associated with defined coagulation abnormalities. Specific abnormalities that might increase the tendency of thrombosis in cancer patients include the following:

- Damage to the vascular endothelium and lowering of levels of the naturally occurring anticoagulant proteins C and S from chemotherapeutic agents[40–44]
- Elevated fibrinogen[43, 45]
- Elevated plasminogen activator inhibitor[43, 46]
- Low antithrombin III[47]
- Splenectomy (in some patients) resulting in thrombocytosis

Therefore, we can say that to decrease the risk of catheter-related thrombosis, we must minimize venous trauma during insertion and ensure perfect positioning of the catheter tip in the RA. If a patient shows a tendency to catheter-related thrombosis and appears to be relatively hypercoagulable, a more aggressive therapy (venous thrombolysis) may be indicated to salvage central veins to prevent depletion of veins for central venous access.

ACQUIRED IMMUNODEFICIENCY SYNDROME

Patients with AIDS are susceptible to infections by opportunistic organisms because of the profound defects of T-cell function; however, because B-cell function is also impaired, bacterial infections are frequent.[48–51] Central venous access is frequently required in AIDS patients. Similar to oncology patients, AIDS patients with central venous catheters are susceptible to catheter-related infections. Skoutelis and colleagues[52] found a higher rate of catheter-related infections in AIDS patients than in oncology patients. The risk of infections, in decreasing order, was AIDS, acute leukemia, lymphomas, chronic leukemias, and solid tumors. Keung and colleagues reported the greatest infection rate in bone marrow transplant recipients (11.5 infections/1000 catheter days), followed by HIV patients (6.6 infections/1000 catheter days), and then other oncology patients (2.4 infections/1000 catheter days). Other studies of AIDS patients yielded rates of catheter infections between 1.9 and 4.7 infections per 1000 catheter days.[52–55]

The role of HIV in defective cell-mediated immunity (and the resulting opportunistic infections and increased prevalence of certain cancers) is that the virus attacks T lymphocytes, the principal agents in cell-mediated immunity. The increased risk of bacterial infections may not be so apparent and is likely multifactorial. First, despite the high concentrations of serum immunoglobulins, the lymphocyte function is impaired. Depletion of T-helper cells may be partially responsible for the impaired B-cell antibody response to microorganisms. Also of great importance is the fact that 20 to 25% of AIDS patients are neutropenic.[56,57] The neutropenia may be due to the virus itself or to myelotoxic drugs, such as chemotherapeutic agents, antiviral agents (zidovudine, ganciclovir), or others (trimethoprim–sulphamethoxazole).[58] In one study, the incidence of bacterial infections during periods of severe neutropenia (neutrophil count less than 500/mm^3) was 230% higher than when the neutrophil count was 500 to 1000/mm^3.[59] Neutrophils also function abnormally and have impaired adherence, chemotaxis, phagocytosis, and defective bactericidal capacity.[56,60,61]

A high prevalence of catheter-related infections due to gram-positive organisms has been demonstrated in AIDS patients.[4,52,55] The early recognition of catheter-related infection may be difficult because of the multiple causes of fever. Nevertheless, if catheter-related infection is suspected, wide-spectrum antibiotics, including antistaphylococcal prophylaxis, must be initiated promptly. AIDS patients may have a higher mortality rate from catheter-related infections (up to 2.5%).[55] Aggressive wound care and dressing changes are also necessary if infection is suspected. Of note, immune function at the time of central venous catheter placement as measured by absolute granulocyte count and CD4 T-cell count are not helpful in predicting infectious complications.[53]

Fungemia also can complicate the presence of central venous catheters. Frequent and protracted manipulation of catheters introduces fungi from skin or from inanimate environmental objects into the bloodstream. The profound impairment of cellular immunity may prevent the clearance of fungal elements and result in fungemia.[62] Colonization of peripheral sites, such as skin, oral mucosa, and the intestinal and respiratory tracts, has been identified as a risk factor for systemic infections.[63] Patients with AIDS frequently are affected with oral or esophageal candidiasis (70–100%). Fungemia frequently develops during the course of ketoconazole or fluconazole therapy (antifungal therapy against oropharyngeal candidiasis, or OPC), which apparently provides minimal protection for infection of the catheter.[62] In cases of fungal infection, catheters must be removed promptly because of the well-documented failure of antifungal therapy to clear the infection.[22,52,64,65] Finally, there have been reports of primary cutaneous *Asperigillus* infection at the dressing site of venous catheters, typically associated with adhesive tape. The infection presents as erythematous macules, papules, or plaques that rapidly evolve, at times via a hemorrhagic bullous stage, to ulcerations with central necrotic eschars.[66] The lesion may involute if the predisposing local factors (occlusive dressings, tape adhesives) are removed; however, delayed healing has been described. Prompt removal of catheter and institution of antifungal therapy, if the local infection is not controlled, are needed.

BURNS

Aggressive surgical approaches to the burn wound have resulted in enhanced survival.[67,68] Central venous access is a major tool in such management but is associated with both morbidity and mortality. Morbidities include suppurative thrombophlebitis, septicemia, pneumothorax, and bacterial endocarditis.[69–71] Infection is the leading cause of morbidity and mortality in patients with burns,[72] and burn patients with venous catheters are considered to be at highest risk of septic complications from the catheters. The National Nosocomial Infection Surveillance (NNIS) System conducted surveillance of intensive care units (ICUs) from 1986 through 1990 and reported rates of central catheter-related bloodstream infections ranging from 2.1 infections per 1000 catheter days in the respiratory ICU to 30.2 infections per 1000 catheter days in the burn ICU.[73] The NNIS report of 1990 through 1995 showed a decrease to 15.6 infections per 1000 catheter days in the burn units.

The patient with thermal injuries is exposed to septic hazards. Burned skin harbors many potentially pathogenic bacteria.[74] *Burn wound colonization* is defined as the presence of microorganisms in a wound that appears clinically noninfected. The Center for Disease Control defines an *invasive wound infection* as microbial growth in the burn wound with invasion into and necrosis of surrounding viable

tissue. Secondary bloodstream infection has been documented in a study where it was found that burn wound manipulation–induced bacteremia occurred in 20.6% of procedures.[75] Burn wound manipulation is a frequent task during debridement, excision of infected wounds, wound closure, and skin grafting. Saski and colleagues[75] further showed that bacteremia occurred more commonly with larger burn wounds and with increased intensity of burn wound manipulation. In another study, bloodstream infection was not present in patients who had less than 30% total body surface area (TBSA) injury, but it was present in 20.8% of patients with 30 to 60% TBSA injury.

Traditional management advocated replacement of catheters in burn patients to new venous access sites every 2 to 3 days as a means to decrease morbidity from catheter-related infections.[69,74,76] The morbidity from insertions of central venous catheters is high, especially in the pediatric burn population. Subsequent studies[77–79] have shown benefit of less frequent catheter placement, and the study by Askew and colleagues[77] demonstrated that frequent catheter change results in increased catheter-related sepsis rates. In another study,[78] central venous catheters that were placed more than 5 cm from the burn wound had a 20% risk of central venous catheter tip bacterial colonization by day 8 after insertion. Under such circumstances (insertion sight more than 5 cm from the burn wound), weekly catheter changes seem reasonable. Additionally, there is no apparent difference in sepsis rates if catheters are changed over a guidewire as opposed to insertion at a new access site with each catheter change.[79] Systematic rotation of catheter sites is an undesirable alternative because eventually it may be necessary to place a catheter through or close to a burn wound as viable access sites become depleted. Finally, there is no significant difference in sepsis rates between upper central and femoral placement of catheters in burn patients.[79–82] Femoral vein catheterization has been presumed to increase the risk of bacteremia because of the proximity to the perineum; however, these studies showed no increase in the sepsis rate in the burn population.

Proximity to burn wounds is one of the prime determinants of bacterial colonization of the central venous catheter.[77–79,83] Kealy and colleagues[78] showed an infection rate of 40 infections per 1000 catheter days if catheters were inserted within 5 cm of burn wounds, whereas catheters inserted through normal skin farther than 5 cm from a burn had an infection rate of 3.5 infections per 1000 catheter days.

Venous thrombosis of the central venous system can occur as with any patient with indwelling central venous catheters.[84] Superinfection of the thrombus is a cause of septic pulmonary emboli in burn patients. Thrombolytic therapy should be initiated as soon as possible once the diagnosis is confirmed. Burn wounds are not a contraindication for thrombolysis. Reports of successful venous thrombolysis in burn patients as early as 6 days following surgical excision and grafting are available.

RENAL FAILURE

Uremia causes acquired platelet dysfunction, and patients frequently have mucocutaneous and serosal bleeding as well as prolonged bleeding times. The cause of platelet dysfunction is unknown, but interference with the platelet membrane receptor is postulated. Although factor VIII/VWF is elevated with no apparent functional abnormalities, cryoprecipitate (which contains significant quantities of factor VIII) and 1-deamino-(8-D-arginine)–vasopressin (DDAVP), which facilitates the release of VWF from endothelial sites, have been shown to correct the bleeding time. Fortunately, the platelet dysfunction is not severe enough to affect venous catheter placement and therapy is unnecessary; however, if the patient has had bleeding problems from previous catheter placements or other procedures, DDAVP may be given by intravenous (IV) infusion to correct the bleeding time within 2 hours before catheter placement.

Patients with chronic renal failure eventually will require surgical placement of upper-extremity arteriovenous grafts or fistulae, and catheter placement must be planned such that the venous access does not impede the venous runoff of the shunts. Many patients with central venous catheters develop stenoses or occlusion of the vein at the site of venous access due to trauma during catheter placement and formation of clot around the catheter (Fig. 9–1).

Therefore, placement of catheters in the subclavian veins (the venous drainage of the arteriovenous fistula, or AVF, in the upper extremity) should be avoided in patients with renal failure. The internal jugular vein is the access of choice and decreases the risk of obstructing the upper-extremity venous drainage. Catheters should be placed in the subclavian veins only as a last option. Similarly, because the arm veins are important for placement of AVF, peripherally inserted central catheters (PICCs) should not be inserted in the arm veins because injury to the vein at the puncture site may cause stenosis. Even if a functioning AVF is present in the contralateral arm, a PICC or subclavian catheter is not recommended because eventually an AVF will likely need to be placed in the ipsilateral arm. A Hohn catheter in an internal jugular vein is a better alternative.

For the same reasons, the treatment of stenoses and thromboses resulting from central catheter placement should be more aggressive than in other patients. In most patients, if a catheter placement results in a stenosis or thrombosis of a central vein, one can remove the catheter and place a new one on the contralateral side. In a patient on dialysis, however, aggressive treatment with angioplasty, thrombolysis, or stenting is necessary to salvage the vein. Every effort should be made to save the extremity as a site for AVF or central catheter placement.

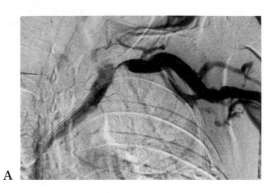
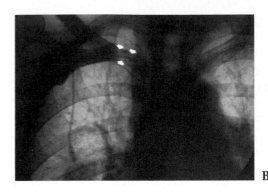

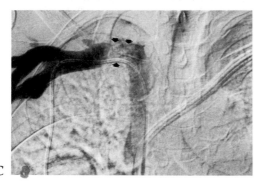

Figure 9–1 Subclavian access in dialysis patients. This patient with chronic renal failure had a portacath placed via the right subclavian vein and a permacath placed via the left subclavian vein. The patient presented with left upper-extremity swelling. The left-arm venogram **(A)** showed a severe stenosis at the puncture site of the left subclavian vein. In addition, thrombus was demonstrated (*arrows*) in the right innominate vein around the indwelling catheter **(B, C)**. Placement of catheters via the subclavian veins in patients on hemodialysis can cause central venous stenosis and limit access options.

LIVER DISEASE

Disorders of blood coagulation in patients with liver disease are complex with multiple causes of hemostatic abnormalities. There is decreased synthesis of clotting factors, synthesis of abnormal clotting factors, and thrombocytopenia. As previously described, the vitamin K–dependent clotting factors (II, VII, IX, and X) as well as factors V, XIII, and fibrinogen are synthesized in the liver, and all may be decreased in patients with liver disease. In addition, the liver may produce abnormal fibrinogen (*dysfibrinogenemia*). Thrombocytopenia is frequently caused by congestive splenomegaly leading to sequestration of platelets. Multiple laboratory tests may be abnormal as a result of these defects. The

PT is prolonged because of the decrease in vitamin K–dependent factors; the PTT also may be prolonged due to dysfibrinogenemia, and the bleeding time can be prolonged secondary to thrombocytopenia or platelet abnormality. As previously discussed, the correction of coagulation abnormalities by administration of blood products should be done only in patients with severe bleeding diathesis. Patients with severe thrombocytopenia due to hypersplenism (platelet count less than $30,000/mm^3$) are at greatest risk for bleeding complications during catheter placement and require prophylactic platelet transfusion. This situation is complicated, however, in that transfused platelets can become quickly sequestered by the enlarged spleen. Therefore, the platelets should be transfused during the procedure, not before. If delayed bleeding occurs in a patient with thrombocytopenia, repeat transfusions of platelets are necessary until hemostasis is obtained. Likewise, patients with multiple coagulation and platelet deficiencies (prolonged PT, prolonged PTT, thrombocytopenia, $\pm$ uremia) also should be treated. If catheter placement is elective, parenteral administration of vitamin K should return the PT to normal in about 6 to 12 hours. On the other hand, if one cannot wait for vitamin K correction of PT, then 3 to 4 U of fresh frozen plasma should be given. We emphasize that only the most severe bleeding diathesis needs to be treated before catheter placement. Goldfarb and LeBrec[37] reported the safe placement of internal jugular vein catheters in patients with liver disease and bleeding diathesis, without prior correction of abnormalities, with no significant bleeding complications. Likewise, Foster and colleagues[38] reported no bleeding complications in 259 internal jugular and subclavian venous catheter placements in liver allograft recipients without correcting coagulopathies.

ANTICOAGULATION

Patients receive anticoagulation for a variety of reasons, such as atrial fibrillation, deep vein thrombosis, cardiac surgery, the presence of artificial heart valves, and prophylactic prevention of thrombosis of vascular bypass grafts. In elective situations, anticoagulation therapy must be discontinued to allow the coagulation systems to return to normal. Alternatively, central catheter placement can be performed while the patient is anticoagulated with no excessive risk of bleeding. Peterson[85] placed internal jugular catheters in anticoagulated patients undergoing cardiac surgery and found no excessive morbidity. The risk of reversing anticoagulation therapy must be balanced against the risk of bleeding in each patient.

For example, in a patient with severe cardiac disease who is undergoing anticoagulation, the risk of inducing a cardiac complication by discontinuing the anticoagulation may outweigh the risk of bleeding during venous catheter placement while the patient is anticoagulated. Careful technique and manual pressure to obtain hemostasis (as long as necessary) should minimize the risk of serious bleeding; nevertheless, there are instances when anticoagulation must be reversed before central venous catheter placement (e.g., an anticoagulated patient with life-threatening gastrointestinal bleeding who requires a venous catheter).

The two most common drugs for anticoagulation are heparin and warfarin. Heparin is a glycosaminoglycan that acts by accelerating the inhibitory effect of antithrombin III on activated serine protease clotting factors (IXa, Xa, XIa, and thrombin). IV infusion of heparin is usually given at a rate to increase the activated partial thromboplastin time 1.5 to 2 times. The anticoagulation effect diminishes rapidly on cessation of administration, with complete reversal in about 4 hours in normal individuals (i.e., the heparin half-life is approximately a half-hour). If immediate neutralization is required, protamine sulfate may be administered. Protamine sulfate is infused intravenously as a dilute solution (2 mg/mL) at a slow rate (no more than 50 mg per 10 minutes). Each milligram of protamine sulfate neutralizes approximately 100 USP heparin units, but the amount required decreases with time as heparin is metabolized. For example, 1 mg of protamine sulfate neutralizes 100 USP heparin immediately after heparin is administered. Thirty minutes after heparinization, only 0.5 mg of protamine sulfate would neutralize 100 USP of heparin.

Warfarin acts by preventing vitamin K from promoting the carboxylation of glutamic acid residues and therefore the formation of gamacarboxy-glutamic acid. The result is an abnormal production of vitamin K–dependent clotting factors

(VII, X, IX, and thrombin) as reflected in a prolonged PT. The PT will not become increased until about 2 days after the first oral dose of warfarin, however. Likewise, the PT will return to normal 2 to 3 days after cessation of the drug. Therefore, for elective procedures, warfarin should be discontinued at least 3 days before catheter placement. Emergent procedures may require reversal of warfarin with parenteral administration of 50 mg of vitamin K (if there is time to wait 6 to 12 hours), or an immediate result is obtained by giving 3 to 4 U of fresh frozen plasma.

TOTAL PARENTERAL NUTRITION

Total parenteral nutrition (TPN) is an important means of providing nutrition to critically ill patients, such as oncology and postsurgical patients. Central venous access is necessary for TPN because the hyperosmolar infusate is sclerosing to the endothelium of veins. TPN into small veins or even the subclavian or brachiocephalic veins will likely cause thrombosis. The catheter tip should be in the proximal RA to avoid TPN complications. Further, these patients may be critically ill and immunocompromised and, therefore, at increased risk for catheter-related infections. In addition, TPN is an important contributing factor for fungemia in pediatric patients.[86] Outbreaks of *Candida parapsilosis* fungemia in the ICU have been associated with TPN.[86–88] The hospital environment and an increased manipulation of catheters in critically ill patients may be contributing factors.

Catheter-related bacterial bloodstream infections are also major complications of TPN therapy. TPN solutions contain dextrose, amino acids, and lipid emulsions, which are media to support growth of certain microbial species. Lipid emulsions are particularly suited for the growth of bacteria and yeast. Growth of bacteria and yeast occurs within 6 hours after inoculation of a lipid emulsion and reaches clinically significant levels (more than 10^6 colony-forming units/mL) within 24 hours. Despite the potential growth characteristics of TPN fluids, most bacterial infections result from contamination of the catheter, not the fluids. Coagulase-negative staphylococci and *Staphylococcus aureus*, which do not grow in TPN fluids, are the predominant pathogens in these situations. Moreover, there is an increased risk of catheter-related infections when catheters used for TPN are used for other purposes. Therefore, a single-lumen TPN catheter never should be used for other purposes, such as transfusion of blood or blood products or administration of fluids. It is necessary to place a double-lumen PICC or Hohn catheter so that one lumen is for TPN and the other one for other uses. Rigorous aseptic catheter care must be followed to decrease the risk of TPN-related infection.

CYSTIC FIBROSIS

Patients with cystic fibrosis (CF) may require repeated courses of IV antibiotics and prolonged IV access for administration of TPN during their lifetime. Repeat venipuncture, especially in young patients, is difficult and traumatic. The medications may be toxic and damage the peripheral veins requiring central venous administration. The frequency of courses of antibiotics is quite variable. Some patients may need several courses of a year or less. Some patients' airway becomes colonized with *Pseudomonas aeruginosa* requiring frequent courses of IV antibiotics. Despite a persistent colonization of the airways with *P. aeruginosa* and *S. aureus*, bacteremia is rare.[90] The combination of diabetes mellitus, corticosteroid therapy, TPN, and the need for extended courses of broad-spectrum antibiotics contributes to catheter colonization. Catheter-related septicemia has been reported in up to 10% of patients,[89] with a relatively high percentage of catheter-related infections due to atypical organisms and fungi, especially *Candida albicans*.[89–91]

Fahy and associates[89] recommend prophylactic antifungal therapy to prevent fungal colonization of portacaths in CF patients, especially those with impaired glucose tolerance or who require corticosteroids. PICCs are useful in patients with CF, especially those who require IV antibiotics infrequently. Furthermore, if TPN is required, a double-lumen catheter should be placed (see previous section). Portacaths are used in patients with CF and may be of benefit in patients requiring more frequent treatments. Studies by Fahy and colleagues[89] and Sola and associates[92] have shown no unusual infectious complications with portacaths in patients with CF; however, Sola and colleagues[92] reported SVC syndrome or deep vein thrombosis in 13.6% of patients. Therefore, because of the high incidence of major thrombotic events and the risk of pulmonary embolism, patients with CF with portacaths can receive aspirin prophylaxis, but it must be remembered that some patients may develop hemoptysis, which would require the aspirin to be stopped.

DEMENTIA

Some patients with dementia or psychosis occasionally require central venous access for therapy of concomitant diseases. Special care must be taken to secure catheters to avoid inadvertent or voluntary removal of the catheter by the patient. Portacaths may be better suited. Extra care should be taken, and the skin incision must be securely sutured and carefully dressed.

PATIENTS ON CRUTCHES

Some patients on crutches may require placement of a PICC. In such circumstances, the PICC should be placed away from the axilla so that the hub of the PICC does not get caught or damaged by the crutch. We propose placement of the PICC in the cephalic vein because the skin entry site is more lateral on the arm and less likely to be traumatized by the crutch.

VASCULAR BYPASS GRAFTS

When a central venous catheter is needed in a patient with a vascular bypass procedure, it is important to know where the bypass graft is located. Venous access should not be obtained in a vein adjacent to an arterial bypass anastomosis because of the risk of infection. Femoral venous catheters should not be placed in patients with aorto-bifemoral bypass grafts or a femoral–distal bypass graft. Patients with axillofemoral bypass grafts should not have subclavian vein catheters on the side of the axillary anastomosis. Infection of an arterial bypass graft can have life-threatening complications.

REFERENCES

1. Howell PB, Walters PE, Donowitz GR, Farr BM. Risk factors for infection of adult patients with cancer who have tunneled central venous catheters. *Cancer.* 1995;75:1367–1375.
2. Uderzo C, D'Angelo P, Rizzari C, et al. Central venous catheter-related complications after bone marrow transplantation in children with hematological malignancies. *Bone Marrow Transplant.* 1992;172:275–279.
3. Moosa HH, Julian TB, Rosenfield CS, Shadduck RK. Complications of indwelling central venous catheters in bone marrow transplant recipients. *Surg Gynecol Obstet.* 1991;172:275–279.
4. Keung YK, Watkins K, Chen SC, Groshen S, Levine AM, Dover D. Increased incidence of central venous catheter-related infections in bone marrow transplant patients. *Am J Clin Oncol.* 1995;18:469–474.
5. Bodey GP. Antibiotics in patients with neutropenia. *Arch Intern Med.* 1984;144:1845–1851.
6. Lazarus HM, Creger RJ, Bloom AD, Shenk R. Percutaneous placement of femoral central venous catheter in patients undergoing transplantation of bone marrow. *Surg Gynecol Obstet.* 1990;170:403–406.
7. Goldman ML, Bibao MK, Rosch J, et al. Complications of indwelling chemotherapy catheters. *Cancer.* 1975;36:1983–1990.

8. Lockich JJ, Bothe A, Benotti P, et al. Complications and management of implanted venous catheters. *J Clin Oncol.* 1985;3:710–712.

9. Hagle ME. Implantable devices for chemotherapy: access and delivery. *Semin Oncol Nurs.* 1987;3:96–105.

10. Gyves JW, Ensminger WD, Niederhuber JE, et al. Totally implanted system for intravenous chemotherapy in patients with cancer. *Am J Med.* 1982;73:841–845.

11. Barrios CH, Zuke JE, Blaes B, Hirsch JD, Lyss AP. Evaluation of an implantable venous access system in a general oncology population. *Oncology.* 1992;49:474–478.

12. Elishoov H, Or R, Strauss N, Engelhard D. Nosocomial colonization, septicemia, and Hickman/Broviac catheter-related infections in bone marrow transplant recipients. *Medicine.* 1998;77:83–101.

13. Morrison VA, Peterson BA, Bloomfield CD. Nosocomial septicemia in the cancer patient: the influence of central venous access devices, neutropenia and type of malignancy. *Med Pediatr Oncol.* 1990;18:209–216.

14. Hathorn JW, Pizzo PA. Infectious complications in the pediatric cancer patient. In: Pizzo PA, Poplack DG, eds. *Principles and Practice of Pediatric Oncology.* Philadelphia, PA: Lippincott; 1989:85–110.

15. Pizzo PA, Meyers J. Infections in the cancer patient. In: DeVita VT, Hellman S, Rosenberg SA, eds. *Cancer: Principles and Practice of Oncology*, 3rd ed. Philadelphia, PA: Lippincott; 1989:460–484.

16. Pizzo PA, Robichaud KJ, Wesley R, Commers JR. Fever in the pediatric and young adult patient with cancer: a prospective study of 1001 episodes. *Medicine.* 1982; 61:153–165.

17. Huges WT, Armstrong D, Bodey GP, et al. Guidelines for the use of antimicrobial agents in neutropenic patients with unexplained fever. *J Infect Dis.* 1990;161:381–396.

18. Engelhard D, Elishoov H, Strauss N, et al. Nosocomial coagulase-negative staphylococcal infections in bone marrow transplantation recipients with central vein catheter. *Transplantation.* 1996;61:430–434.

19. Decker MD, Edwards, KM. Central venous catheter infections. *Pediatr Clin North Am.* 1988;35:579–612.

20. Riikonen P, Saarinen UM, Lahteenoja KM, Jalanko H. Management of indwelling central venous catheters in pediatric cancer patients with fever and neutropenia. *Scand J Infect Dis.* 1993;25:357–364.

21. Hiemenz J, Skelton J, Pizzo PA. Perspective on the management of catheter-related infections in cancer patients. *Pediatr Infect Dis J.* 1986;5:6–11.

22. Darbyshire PJ, Weightman NC, Speller DCE. Problems associated with indwelling central venous catheters. *Arch Dis Child.* 1985;60: 129–134.

23. Raad II, Bodey GP. Infectious complications of indwelling vascular catheters. *Clin Infect Dis.* 1992;15:197–208.

24. Benezra D, Kiehn TE, Gold JWM, Brown AE, Turnbull ADM, Armstrong D. Prospective study of infections in indwelling central venous catheters using quantitative blood cultures. *Am J Med.* 1988;85:495–498.

25. Groeger JS, Lucas AB, Thaler HT, Friedlander-Klar H, et al. Infectious morbidity associated with long-term use of venous access devices in patients with cancer. *Ann Intern Med.* 1993;119:1168–1174.

26. Sanders JE, Hickman RO, Aker S, et al. Experience with double-lumen right atrial catheters. *JPEN J Parenter Enter Nutr.* 1982;6: 95–99.

27. Jansen RFM, Wiggers T, Van Geel BN, Van Putten WLJ. Assessment of insertion techniques and complication rates of dual-lumen central venous catheters in patients with hematologic malignancies. *World J Surg.* 1990;14:101–106.

28. Petersen FB, Clift RA, Hickman RO, Sanders JE, et al. Hickman catheter complications in marrow transplant recipients. *JPEN J Parenter Enter Nutr.* 1986;10:58–62.

29. Sayer HG, Longton G, Bowden R, Pepe M, Storb R. Increased risk of infection in marrow transplant patients receiving methylprednisolone for graft-versus-host disease prevention. *Blood.* 1994;84:1328–1332.

30. Wade JC, Schimpff SC, Newman KA, Wiernik PH. *Staphylococcus epidermidis*: an increasing cause of infection in patients with granulocytopenia. *Ann Intern Med.* 1982;97: 503–508.

31. DeLoughery TG, Liebler JM, Sionds V, Goodnight SH. Invasive line placement in critically ill patients: do hemostatic defects matter? *Transfusion.* 1996;36:827–831.

32. Bernard RW, Stahl WM. Subclavian vein catheterizations: a prospective study. 1. Non-

infectious complications. *Ann Surg.* 1971;173: 184–190.

33. Doerfler ME, Kaufman B, Goldenberg AS. Central venous catheter placement in patients with disorders of hemostasis. *Chest.* 1996;110:185–188.

34. Yurtkuran M. Catheterization of the femoral vein for chronic hemodialysis. *Angiology.* 1987;38:847–850.

35. Vanherweghem JL, Cabolet P, Dhaene M, et al. Complications related to subclavian catheters for hemodialysis. *Am J Nephrol.* 1986;6:339–345.

36. Christensen KH, Nerstom B, Baden H. Complications of percutaneous catheterization of the subclavian vein in 129 cases. *Acta Chir Scand.* 1967;133:615–620.

37. Goldfarb G, Lebrec D. Percutaneous cannulation of the internal jugular vein in patients with coagulopathies: an experience based on 1,000 attempts. *Anesthesiology.* 1982;56: 321–323.

38. Foster PF, Moore LR, Sankary HN, et al. Central venous catheterization in patients with coagulopathy. *Arch Surg.* 1992;127: 273–275.

39. Gewitz AS, Miller ML, Keys TF. The clinical usefulness of the preoperative bleeding time. *Arch Pathol Lab Med.* 1996;120:353–356.

40. Rogers JS, Murgo AJ, Fontana JA, Raich PC. Chemotherapy for breast cancer decreases plasma protein C and protein S. *J Clin Oncol.* 1988;6:276–281.

41. Cantwell BMJ, Carmichael J, Ghani SE, Harris AL. Thromboses and thromboemboli in patients with lymphoma during cytotoxic chemotherapy. *BMJ.* 1988;297:179–180.

42. Levine MN, Gent M, Hirsh J, et al. The thrombogenic effect of anticancer drug therapy in women with Stage II breast cancer. *N Engl J Med.* 1988;318:404–407.

43. Conlan MG, Haire WD, Lieberman RP, Lund G, et al. Catheter-related thrombosis in patients with refractory lymphoma undergoing autologous stem cell transplantation. *Bone Marrow Tranplant.* 1991;7:235–240.

44. Kaufman PA, Jones RB, Greenberg CS, Peters WP. Autologous bone marrow transplantation and factor XII, factor VII and protein C deficiencies: report of a new association and its possible relationship to endothelial cell injury. *Cancer.* 1990;66:515–521.

45. Seifter EJ, Parker RI, Gralnick HR, et al. Abnormal coagulation results in patients with Hodgkin's disease. *Am J Med.* 1985;78: 942–950.

46. Kluft C, Verheijen JH, Jie AFH, et al. Postoperative fibrinolytic shutdown: a rapidly reverting acute phase pattern for the fast-acting inhibitor of tissue-type plasminogen activator after trauma. *Scand J Clin Lab Invest.* 1985;45:605–610.

47. Lokich JJ, Becker B. Subclavian vein thrombosis in patients treated with infusion chemotherapy for advanced malignancy. *Cancer.* 1983;52:1586–1589.

48. Polsky B, Gold JWM, Whimbey E, et al. Bacterial pneumonia in patients with the acquired immunodeficiency syndrome. *Ann Intern Med.* 1986;38–41.

49. Whimbey E, Gold JWM, Polsky B, et al. Bacteremia and fungemia in patients with the acquired immunodeficiency syndrome. *Ann Intern Med.* 1986;104:511–514.

50. Witt DS, Craven DE, McCabe WR. Bacterial infections in adult patients with the acquired immunodeficiency syndrome (AIDS) and AIDS-related complex. *Am J Med.* 1987;82: 900–906.

51. Jacobson MA, Gellermann H, Chambers H. *Staphylococcus aureus* bacteremia and recurrent staphylococcal infection in patients with acquired immunodeficiency syndrome and AIDS-related complex. *Am J Med.* 1988; 85:172–176.

52. Skoutelis AT, Murphy RL, MacDonell KB, Von Roenn JH, et al. Indwelling central venous catheter infections in patients with acquired immunodeficiency syndrome. *J Acquir Immune Defic Syndr Hum Retrovirol.* 1990;3:335–342.

53. Gleason-Morgan D, Church JA, Bagnall-Reeb H, Atkinson J. Complications of central venous catheters in pediatric patients with acquired immunodeficiency syndrome. *Pediatr Int Dis J.* 1991;10:11–14.

54. Henry K, Thurn J, Johnson S. Experience with central venous catheters in patients with AIDS. *N Engl J Med.* 1989;320:1496.

55. Raviglione MC, Battan R, Pablos-Mendez A, et al. Infections associated with Hickman catheters in patients with acquired immunodeficiency syndrome. *Am J Med.* 1989;86: 780–786.

56. Murphy PM, Clifford LH, Fauci AS, Gallin JI. Impairment of neutrophil bactericidal capacity in patients with AIDS. *J Infect Dis.* 1988;158:627–630.

57. Clement M. General approach to the human immunodeficiency virus-infected patient. In: Leoung G, Mills G, eds. *Opportunistic Infections in Patients with the Acquired Immunodeficiency Syndrome.* New York, NY: Marcel Dekker; 1989:88–101.

58. Meynard JL, Guiguet M, Arsac S, Frottier J, Meyohas MC. Frequency and risk factors of infectious complications in neutropenic patients infected with HIV. *AIDS.* 1997; 11:995–998.

59. Shaunak S, Bartlett JA. Zidovudine-induced neutropenia: are we too cautious? *Lancet* 1989;2:91–92.

60. Lazzarin A, Uberti Foppa C, Galli M, et al. Impairment of polymorphonuclear leukocyte function in patients with acquired immunodeficiency syndrome and with lymphadenopathy syndrome. *Clin Exp Immunol.* 1986;65:105–111.

61. Ellis M, Gupta S, Galant S, et al. Impaired neutrophil function in patients with AIDS or AIDS-related complex; a comprehensive evaluation. *J Infect Dis.* 1988;158:1268–1275.

62. Gonzalez CE, Venzon D, Lee S, Mueller B, Pizzo PA, Walsh TJ. Risk factors for fungemia in children infected with human immunodeficiency virus: a case control study. *Clin Infect Dis.* 1996;23:515–521.

63. Karabinis A, Hill C, Leclercq B, Tancrede C, Baume D, Andremont A. Risk factors for candidemia in cancer patients: a case control study. *J Clin Microbiol.* 1988;26:429–432.

64. Prince A, Heller B, Levy J, Heird WC. Management of fever in patients with central vein catheters. *Pediatr Infect Dis.* 1986;5:20–24.

65. Abraham JL, Muller JL. A prospective study of prolonged central venous access in leukemia. *JAMA.* 1982;248:2868–2873.

66. Hunt SJ, Nagi C, Gross KG, Wong DS, Mathews WC. Primary cutaneous aspergillosis near central venous catheters in patients with the acquired immunodeficiency syndrome. *Arch Dermatol.* 1992;128: 1229–1232.

67. Burke JF, Tompkins R, Remensnyder JP, et al. Significant reductions in mortality for children with burn injuries through the use of prompt eschar excision. *Ann Surg.* 1988;208: 577–585.

68. Tompkins RG, Burke JF, Schoenfeld DA, et al. Prompt eschar excision: a treatment system contributing to reduced burn mortality: a statistical evaluation of burn care at the Massachusetts General Hospital (1974–1984). *Ann Surg.* 1986;204:272–281.

69. Pruitt BA Jr, McManus WH, Kim SH, Treat RC. Diagnosis and treatment of cannula-related intravenous sepsis in burn patients. *Ann Surg.* 1980;191:546–554.

70. Alexander JW. Control of infection following burn injury. *Ann Surg.* 1971;103:435–441.

71. Baskin TW, Rosenthal A, Pruitt BA. Acute bacterial endocarditis: a silent source of sepsis in the burn patient. *Ann Surg.* 1997;184:618.

72. Peck MD, Heimbach DM. Does early excision of burn wounds change the pattern of mortality? *J Burn Care Rehabil.* 1989;10:7–10.

73. Pearson ML, Hierholzer WJ, Garner JS, Mayhall CG, et al. Special Communication. Guideline for prevention of intravascular device-related infections. Part I. Intravascular device-related infections: an overview. *Am J Infect Control.* 1996;24:262–293.

74. Michel L, Marsh M, McMichan J, et al. Infection of pulmonary artery catheters in critically ill patients. *JAMA.* 1981;245: 1032–1036.

75. Saski TM, Welch GW, Herndon DN, et al. Burn wound manipulation-induced bacteremia. *J Trauma.* 1979;19:46–49.

76. Bozzetti F, Terno G, Bofanti G, et al. Prevention and treatment of central venous catheter sepsis by exchange via a guide wire. *Ann Surg.* 1983;198:48–52.

77. Askew AA, Tuggle DW, Judd T, Smith EI, Tunell WP. Improvement in catheter sepsis rate in burned children. *J Pediatr Surg.* 1990; 25:117–119.

78. Kealey GP, Chang P, Heinle J, Rosenquist MD, Lewis RW. Prospective comparison of two management strategies of central venous catheters in burn patients. *J Trauma.* 1995;38:344–349.

79. Goldstein AM, Weber JM, Sheridan RL. Femoral venous access is safe in burned children: an analysis of 224 catheters. *J Pediatr.* 1997;130:442–446.

80. Still JM, Law E, Thiruvaiyaru D, Belcher K, Donker K. Central line-related sepsis in acute burn patients. *Am Surg.* 1998;64:165–170.

81. Purdue GF, Hunt JL. Vascular access through the femoral vessels: indications and complications. *J Burn Care Rehabil.* 1986;7:498–500.

82. Murr MM, Rosenquist MD, Lewis RW, Heinle JA, Kealey GP. A prospective safety study of femoral vein versus non-femoral

vein catheterization in patients with burns. *J Burn Care Rehabil.* 1991;12:576–578.

83. Franceschi D, Gerding RL, Phillips G, Fratianne RB. Risk factors associated with intravascular catheter infections in burned patients: a prospective, randomized study. *J Trauma.* 1989;29:811–816.

84. Germann G, Kania NM. Extensive thrombosis of the caval venous system after central venous catheters in severely burned patients. *Burns.* 1995;21:389–391.

85. Petersen GA. Does systemic anticoagulation increase the risk of internal jugular vein cannulation? *Anesthesiology.* 1991;75:1124–1127.

86. Weese-Meyer DE, Fondriest DW, Brouillette RT, Shulman ST. Risk factors associated with candidemia in the neonatal intensive care unit: a case control study. *Pediatr Infect Dis.* 1987;6:190–196.

87. Taylor GD, Buchanan-Chell M, Kirkland T, McKenzie M, Wiens R. Trends and sources of nosocomial fungemia. *Mycoses.* 1994;37:187–190.

88. Sanchez V, Vazquez JA, Barth-Jones D, Dembry L, Sobel JD, Zervos MJ. Nosocomial acquisition of *Candida parapsilosis:* an epidemiologic study. *Am J Med.* 1993;94:577–582.

89. Fahy JV, Keoghan MT, Crummy EJ, Fitzgerald MX. Bacteremia and fungemia in adults with cystic fibrosis. *J Infect.* 1991;22:241–245.

90. Morris JB, Occhionero ME, Gauderer MWL, Stern RC, Doershuk CF. Totally implantable vascular access devices in cystic fibrosis: a four-year experience with fifty-eight patients. *J Pediatr.* 1990;117:82–85.

91. Bhargava V, Tomashefski JF, Stern RC, Abramowski CR. The pathology of fungal infection and colonization in patients with cystic fibrosis. *Hum Pathol.* 1989;20:977–986.

92. Sola JE, Stone MM, Wise B, Colombani PM. Atypical thrombotic and septic complications of totally implantable venous access devices in patients with cystic fibrosis. *Pediatr Pulmonol.* 1992;14:239–244.

Chapter 10

Alternative Routes of Catheter Placement

John A. Kaufman

Patients who require chronic long-term central venous access are at risk for occlusion of the central access veins. The risk of catheter-related central venous thrombosis is related to the patient's underlying disease, the access site, and the device characteristics. The rate of catheter-related central venous thrombosis is therefore difficult to determine but approaches 30% in some populations.[1] As more access sites become occluded, the provision of a secure, functional long-term central venous access becomes challenging. This chapter reviews the techniques that have been devised for insertion of central venous access devices in the patient with limited access options.

PATIENT ASSESSMENT

Patient assessment should begin with a clinical history, physical examination, and review of prior imaging studies and procedural records. Some patients may present with a history of multiple prior central venous catheters, failed attempts at central venous access, infusion of sclerosing medications through peripheral intravenous lines, intravenous drug abuse, dialysis, plasmapheresis, or surgical interruption of the central veins. Specific questions should be asked regarding past episodes of extremity swelling or known hypercoagulable conditions. Additional risk factors include mediastinal masses or adenopathy, fibrosing mediastinitis, and mediastinal radiation therapy. The number and location

of previous central venous catheters should be determined. In addition, the presence and location of devices such as pacemakers, venous stents, and vena cava filters are important when planning venous access procedure.[2]

On physical examination, a swollen extremity with prominent superficial veins may be noted (Table 10–1). Dilated veins should be traced from their origin to their termination. Upper-extremity veins that are confluent with abdominal wall veins are highly suggestive of superior vena cava (SVC) occlusion. Scars from prior central venous catheters, dialysis access, or other surgical procedures are important clues to the patient's condition. The extent of a radiation portal sometimes can be estimated from the small permanent tattoos applied by therapists to guide therapy or from changes in skin appearance.

The amount of information available from prior imaging studies is always surprising. The extent and age of an occlusion sometimes can be determined. Important anatomic variants or pathology in adjacent structures may be found when old studies are reviewed prior to a venous access procedure.

When prior imaging studies are not available, a thorough evaluation of all possible alternative venous access routes is essential. This evaluation should include both the peripheral and central veins. In particular, the status of the SVC and inferior vena cava (IVC) is critical information because these are the target vessels for most

Table 10–1   Patient Assessment

History	Findings at Physical Examination
Prior catheters	Scars from prior accesses
Prior DVT	Edema, dilated superficial veins, cords
Dialysis accesses, shunts/fistulas	Scars, functioning or old
Radiation	Simulation tattoos, erythema
Hypercoagulable conditions	Adenopathy, surgical scars, cords

DVT, deep venous thrombosis.

alternative access strategies. Cross-sectional vascular imaging modalities as well as conventional venography may be required.

Ultrasound (US) can determine the patency of the veins of the upper and lower extremity and the deep veins of the neck. Gray-scale compression US can provide definitive information regarding the presence of venous thrombosis.[3,4] The addition of Doppler waveform analysis and color-flow imaging improves the identification of patent venous segments. Unfortunately, because of the thickness of the overlying structures,[4] this modality is of limited utility for assessing the central veins of the chest and abdomen. Patency of the central veins can be inferred from gray-scale or Doppler waveforms in the peripheral vessels, but cross-sectional imaging with computed tomography (CT) or magnetic resonance (MR) is preferable.

Both CT and MR can provide useful information when evaluating a patient for central venous occlusion or planning an alternative access.[5,6] Contrast enhancement is essential for venous imaging with CT, with attention to the route of access (i.e., the nonsymptomatic side) and acquisition of a delayed scan to visualize veins. Venous studies with MR can be performed without contrast, although gadolinium-enhanced acquisitions are optimal. Both these modalities produce data that can be manipulated with image postprocessing tools to depict the venous structures better.

A major advantage of both CT and MR is the ability to image clearly the deep central veins of the chest and abdomen. In addition, the anatomy of adjacent structures and the presence of pathology can be evaluated.

Conventional venography remains essential in the evaluation of patients with limited venous access. This simple and safe procedure provides an enormous amount of information regarding the nature and extent of the venous occlusions. Perhaps most important, collateral pathways are preferentially filled, showing the site of reconstitution and allowing the operator to select targets for central venous access. Bilateral upper-extremity venograms should be performed when evaluating the central veins. The jugular veins are not normally opacified during upper-extremity injections, an important limitation of this technique; however, jugular veins can be evaluated with ultrasound in conjunction with the upper-extremity venograms.

PREVENTION OF CATHETER-RELATED CENTRAL VENOUS THROMBOSIS

The best strategy for patients with limited central venous access is prevention of the problem in the first place. Therefore, reasonable attempts should be made to minimize venous trauma during insertion

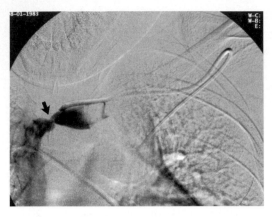

Figure 10–1 Injection through a left subclavian Hickman catheter. The catheter tip has withdrawn into the proximal left brachiocephalic vein. A stenosis (*arrow*) is present distal to the catheter tip, and a fibrin cap is present on the catheter itself. The catheter, in place for about 1 year, has malfunctioned for several months.

of catheters. The smallest diameter catheter for a particular need should be inserted, and a central location of the catheter tip should be ensured (Fig. 10–1). Administration of 1 mg of oral warfarin (Coumadin) daily significantly decreases catheter-related central venous thrombosis in oncology patients.[1] Administration of low-molecular-weight heparin, 2500 IU subcutaneously daily, may prove equally beneficial.[7] Catheters coated with heparin or other medications, which may render catheters less thrombogenic, are not yet available.

TECHNIQUES FOR ALTERNATIVE CENTRAL VENOUS ACCESS

Alternative access procedures should be performed with the same attention to detail as conventional access procedures. Patient monitoring, conscious sedation, surgical scrub technique, and prophylactic antibiotics are used. Usually, alternative access procedures are longer and more complicated and difficult than standard catheter placements, and so a conscious effort to maintain sterile technique is necessary.

Recanalization

Inserting a long-term central venous access catheter through a vein that is already occluded is the ideal procedure in patients with limited access for the simple reason that no new veins are placed at risk and are saved for future use.[8] At our institution, this is the preferred technique for patients with limited access. The objective of this approach is only to place a catheter, not to recanalize the vein in the usual sense of relieving an obstruction, but both goals can be accomplished simultaneously if desired.[9] This approach uses familiar access routes and recanalization tools (Fig. 10–2). There is a risk, however, that this approach will fail after expenditure of much time and effort, requiring a different approach. Therefore, before undertaking this method, the location, duration, and length of the occlusion and the status of the collateral venous drainage must be considered.

The location of the occlusion dictates the initial approach to access. In most instances, puncture of a patent segment of vein peripheral to the occluded segment is desirable. This provides a good target for the initial puncture and a secure footing for catheter exchanges and venograms (Fig. 10–3). Occasionally, it will be necessary to puncture the occluded vein directly. We reserve this approach for relatively recent occlusions when the vein, distended by thrombus, is easily identified with US.

The duration of the occlusion is important when deciding whether to attempt recanalization. Chronic occlusions are more difficult to cross, with a higher risk of perforation. This is particularly the case with long occlusions. Recent occlusions, whether long or short, are less difficult to traverse; however, it is difficult to predict the success of crossing an occlusion without trying.

The collateral drainage around an obstruction is an important consideration when contemplating a simple recanalization. Peripheral propagation of thrombus is a risk with this strategy and could occlude the collaterals and lead to decompensation

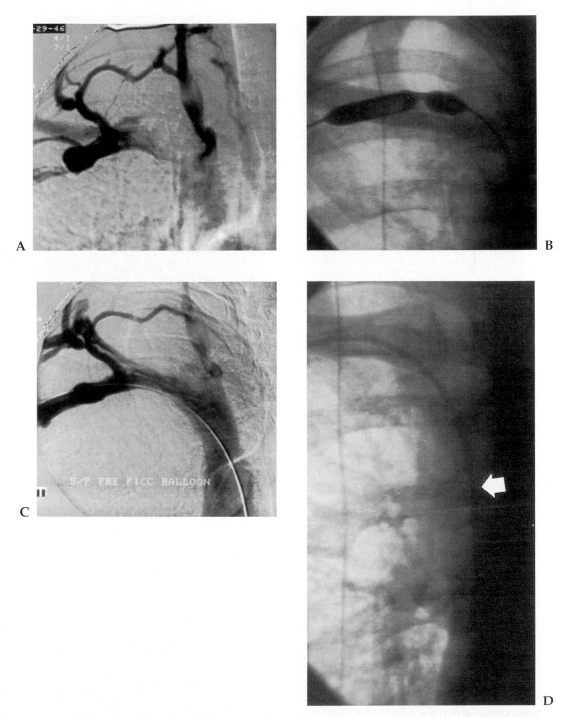

Figure 10–2 Angioplasty of a subclavian vein stenosis during insertion of a peripherally inserted central catheter line. **(A)** Arm venogram shows stenosis of the right subclavian vein at the junction with the internal jugular vein. Prominent collateral drainage is present. The patient was asymptomatic. **(B)** Image during the angioplasty shows a tight "waist" in the balloon at the stenosis. **(C)** Venogram after the angioplasty. The catheter was easily advanced over a hydrophilic guidewire. **(D)** Successful placement of the catheter (*arrow*).

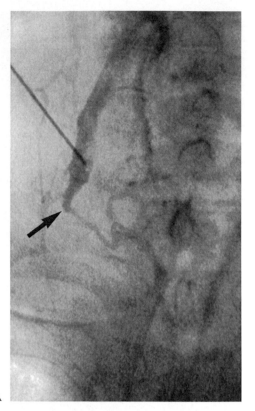
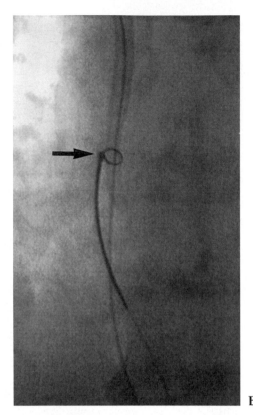

A

B

Figure 10–3 Recanalization of an occluded right brachiocephalic vein. **(A)** Injection of contrast in the right internal jugular vein shows distal occlusion (*arrow*). This was crossed with a straight hydrophilic guidewire and dilated progressively. **(B)** After removal of the peel-away sheath, the catheter could not be advanced into the right atrium. A loop snare (*arrow*) inserted via the common femoral vein was used to pull the catheter tip into the final position.

of the venous drainage. This is more likely to occur in patients with poor collaterals and an uncontrolled hypercoagulable diathesis. In this situation, a different access site rather than recanalization is appropriate. Alternatively, in some instances, enlarged collateral actually may offer a suitable conduit for catheter placement.[10]

Ultrasound, venography, and rarely CT can be used to guide the initial access. Micropuncture kits (Cook, Inc., Bloomington, IN, U.S.A.) that allow puncture with a 21-gauge needle, access with an 0.018-inch mandril wire, and insertion of a coaxial dilator that converts the access to an 0.035-inch or larger system are invaluable for this approach. After initial access is obtained peripheral to the occlusion, an angled hydrophilic cath-

eter such as an H-1 or C-2 should be advanced to the site of obstruction. We prefer a 5 French (F) braided catheter (Slip Cath, Cook, Inc.) with a tapered tip. Injection of contrast at this location may reveal a tiny residual lumen (the best possible case) or perhaps a small "nipple" that marks the former lumen. The occlusion is probed with a 0.038- to 0.035-inch hydrophilic guidewire while using the angled catheter to direct the effort. A straight hydrophilic guidewire is preferable because an angled guidewire may enter small tributaries as it is advanced. In difficult cases, progressively stiffer guidewires (including the back end of an Amplatz guidewire) can be used as necessary to initiate crossing the lesion. Sharp recanalization with a needle from a transjugular intrahepatic portocaval shunt (TIPS) kit has been described.[11]

When antegrade attempts to cross obstruction fail, a retrograde approach, from a femoral vein, should be considered. An H-1 or other slightly angled catheter is used in conjunction with a hydrophilic guidewire to cross the lesion. Larger, stiffer catheters such as 6 and 7 F can be useful in the beginning, although frequently 5 F hydrophilic catheters are needed to traverse the lesion completely.

HELPFUL HINT
Long sheaths (40–60 cm) provide support for the catheter while working through the lesion and exchange-length guidewires are essential to avoid losing access during catheter exchanges.

Once through the lesion, the guidewire may be snared through the upper extremity access site and brought out of the arm through a sheath. Ultimately, an exchange-length 0.035-inch Amplatz guidewire should be inserted across the two access sites, bridging the occlusion. This is a very secure situation because the guidewire can be controlled from both ends during the introduction of dilators, sheaths, and catheters (so-called body floss).

When the goal is limited to placing a catheter, the occlusion may be dilated with progressively larger vascular dilators. For large catheters, angioplasty of the entire occluded segment with a 6- to 8-mm balloon results in a channel that will easily accommodate most catheters. More lasting recanalization is rarely necessary in this setting but can be accomplished with placement of a stent immediately before catheter insertion. Prophylactic low-dose Coumadin is strongly recommended in this setting to promote stent patency. Catheter-directed thrombolysis of an acute central venous occlusion, before placement of a long-term central venous access catheter, significantly lengthens the procedure.[10]

Once the occlusion has been crossed and dilated, the introducer peel-away sheath for the catheter should be placed so that it is completely across the occlusion. This ensures the ability to place the catheter after the guidewire is removed. In some cases, the peel-away sheath provided with the access catheter is not long enough. Either a longer peel-away sheath should be inserted or the catheter placed over one or two guidewires. In the latter case, angioplasty of the occlusion with a balloon several millimeters larger in diameter than the catheter is helpful. Pinching the external end of the peel-away sheath tightly while loading the catheter on to the guidewires reduces the serious risk of air embolism and reduces blood loss. Valved sheaths can be used when inserting ports that are supplied with detached catheters. Occasionally, a snare introduced from below may be needed to pull a catheter into position.

Translumbar Cannulation of the Inferior Vena Cava

Translumbar placement of central venous catheters was first described in 1985.[12–17] Infection and occlusive IVC thrombosis rates are less than 5%, respectively, although catheter malfunction is common.[14,15] All types of long-term central venous access catheters can be inserted using this approach, including large-bore dialysis and plasmapheresis catheters. Procedural complications such as arterial puncture and retroperitoneal hematoma have been reported.[15] Catheter tip migration can occur due to respiratory motion, patient movement, or accidental dislodgment.[16] Nevertheless, this access is straightforward, safe, durable, and reliable (Table 10–2).

Patient evaluation begins with an assessment of the skin of the back and abdomen of the right side. Open wounds, surgical drains, infection, or tumor involvement of these areas are contraindications to this approach. Because the catheter is tunneled from the back to the abdomen overlying the anterior aspect of the lower ribs, a clear pathway must exist. Also, patients must be able to cooperate and lie in a decubitus or semiprone position for

Table 10–2   Translumbar Inferior Vena Cava Catheter Placement

1.   Review prior abdominal imaging studies

2.   Examine skin of right lower back and abdomen

3.   Check coagulation studies, platelets

4.   Consider pigtail catheter in IVC via femoral approach

5.   Position patient left lateral decubitus or partially supine with right side elevated

6.   Wide skin prep

7.   Use long 21-gauge micropuncture needle or translumbar aortography set

8.   Puncture just above right iliac crest 8–10 cm from midline

9.   Advance needle to just anterior to L2–3 to L3–4 interspace

10. Aspirate blood

11. Inject contrast to confirm position

12. Use 0.035-inch Amplatz super-stiff guidewire for dilatation

13. Tunnel around curve of flank to lower chest/upper abdomen

14. Locate port pockets over lower ribs anteriorly

15. Place catheter tip above renal veins, preferably in right atrium

IVC, inferior vena cava.

the procedure. Review of cross-sectional imaging may reveal important information, such as a left-sided IVC.[17] An abdominal CT scan with oral and intravenous (IV) contrast or an MRI should be obtained before the procedure is performed if there is any question of IVC patency, unusual caval anatomy, or retroperitoneal pathology.

There are relatively few contraindications to translumbar access to the IVC. Coagulopathies should be corrected before the procedure is done because puncture of lumbar and accessory renal arteries as well as the aorta can occur. In patients with large abdominal aortic aneurysms, the IVC may be displaced and compressed so that percutaneous access is not feasible. This procedure can be performed safely with an IVC filter in place.[17]

It may be helpful to insert a catheter or guidewire through a femoral vein into the IVC to serve as a target (Fig. 10–4). Also, an initial cavogram or road mapping can be used for puncture of the IVC.

HELPFUL HINT
Even if both femoral veins are thrombosed, a collateral vein in the groin region usually can be catheterized using ultrasound and a micropuncture set. A venogram can be performed via the collateral vein and the patency of the IVC assessed. The collateral vein can also be used to inject contrast for a roadmap during the definitive puncture of the IVC.

The femoral catheter is inserted with the patient supine at the level of the L2–3 interspace and secured in place with sterile adhesive and connected to a continuous flush. Although individuals experienced in translumbar IVC access usually skip this step, we continue to use it in all cases.

The patient is turned to either the oblique prone (right side elevated) or left lateral decubitus position with a small towel roll

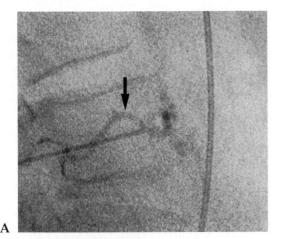

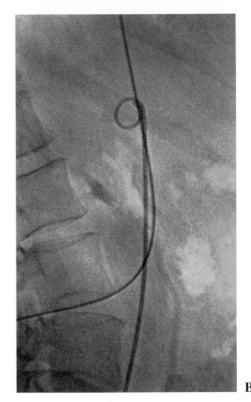

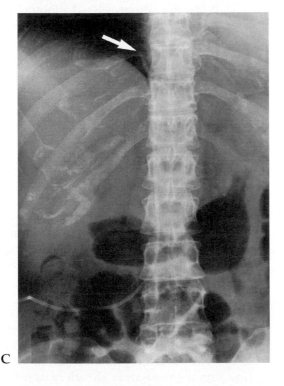

Figure 10–4 Translumbar inferior vena cava (IVC) catheter placement. (A) Lateral view during puncture shows opacification of a lumbar artery (*arrow*). The needle was redirected anteriorly toward the catheter that had been placed in the IVC from the femoral approach. (B) Lateral view after entry into the IVC shows the super-stiff guidewire in relation to the femoral catheter. (C) Completion radiograph showing the catheter entering the IVC at the L3–4 interspace. The tip of the catheter (*arrow*) is in the right atrium.

between the left ribs and iliac crest to maintain a straight orientation of the lumbar spine. The sterile field extends from the table posteriorly across the flank and abdomen to the midline anteriorly and from below the iliac crest to the nipples. The right arm is placed across the chest in order to maximize the size of the field. Such a large area is required because the catheter will be tunneled from a posterior puncture site to an anterior exit site. The patient is draped to allow access to both the right lower back and the right abdomen during the case. Fluoroscopy is then performed to localize the L2–3 interspace.

Translumbar puncture of the IVC is similar to translumbar puncture of the aorta in that the needle is inserted into the skin lateral and inferior to the desired entry site in the vessel. The trajectory of the needle is therefore cephalad, anterior and medial to enter the IVC between the L2–3 and L3–4 vertebral interspace. The skin puncture is just over the right iliac crest 8 to 10 cm lateral to the spinous processes. After injection of 1 to 2% Xylocaine into the skin and subcutaneous tissues, a small dermatome is made and the deep tissues spread with a hemostat. Local anesthetic can be deposited along the anticipated path of the access needle with a spinal needle or with the access needle. Discomfort and pain are common as the retroperitoneal tissues are traversed with the access needle and dilators.

The choice of access needle varies with the operator. The needle must be long enough to reach the IVC. Long micro-access kits with 21-gauge needles and 0.018-inch platinum-tipped mandril guidewires are available (Neff set, Cook, or AccuStick, Boston Scientific). The thin needle may be difficult to control when traversing the tough retroperitoneal tissues in some patients; so a larger conventional translumbar aortography set may be used.

The needle is advanced toward the L2–3 level just anterior to the spine. If a catheter already has been placed in the IVC from a femoral approach, this is used as the target.

HELPFUL HINT
Rotate the C-arm so that the target catheter that has been placed in the IVC (or the IVC on a roadmap) is free of the spine (i.e., there is no overlap of the IVC and the spine on the image). This ensures a straight shot at the IVC without hitting the spine with the needle. The view then should be "down the barrel" of the needle so that the initial puncture of the skin is over the IVC on the fluoroscopic image and the needle remains over the IVC as it is advanced toward the IVC.

The patient may feel back pain as the needle is advanced, and this pain is treated with injection of additional small amounts of lidocaine (Xylocaine). Deflection of this catheter can be visualized just as the IVC is entered, or a faint click may be felt transmitted along the needle. A 20-mL syringe

is used to aspirate as the needle is withdrawn until blood is obtained. Injection of contrast is essential to document the position of the needle tip. Arterial puncture is no cause for alarm as long as it is recognized. Simply withdraw the needle and change the angle of approach.

A soft-tipped guidewire is advanced into the IVC, the coaxial dilator is advanced over the guidewire, and the access guidewire is removed. If any question remains as to the identity of the vessel that has been entered, contrast is injected again at this time. A 180-cm-long 0.035-inch Amplatz superstiff guidewire is inserted with the tip in the SVC, if possible. Progressive dilatation to at least one French size larger than the peel-away sheath is done. Dilatation of the tract and IVC wall with a small-diameter angioplasty balloon may be necessary in some patients.

The point at which the catheter is inserted depends on the type of device. For example, with detached ports, the catheter is inserted at this time, whereas for one-piece Hickman catheters, the tunneling is completed first. In either case, a peel-away sheath is inserted over the guidewire. This sheath must be long enough to provide secure access to the IVC. When a relatively flat trajectory has been used, the sheath may kink at the IVC entry site once the dilator is removed.

HELPFUL HINT
Insertion of the catheter over a guidewire or preloading one or two hydrophilic guidewires into the catheter before insertion into the peel-away sheath is useful in this situation. This guidewire usually can be advanced through the kink, which sometimes straightens the sheath enough to allow passage of the catheter. If the guidewire fails to straighten the kink, the sheath can be withdrawn slightly over the guidewire to reposition the kink in a straight segment of the tract. In general, the peel-away sheath should be at least one French size larger than the catheter to minimize friction and facilitate insertion.

The catheter tip should be positioned as high as possible, preferably in right atrium. At the very least, the catheter tip should be above the renal veins to take advantage of the copious renal inflow.

The tunnel from the puncture site to the skin exit site or pocket then is anesthetized with 1 to 2% subcutaneous Xylocaine. Long tunnels around the flank may be difficult to make. Therefore, small access incisions can be made to divide the tunnel into segments. This process is necessary because the tunneling devices supplied with venous access devices are not long or malleable enough to tunnel around the curve of the flank. Ports must be placed over the lower aspect of the anterior ribs to provide support during access. External catheters should exit the skin above the belt line for comfort and ease of care. Routine flushing, closure techniques, and dressings should be applied at the completion of the procedure.

Trans-hepatic Catheter Placement

Complete occlusion of both the SVC and infrarenal IVC occurs in a small number of patients with chronic venous access. Usually, the intrahepatic portion of the IVC remains patent. In these patients, central venous catheters can be placed through a hepatic vein or directly into the intrahepatic IVC.[18,19] Catheters of all types have been placed in this manner, including the dialysis catheter.[20] This approach appears to be successful in the pediatric population.[21,22] Some investigators advocate the trans-hepatic route for diagnostic and interventional procedures in addition to chronic venous access.[23] The trans-hepatic approach for long-term central venous access usually is reserved for patients with no other access options (Table 10–3).

Experience with this approach is limited. Only a few case reports and small series have been published. We believe that this approach is durable, and we maintained one in a patient for 7 years. Several catheter changes have been required over the years,

but the same access has been preserved. Complications of this method include catheter dislodgment with bleeding from the hepatic tract and thrombosis of the hepatic vein with the catheter.[24] Contraindications to this approach include coagulopathy, massive ascites, active hepatic or biliary infection, vascular hepatic tumors along the anticipated path of the catheter, and inability to puncture or tunnel through normal skin. Prior partial hepatectomy, small amount of ascites, and polycystic liver disease are relative contraindications.

Limited data are available for the selection of either a hepatic vein or the intrahepatic IVC for puncture. Direct puncture of the intrahepatic IVC provides the longest path through the hepatic parenchyma, which may help to stabilize the catheter in patients with major excursion of the liver during respiration. Puncture of a hepatic vein (usually the middle hepatic vein) results in a longer intravascular portion of the catheter, an important consideration in children, who eventually might outgrow the catheter. This approach places the hepatic vein at risk for thrombosis, a complication that is usually asymptomatic as long as the other hepatic veins are patent.

Before the procedure is done, review of hepatic imaging, preferably a contrast enhanced CT scan, is important. The liver, hepatic veins, intrahepatic IVC, subphrenic space, and the perihepatic peritoneal cavity should be inspected. Trans-hepatic placement of a central venous catheter should not be undertaken without preprocedural cross-sectional imaging. The skin of the right upper quadrant must be free of infection and tumor.

The patient is positioned supine on the fluoroscopy table. For a right lateral intercostal approach, the right arm is positioned on an arm board and abducted to 90 degrees. For an anterior subcostal approach, the arm remains at the patient's side. The skin is prepped from the table on the right to the midline of the abdomen and from the iliac crest to the nipple.

Table 10–3   Transhepatic Catheter Placement

1. Review prior abdominal imaging

2. Examine skin of right flank and upper abdomen

3. Check coagulation studies, platelets

4. Position patient supine

5. Wide skin prep

6. Select lateral intercostal (midaxillary line) or anterior subcostal puncture

7. Consider US guidance for subcostal puncture

8. Use long 21-gauge micropuncture needle

9. Do not cross midline with needle tip

10. Target is intrahepatic IVC or middle hepatic vein (latter preferred in children)

11. Aspirate blood

12. Inject contrast to confirm location

13. Use 0.035-inch Amplatz super-stiff guidewire for dilatation

14. Locate port pockets over lower ribs anteriorly

15. Place catheter tip in right atrium

US, ultrasound; IVC, inferior vena cava.

The lateral access is through the 10th or 11th intercostal space in the midaxillary line. Fluoroscopy in inspiration and expiration is essential to determine the location of the pleural cavity. Local anesthetic is injected subcutaneously and over the top edge of the rib. A 21-gauge needle can be used to anesthetize the liver capsule. Through a 1-cm skin incision, a 21-gauge micro-access needle is advanced over the top of the rib in a horizontal plane toward the spine. The patient must suspend respiration. The needle should not pass beyond the midline. Aspiration of blood during withdrawal of the needle is followed by injection of contrast material to identify the vessel. The entry site can be either the middle hepatic vein or IVC. Ultrasound guidance is occasionally necessary.

The anterior access is usually subcostal. Preparation is identical to the lateral inter-costal approach; however, ultrasound guidance is needed for this approach. The planned entry site is the middle hepatic vein.

Once venous access is achieved, a 0.018-inch platinum-tipped guidewire is advanced into the right atrium, the coaxial dilator is advanced into the IVC, and the guidewire exchanged for a standard length 0.035-inch Amplatz super-stiff guidewire. If possible, the tip of this guidewire should be positioned in the SVC to avoid arrhythmias. Serial dilatation allows insertion of the peel-away sheath and ultimately the access catheter with its tip ideally in the right atrium (Fig. 10–5).

Timing of insertion of the catheter is determined by the type of device; one-piece Hickman catheters are inserted after tunneling, whereas catheters detached from ports are inserted first and then tunneled back to the pocket.

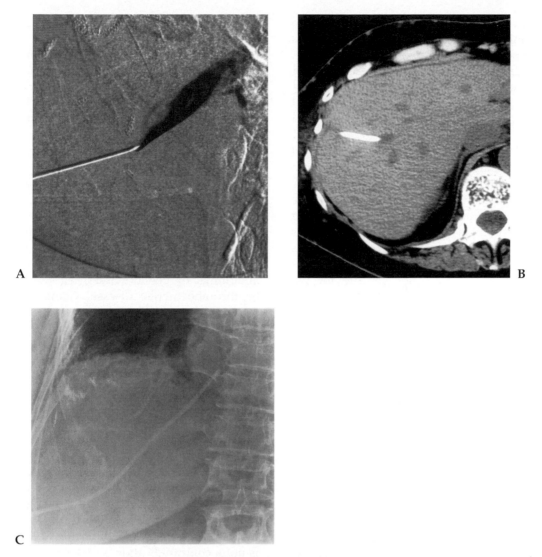

Figure 10–5 Trans-hepatic cannulation of the inferior vena cava (IVC) via the middle hepatic vein in a patient with occlusions of the superior vena cava (SVC) and infrarenal IVC. **(A)** Digital subtraction venogram performed through the micro-access needle confirms puncture of a hepatic vein. **(B)** Postprocedural computed tomography scan shows the catheter as it enters the middle hepatic vein. **(C)** Chest radiograph shows the tip of the catheter in the right atrium. The course of the catheter conforms to that of the middle hepatic vein. (Reproduced from Kaufman JA, et al. Long-term central venous catheterization in patients with limited access. *AJR Am J Roentgenol.* 1996;167:1327–1333, with permission.)

HELPFUL HINT

If a difficult catheter insertion is anticipated, preloading a hydrophilic guidewire into the catheter or insertion over a guidewire may be necessary. Standard-length peel-away sheaths may not be long enough to reach the venous entry site in some patients.

Catheters should be tunneled away from the puncture site. A short redundancy in the subcutaneous tissue at the entry site helps to prevent movement of the catheter tip with respiration. Excursion of the catheter with respiration can be assessed during the procedure by having the patient inhale and exhale deeply under fluoroscopy. Catheters placed through a lateral access are tunneled anteriorly in a manner similar to translumbar catheters. Pockets for ports should be created over the anterior ribs, when possible, to provide a firm target during access. Standard suture techniques, catheter flushing, and dressings are done.

When no longer needed, removal of trans-hepatic catheters is different from other venous catheters. The major risk is intraperitoneal or subcapsular hemorrhage from an immature track. Catheters that have been in place for several weeks or more have a well-developed fibrous tunnel that separates the peritoneal space (although this may not be true for patients with ascites). Embolization of the track with Gelfoam pledgets should be considered for early removal of a large non-infected catheter.[23] This step can be performed by cutting down on the catheter at the puncture site, gaining control of the exposed catheter, transecting the catheter, placing a hydrophilic guidewire through the intravascular portion of the catheter, and exchanging for an appropriate-sized sheath through which Gelfoam particles or torpedoes can be deposited.

Femoral Vein

Long-term central venous access through the femoral vein is being done more frequently, but it remains controversial.[25–28] This access is frequently used in children in the acute care setting.[29,30] All types of chronic access catheters can be placed.[28]

Patients who are candidates for the femoral approach also could have trans-lumbar catheters. Advantages of femoral vein catheters are ease of access and tunneling.[25–28] Disadvantages are the increased risks of iliofemoral vein thrombosis and infection.[28,29] In one series of acute femoral vein catheters in adults, the rate of ultra-sonographically diagnosed femoral vein thrombosis was 25%.[30] The rate of IVC and iliofemoral thrombosis is much lower with chronic access catheters, approaching

10% in some series.[26,28] Most investigators have used the right common femoral vein for access; so no data are available on the relative risk of thrombosis and side of access. Because a comprehensive surveillance for venous thrombosis has not been routinely performed, the rate of asymptomatic thrombosis may be higher. The infection rates follow a similar incidence, being higher with nontunneled catheters.[27] The infection rate with tunneled femoral dialysis catheters was 5.2/1000 days.[28]

The status of the iliofemoral veins and IVC should be checked before femoral vein catheter placement in patients with a past history of venous instrumentation, abdominal or pelvic masses, leg swelling, or thromboembolic disease. Compression ultrasound with Doppler evaluation of femoral venous flow during respiration and Valsalva maneuver should be obtained. A compressible common femoral vein with normal Doppler flow signal implies a patent access site and central veins. Further evaluation with CT or MR venography may be useful in difficult cases. The skin in the inguinal region, upper thigh, and lower abdomen must be checked (Table 10–4).

Contraindications include coagulopathy, infection or other dermatologic conditions in the intertriginous fold, and open wounds. Prior iliofemoral deep venous thrombosis is a relative contraindication. An IVC filter is not a contraindication.

With the patient supine, the skin should be prepped from the greater trochanter to the midline of the abdomen and from the midthigh to the costal margin. The right common femoral vein approach is preferred because of less iliac vein tortuosity. In addition, compression of the left common iliac vein by the right common iliac artery may increase the rate of thrombosis from left-sided approaches.

After infiltration of the skin with local anesthetic, the common femoral vein is punctured over the femoral head with either a micro-access or a standard angiographic needle. If there is any question of venous patency or anatomy, contrast can

Table 10–4   Femoral Catheter Placement

1.	Review prior abdominal imaging
2.	Right common femoral vein access is preferred
3.	Examine skin of right groin, thigh, and lower abdomen
4.	Check coagulation studies, platelets
5.	Position patient supine
6.	Wide skin prep
7.	Puncture common femoral vein with 21-gauge micropuncture kit or angiographic needle
8.	Consider US guidance for difficult punctures
9.	Aspirate blood
10.	Inject contrast to confirm location and venous patency, if necessary
11.	Use 0.035-inch Amplatz super-stiff guidewire for dilatation
12.	Tunnel onto thigh or lateral lower abdomen
13.	Use subcuticular closure for groin incision

be injected through a dilator. Ultrasound guidance for puncture is optional. Serial dilation to the size of the introducer sheath is accomplished over a standard-length 0.035-inch Amplatz super-stiff guidewire. The catheter is inserted through a peel-away sheath, with the tip positioned as high as possible in the IVC (ideally at the right atrium). Long catheters (60 cm or longer) are used. Sheath kinking is rarely a problem (Fig. 10–6).

The catheters can be tunneled either down to the lateral thigh or up onto the abdomen.[28] These approaches show good clinical results and patient acceptance. The advantages of having the skin exit or port on the abdomen, above the belt line, are easier access and care. Abdominal tunnels should swing laterally for a gentle curve at the insertion site.

The groin incision should be closed with subcuticular sutures (such as 4.0 Dexon) to minimize the risk of infection. External sutures are difficult to keep clean in this area and may provide a pathway for bacteria to enter the subcutaneous tissues. Routine catheter flushing, wound care, and dressing protocols are followed. Prophylactic therapy with Coumadin, 1 mg daily, is recommended to prevent catheter-related iliofemoral thrombosis. Thrombosis is treated with full anticoagulation.[28]

Collateral Veins

Enlarged upper-extremity collateral veins sometimes can be successfully negotiated to allow central positioning of a catheter[10,31,32] with percutaneous techniques or combined with surgery.[32] Lower truncal collateral veins also have been used for venous access, although experience with this approach is limited.[33] In general, these have been patients in whom other alternative access was not available or in whom an enlarged collateral vein was encountered during an access procedure that was then used.

Contrast venography is useful in allowing the interventionist to determine the quality of the collateral vein and the reconstituted

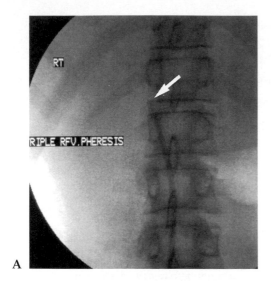
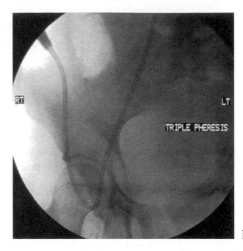

Figure 10–6 Femoral vein plasmapheresis catheter in a child with obstruction of the superior vena cava by lymphoma. **(A)** The catheter tip (*arrow*) is just above the renal veins. Ideal location would be in the right atrium. **(B)** The catheter is tunneled superiorly and laterally.

central vein. Simultaneous bilateral upper-extremity venograms or direct injection of an enlarged superficial neck or chest vein may be necessary (Fig. 10–7). Although CT and MR may reveal more collateral veins, they may not be usable due to size, location, tortuosity, or stenoses. Direct puncture of intercostal and hemiazygous veins and catheterization of chest wall collateral veins from the basilic vein to reach the intercostal veins can be successful.[10,31,32] The full range of angiographic tools may be required, including hydrophilic selective catheters and expensive torque-control guidewires. Catheters have been placed in the SVC or left within an enlarged azygous vein.[31,32] An important consideration with this approach is the status of other collateral veins because occlusion of a major isolated draining vein may precipitate severe symptoms. This particular approach to venous access allows for maximal creativity on the part of the interventionist.

Miscellaneous and Surgical Approaches

Almost any vein that drains centrally potentially can be used for percutaneous access. For example, insertion of 2 F PICCs through scalp veins in infants allowed central (i.e., SVC) placement in 48% of attempts in one report.[34] Cannulation of small peripheral veins and negotiation into central veins may require sophisticated angiographic tools, excellent imaging, and small access devices and may be time consuming. With the combined use of fluoroscopy and cross-sectional imaging, it is possible to puncture veins that would be difficult to opacify directly, such as gonadal veins. Whenever attempting a new or unusual approach, it is important to review prior imaging studies as well as relevant cross-sectional anatomy to avoid inadvertent puncture of adjacent structures.

Numerous surgical options are available for alternative venous access, such as ovarian, iliac, internal mammary, azygous vein, and direct cannulation of the right atrium.[35-39] Combined surgical and percutaneous techniques can recanalize occluded central veins, but these occurred before the development of current angiographic tools, imaging techniques, and radiologic interest in central venous access.[40] Some of these approaches may

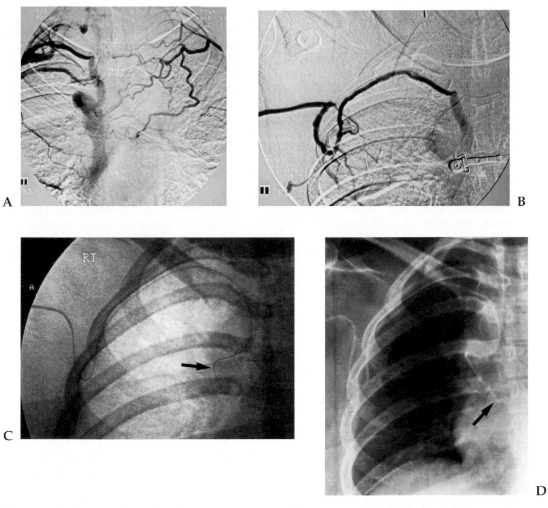

Figure 10–7 Transcollateral catheter in a 27-year-old woman with Hodgkin's disease who was referred for placement of an implantable venous access device. **(A)** Digital subtraction venogram of both upper extremities shows occlusion of the major central thoracic veins with the exception of the azygous vein and the infra-azygous superior vena cava (SVC). **(B)** Digital subtraction venogram of an injection into a right lateral chest-wall vein. The right third intercostal vein is opacified and drains through a patent azygous vein into the SVC. **(C)** The course of a hydrophilic guidewire (*arrow*) used to negotiate the collateral vein to the SVC is demonstrated. **(D)** Chest radiograph after the procedure shows the tip of catheter (*arrow*) in the SVC, below the azygous arch. (Reproduced from Kaufman JA, Crenshaw WB, Kuter I, Geller SC. Percutaneous placement of a central venous access device via an intercostal vein. *AJR Am J Roentgenol.* 1995;165:459–460, with permission.)

now be feasible as wholly percutaneous techniques with appropriate image guidance.

SUMMARY

Prevention of catheter-related central venous occlusion would reduce the utilization of the techniques described; however, this goal remains elusive. Patients with limited options for long-term central venous access require careful evaluation of the available veins and access needs, thorough preprocedural planning, and innovation. Successful catheter placement is of great benefit and is sometimes life-saving.

REFERENCES

1. Bern MM, Lokich JJ, Wallach SR, et al. Very low dose warfarin can prevent thrombosis in central venous catheters: a randomized prospective trial. *Ann Intern Med.* 1990;112: 423–428.
2. Spence LD, Gironta MG, Malde HM, Mickolick CT, Geisenger MA, Dolmatch BL. Acute upper extremity deep venous thrombosis: safety and effectiveness of superior vena caval filters. *Radiology.* 1999;210:53–58.
3. Fraser JD, Anderson DR. Deep venous thrombosis: recent advances and optimal investigation with US. *Radiology.* 1999;211: 9–24.
4. Passman MA, Criado E, Farber MA, et al. Efficacy of color flow duplex imaging for proximal upper extremity venous outflow obstruction in hemodialysis patients. *J Vasc Surg.* 1998;28:869–875.
5. Qanadli SD, Hajjam ME, Bruckert F, et al. Helical CT phlebography of the superior vena cava: diagnosis and evaluation of venous obstruction. *AJR Am J Roentgenol.* 1999; 172:1327–1333.
6. Li W, David V, Kaplan R, Edelman RR. Three-dimensional low dose gadolinium-enhanced peripheral MR venography. *J Magn Reson Imaging.* 1998;8:630–633.
7. Monreal M, Alastrue A, Rull M, et al. Upper extremity deep venous thrombosis in cancer patients with venous access devices: prophylaxis with a low molecular weight heparin (Fragmin). *Thromb Haemost.* 1996;75:251–253.
8. Ferral H, Bjarnson H, Wholey M, Lopera J, Maynar M, Castaneda-Zuniga WR. Recanalization of occluded veins to provide access for central catheter placement. *J Vasc Interv Radiol.* 1996;7:681–685.
9. Funaki B, Zaleski GX, Leef JA, Rosenblum JD. Radiologic placement of long-term hemodialysis catheters in occluded jugular or subclavian veins or through patent thyrocervical collateral veins. *AJR Am J Roentgenol.* 1998;170:1194–1196.
10. Kaufman JA, Crenshaw WB, Kuter I, Geller SC. Percutaneous placement of a central venous access device via an intercostal vein. *AJR Am J Roentgenol.* 1995;165:459–460.
11. Farrell T, Lang EV, Barnhart W. Sharp recanalization of central venous occlusions. *J Vasc Interv Radiol.* 1999;10:49–54.

12. Kenney PR, Dorfman GS, Denny DF Jr. Percutaneous inferior vena cava cannulation for long-term parenteral access. *Surgery.* 1985;97:602–605.
13. Denny DF Jr, Greenwood LH, Morse SS, Lee GK, Baquero J. Inferior vena cava: translumbar catheterization for central venous access. *Radiology.* 1989;170:1013–1014.
14. Lund GB, Lieberman RP, Haire WD, Martin VA, Kessinger A, Armitage JO. Translumbar inferior vena cava catheters for long-term venous access. *Radiology.* 1990;174:31–35.
15. Bennett JD, Papadouris D, Rankin RN, et al. Percutaneous inferior vena caval approach for long-term central venous access. *J Vasc Interv Radiol.* 1997;8:851–855.
16. Rajan DK, Crouteau DL, Sturza SG, Harvill ML, Mehall CJ. Translumbar placement of inferior vena caval catheters: a solution for challenging hemodialysis access. *Radiographics.* 1998;18:1155–1167.
17. Cazenave FL, Glass-Royal MC, Teitelbaum GP, Zuurbier R, Zeman RK, Silverman PM. CT analysis of a safe approach for translumbar access to the aorta and inferior vena cava. *AJR Am J Roentgenol* 1991;156:395–396.
18. Crummy AB, Carlson P, McDermott JC, Andrews D. Percutaneous transhepatic placement of a Hickman catheter [letter]. *AJR Am J Roentgenol.* 1989;153:1317–1318.
19. Kaufman JA, Greenfield AJ, Fitzpatrick GF. Transhepatic cannulation of the inferior vena cava. *J Vasc Interv Radiol.* 1991;2:331–334.
20. Po CL, Koolpe HA, Allen S, Alvez LD, Raja RM. Transhepatic PermCath for hemodialysis. *Am J Kidney Dis.* 1994;24:590–591.
21. Azizkhan RG, Taylor LA, Jaques PF, Mauro MA, Lacey SR. Percutaneous translumbar and transhepatic inferior vena caval catheters for prolonged access in children. *J Pediatr Surg.* 1992;27:165–169.
22. Bergey EA, Kaye RD, Reyes J, Towbin RB. Transhepatic insertion of vascular dialysis catheters in children: a safe, life-prolonging procedure. *Pediatr Radiol.* 1999;29:42–45.
23. Johnson JL, Fellows KE, Murphy JD. Transhepatic central venous access for cardiac catheterization and radiologic intervention. *Cathet Cardiovasc Diagn.* 1995;35:168–171.
24. Pieters PC, Dittrich J, Prasad U, Berman W. Acute Budd-Chiari syndrome caused by percutaneous placement of a transhepatic inferior vena cava catheter. *J Vasc Interv Radiol.* 1997;8:587–590.

25. Friedman B, Kanter G, Titus D. Femoral venous catheters: a safe alternative for delivering parenteral nutrition. *Nutr Clin Pract.* 1994;9:69–72.

26. Bertoglio S, Di Somma C, Meszaros P, Gipponi M, Cafiero F, Percivale P. Long-term femoral vein central venous access in cancer patients. *Eur J Surg Oncol.* 1996;22:162–165.

27. Harden JL, Kemp L, Mirtallo J. Femoral catheters increase risk of infection in total parenteral nutrition patients. *Nutr Clin Pract.* 1995;10:60–66.

28. Zaleski GX, Funaki B, Lorenz JM, et al. Experience with tunneled femoral hemodialysis catheters. *AJR Am J Roentgenol.* 1999; 172:493–496.

29. Pippus KG, Giacomantonio JM, Gillis DA, Rees EP. Thrombotic complications of saphenous central venous lines. *J Pediatr Surg.* 1994;29:1218–1219.

30. Trottier SJ, Veremakis C, O'Brien J, Auer AI. Femoral deep vein thrombosis associated with central venous catheterization: results from a prospective, randomized trial. *Crit Care Med.* 1995;23:52–59.

31. Andrews, JC. Percutaneous placement of a Hickman catheter with use of an intercostal vein for access. *J Vasc Interv Radiol.* 1994; 5:859–861.

32. Meranze SG, McLean GK, Stein EJ, Jordan HA. Catheter placement in the azygous system: an unusual approach to venous access. *AJR Am J Roentgenol.* 1985;144:1075–1076.

33. Denny DF Jr. Central venous access via the hemiazygous vein. In: Trerotola SO, Savader SJ, Durham JD, eds. *Venous Interventions.* Fairfax, VA: SCVIR; 1995:507–510.

34. Racadio JM, Johnson ND, Doellman DA. Peripherally inserted central venous catheters: success of scalp-vein access in infants and newborns. *Radiology.* 1999;210: 858–860.

35. Ikeda S, Sera Y, Oshiro H, et al. Transiliac catheterization of the inferior vena cava for long-term venous access in children. *Pediatr Surg Int.* 1998;14:140–141.

36. Chang MY, Morris JB. Long-term central venous access through the ovarian vein. *JPEN J Parenter Enteral Nutr.* 1997;21:235–237.

37. Jaime-Solis E, Anaya-Ortega M, Moctezuma-Espinosa J. The internal mammary vein: an alternative route for central venous access with an implantable port. *J Pediatr Surg.* 1994;29:1328–1330.

38. Malt RA, Kempster M. Direct azygous vein and superior vena cava cannulation for parenteral nutrition. *JPEN J Parenter Enteral Nutr.* 1983;7:580–581.

39. Oram Smith JC, Mullen JL, Harken AH, et al. Direct right atrial catheterization for total parenteral nutrition. *Surgery.* 1978;83: 274–276.

40. Torosian MH, Meranze S, Mullen JL. Central venous accesses with occlusive central venous thrombosis. *Ann Surg.* 1986;203: 30–33.

Chapter *11*

Catheter Malfunction: Diagnosis and Treatment

Philip C. Pieters

The widespread use of long-term central venous access devices has been emphasized throughout this book. Proficiency in the placement of these catheters is important because the catheter will function well only if it is placed well. Catheter care is also important because even a well-placed catheter is of little use if it becomes infected and must be removed. Equally important are the follow-up and maintenance of malfunctioning catheters because most central venous catheters eventually will malfunction.

Multiple noninfectious complications can threaten catheter longevity. Fibrin sheath formation at the catheter tip is ubiquitous. The effects of fibrin sheath or thrombus formation at the catheter tip can range from the inconvenience of persistent withdrawal occlusion in portacaths and nondialysis tunneled catheters to rendering catheters clinically useless, especially if high flow rates are required, such as in dialysis. Major efforts of catheter maintenance are required to maintain flow rates adequate for hemodialysis, that is, greater than 250 to 300 mL per minute. Silastic cuffed hemodialysis catheters have been used increasingly for providing long-term vascular access and now account for 10 to 15% of access in most dialysis facilities.[1] Dialysis catheter malfunction is common, occurring in 87% of catheters before they were removed in a study by Suhocki and colleagues.[2] The mean time from catheter insertion to the first malfunction was 2.8 months. In another study, the primary patency of hemodialysis catheters at 3 and 6 months was 54% and 33%, respectively, with a median time to initial failure of 3.5 months.[3]

Historically, catheter failure was managed by placement of a new catheter via a new access site.[4] The use of other central veins for access can compromise future access sites, however, and access sites quickly become depleted. Repeated placement of hemodialysis catheters at different sites carries several risks, including the inherent risk of placing a new catheter and venous stenoses or occlusions. Cimochowski and co-workers[5] showed marked venous stenoses in 50% of patients who previously had temporary subclavian vein or internal jugular vein dialysis catheters; mean catheter dwell time was just 11.5 days. Subclavian vein or innominate vein stenosis or occlusion threatens the outflow of an existing ipsilateral access graft or arteriovenous fistula or precludes its surgical placement. As the life expectancy of patients with chronic renal failure increases, preservation of existing central venous catheter sites becomes of paramount importance.[6]

HISTORY AND EXAMINATION

A "simple catheter check" can provoke nonchalance and disinterest of vascular and interventional radiologists even to the extreme that the study is done by a nonphysician member of the venous access team and may be checked by the radiologist afterwards. This situation should be discouraged. The vital importance of the access to the patient must be kept in mind, and everything possible must be done to keep these catheters functional. The vascular and interventional radiologist should be involved from the start. The history and examination can give valuable clues for making a correct diagnosis. Certain symptoms or signs can point to the underlying problem with the catheter.

Pain

Pain during infusion suggests an extravasation of the infused solution into the soft tissues. The location of the pain is a guide as to where the problem lies. There are several causes of extravasation from a venous access device:

- The portacath is not adequately accessed with the access needle.

- The catheter has become disconnected from the port.
- The catheter is fractured (Fig. 11–1).
- The catheter is poorly positioned and has migrated out of the vein.
- Venous thrombosis has developed.
- Fibrin sheath has formed around the catheter.

Inability to Aspirate

Persistent withdrawal occlusion (PWO) is a common presentation of a catheter with fibrin sheath or thrombus at the tip of the catheter acting as a one-way valve. This usually occurs several weeks after placement. If PWO occurs immediately after catheter placement, the problem is most likely due to the catheter being malpositioned with the catheter tip against the wall of the vein. In non–high-flow catheters, PWO can prove to be inconvenient by preventing blood aspiration and yet allowing infusions. In high-flow catheters, however,

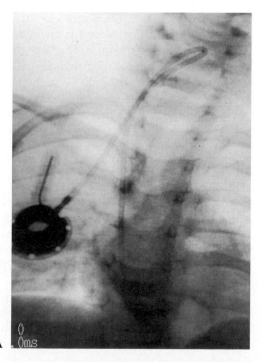
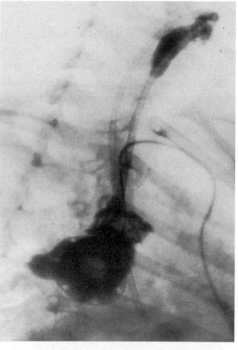

Figure 11–1 **(A)** High puncture has resulted in kinking of the catheter. **(B)** The kinked catheter has broken, causing extravasation into the soft tissues. There is also leakage from the port, possibly due to high resistance to injection (due to the kink) causing leakage around the needle.

PWO can quickly lead to complete loss of catheter function because of the inability to sustain necessary high flow rates.

Poor Flow Rates

When poor flow rates occur shortly after catheter placement, they are usually due to improper tip position, subcutaneous kinking of the catheter, or extrinsic compression of the catheter owing to tight fixation device or sutures around the catheter, constricting the lumen. Catheters that are too short or too long or kinked in the subcutaneous tunnel will not function well and will require correction or replacement. Misplacement of catheters is more likely to occur when inserted without imaging guidance. The rate of catheter malposition is as high as 29% on postprocedure radiographs when fluoroscopy is not used for placement.[7] With the use of fluoroscopic guidance, primary misplacement occurs in fewer than 2% of cases.[2]

Swelling

Swelling of an extremity, both extremities, or the head and neck may indicate venous thrombosis and possibly the superior vena cava (SVC) syndrome. Venography or sonography is needed to evaluate venous thrombosis. Often, the indwelling catheter will function adequately in such circumstances because the thrombus is present at the catheter insertion site or along the intravenous portion of a catheter and not necessarily at the catheter tip. Likewise, a catheter check—injecting contrast through the indwelling catheter and obtaining radiographs—may be perfectly normal even in the face of widespread venous thrombosis. Venous thrombosis is discussed in Chapter 13.

TECHNIQUE FOR CHECKING CATHETERS

Before performing digital subtraction imaging, the catheter dressing should be removed and the skin site and external portion of the catheter examined. The dressing should be checked for drainage. Examining the skin for signs of infection, such as erythema and tenderness, is an important step if catheter exchange over a guidewire is being considered, because a new catheter should not be placed in an infected tunnel or exit site. It is also important to examine the portion of the catheter that is used for clamping the catheter. Occasionally, the stiff plastic may become kinked as a result of repeated clamping, limiting the flow. One must ensure that a suture or fixation device has not been placed too tightly around the external portion of the catheter, compressing the lumen and restricting flow.

The catheter hub should be prepared with Betadine and laid on sterile towels. The indwelling heparin must be discarded. The ability to aspirate is an important finding and should be reported. As previously discussed, the ability to inject but not aspirate through a catheter indicates a one-way valve-like mechanism, usually due to one of three causes: (1) fibrin sheath at the catheter tip, (2) thrombus at the catheter tip, or (3) catheter tip against the wall of the vein. Removal of the heparin is very important. Typically, dialysis catheters are blocked with 5000 U of heparin in each lumen. Injection of 10,000 U of heparin into the bloodstream can cause systemic heparinization, making removal of the catheter and placement of a new catheter dangerous.

HELPFUL HINT

If one port will not aspirate and heparin cannot be removed, avoid injecting contrast through this lumen and use the other lumen to check the catheter. In most instances, injection of a single lumen will provide adequate information. Even if the injection through the one lumen is not diagnostic, it can be assumed that a problem is present, and correction is done based on this information.

The entire length of the catheter must be checked fluoroscopically. Occasionally, constriction of the catheter by a tight suture or fixation device will be evident by fluoroscopy even if it is not noticed by visual inspection. Also, a mechanical kink in the catheter, which is most often (but not always) present at the site of transition from the subcutaneous tunnel into the vein, may be found. Occasionally, when the jugular vein has been used for venous access, a mechanical kink becomes evident only in a particular head position. Therefore, the venous entry site is examined fluoroscopically while the patient rotates his or her head. The position of the tip of the catheter should also be evaluated with fluoroscopy. Contrast should be injected while obtaining digital images (Fig. 11–2). The examination should be tailored to the suspected problem, based on the history. Specifically, if the history indicates extravasation into the soft tissues, a small amount of contrast should

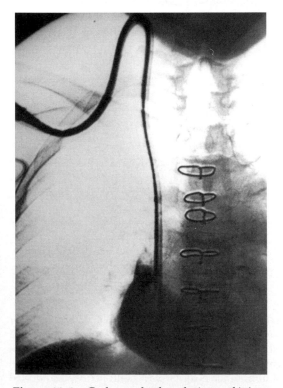

Figure 11–2 Catheter check technique of injecting contrast while obtaining images at a rapid rate. Fibrin sheath and thrombus can be seen better if the image is magnified and collimated over the catheter tip.

be slowly injected under fluoroscopy or digital imaging of the entire length of the catheter. Only a small amount of contrast is needed to visualize leakage into the soft tissues from a rupture of the catheter or to visualize a retrograde "backtracking" along the outer wall of the catheter caused by fibrin sheath or thrombus around the catheter. On the other hand, if the clinical history indicates PWO, a larger injection of contrast is necessary and imaging should focus on the catheter tip. Using a 20-mL syringe filled with contrast, injection should be done as rapidly as possible with images of the catheter tip obtained at a rapid filming rate of two or three frames per second. Use of the 20-mL syringe should eliminate the risk of catheter rupture because of the low-pressure injection generated by this syringe. The contrast should be flushed from the catheter as soon as possible and the catheter blocked with heparin to avoid thrombosis.

HELPFUL HINT
In patients with a history of allergic reaction to iodinated contrast or in patients with renal insufficiency but who are not on dialysis, gadolinium with digital subtraction imaging may be used as an alternative to iodinated contrast.

It is our opinion that a catheter injection with imaging should be performed every time a catheter exchange is performed. Venous thrombosis must be diagnosed if a new catheter is to be placed. It is especially important to check catheters placed by other services before exchange is performed to ensure adequate intravenous location of the catheter to avoid serious complications (Fig. 11–3).

CATHETER CHECK: FINDINGS OF PERSISTENT WITHDRAWAL OCCLUSION

The angiographic signs of fibrin sheath at the catheter tip are variable and are often difficult to interpret. The "classic" well-described signs include the following:

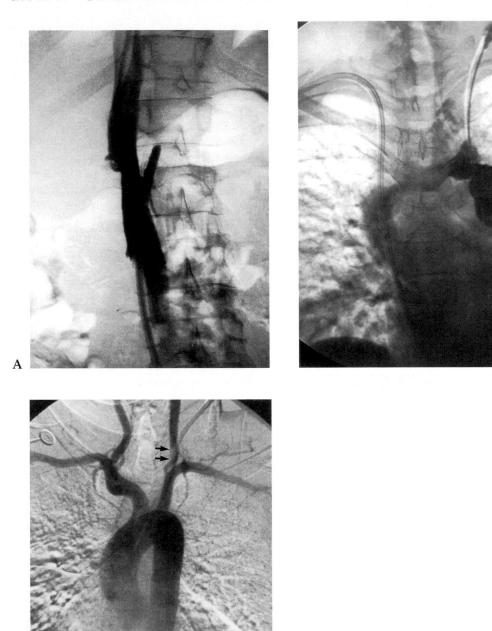

Figure 11–3 Several examples of why a catheter check should be performed before catheter exchange over a guidewire is done. **(A)** The inferior vena cava (IVC) catheter was found to be outside of the IVC, either through the IVC wall or in a small side branch of the IVC. **(B)** Contrast injection of a surgically placed malfunctioning catheter revealed extravasation caused by the extraluminal position of the catheter tip. **(C)** A permacath placed at another hospital had malfunctioned and bled for more than a month, and we were asked to exchange the catheter. Contrast injection, however, showed the catheter to be intra-arterial. Thrombus was present at the entrance site in the left common carotid artery (*arrows*). The vascular surgeons removed the catheter by a cut-down to protect the carotid artery distribution, and the common carotid artery was thrombectomized. If this catheter had been exchanged over a wire, the thrombus would likely have embolized to the brain.

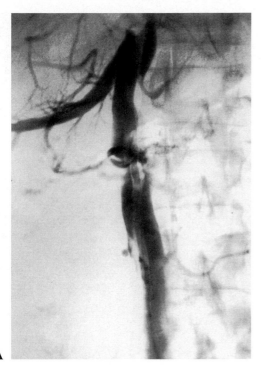

A

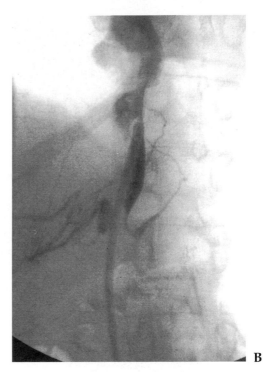

B

Figure 11–4 (A, B) Appearance of fibrin sheath. Filling defects are seen surrounding the catheter tips. A "halo" can be appreciated around the catheter.

- Filling defects associated with either port of the catheter (Fig. 11–4)
- Reflux of contrast material along the proximal shaft of the catheter with efflux from defects in the fibrin sleeve (Fig. 11–5)
- Excessive ejection of contrast from side holes when injecting the proximal port
- Lack of contrast material jet flowing into the right atrium (RA) (Fig. 11–6)

It is quite possible, however, that the angiogram done to check the catheter may not show any abnormality. As stated, interpretation of the study is often difficult because of motion of the catheter caused by cardiac motion and because the sleeve of fibrin can be thin and difficult to see. If no problems are found (kinking, malposition, thrombus, or obvious fibrin sheath) in a patient with PWO, fibrin sheath at the tip can be assumed to be the cause of catheter malfunction and should be treated accordingly.

The findings of thrombus formation at the catheter tip depend on the amount of the thrombus. If nonocclusive thrombus is present, a filling defect or defects should be evident on the angiogram, adhering to the catheter or the wall of the vein (Fig. 11–7). At the other end of the spectrum, the entire SVC may be thrombosed. In this case, one often sees retrograde flow into the azygous arch and azygous vein draining to below the diaphragm, into the inferior vena cava (IVC) (Fig. 11–8).

TREATMENT

Early Catheter Malfunction

Catheters must be inserted correctly to function satisfactorily. Catheter malfunction within the first several days of placement is usually due to improper catheter tip position, subcutaneous kinking, or extrinsic compression resulting from excessive tightening of sutures or fixation devices around

213

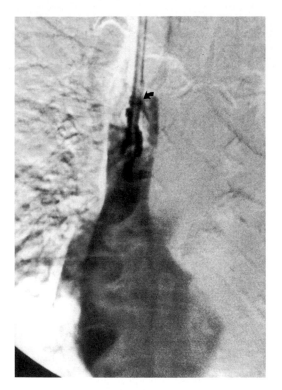

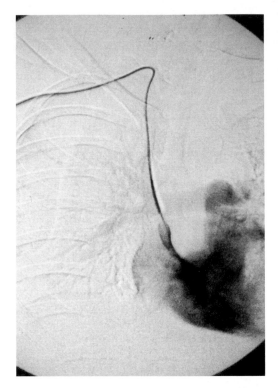

Figure 11–5 Appearance of fibrin sheath. Contrast refluxes along the catheter, within the fibrin sheath, until it effluxes through a defect in the sheath (*arrow*).

Figure 11–6 Appearance of fibrin sheath. The contrast fills a fibrin sheath extending from the tip of the catheter, causing a "wind sock" appearance.

the catheter. Finally, a new catheter placed into existing thrombus or fibrin sheath, which is a residual from a previously placed catheter, will malfunction early.

Suture Constriction

Sutures or fixation devices that impinge on the lumen of the catheter should be removed and a new suture or fixation device placed. Great care must be taken when removing the sutures to avoid cutting the catheter. Removal is done as follows:

1. With an assistant applying counter-resistance to the catheter, firmly grasp and pull the knot with pick-ups or a clamp.
2. Use a scalpel or scissors to cut the knot as close to the catheter as possible without cutting the catheter. One need not cut against the catheter because

suture material with "memory" will unravel when the knot is cut. For example, if the knot has been tied with three or four throws, attempt to cut between the first and second throws (closest to the catheter), which should allow unraveling of the final throw. This process may need to be repeated if more than one knot was tied.
3. Place a new suture or fixation device.

Catheter Kinking

Catheter kinking is frequently the result of a venous puncture too high in the neck or the result of improper subcutaneous tunneling, which results in too acute of an angle at the venous entry site (Fig. 11–9). Placing a guidewire can straighten the kink for temporary relief only; the kink often will reappear when the guidewire is removed because the underlying

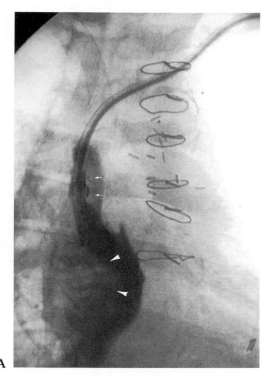
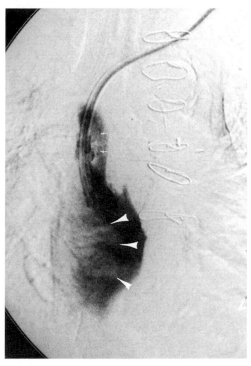

A

B

Figure 11–7 (A, B) Fibrin sheath and thrombus are seen as filling defects along the catheter (*small arrows*) with a large thrombus extending into the right atrium (*arrowheads*).

problem (poor tunneling or poor access site) has not been corrected. Likewise, catheter exchange over a guidewire is unlikely to solve the problem because, even though a new catheter has been placed, the underlying problem of poor tunnel angulation is still present. The best solution is either placement of a new catheter de novo or retunneling using the same venous puncture site (Fig. 11–10). The retunneling procedure is done as follows:

1. After sterile preparation, use a no. 10 or no. 15 scalpel to reopen the incision at the venous entry site.
2. Use a clamp to retrieve the catheter at the incision.
3. Clamp the catheter and cut on the subcutaneous tunnel side of the catheter (i.e., away from the vein).
4. Advance a guidewire through the venous segment of the catheter, which is removed over the guidewire.

5. Insert a peel-away sheath of the appropriate size over the guidewire.
6. Remove the remaining catheter from the subcutaneous tunnel.
7. Create a new subcutaneous tunnel so that the angulation at the venous entry site is less acute.
8. Then insert the catheter in the usual fashion.

Placement of a new catheter can be performed at a different access site or in the same vein. The latter technique is useful when the original venous puncture was too high in the neck, causing catheter kinking and malfunction. Replacement of the catheter via the same venous puncture site may not resolve the problem associated with the catheter, and it is usually better to perform a new puncture, lower in the neck, under sonographic guidance or under fluoroscopic guidance using the indwelling catheter as a landmark (Fig. 11–11). This can be performed even if the vein is thrombosed.

215

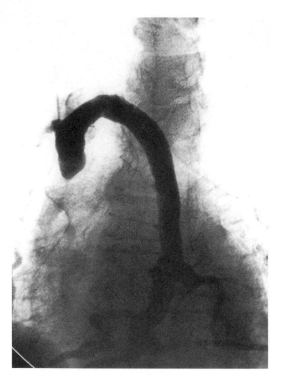

Figure 11–8 There is complete thrombosis of the superior vena cava (SVC) with collateral flow into the azygous arch.

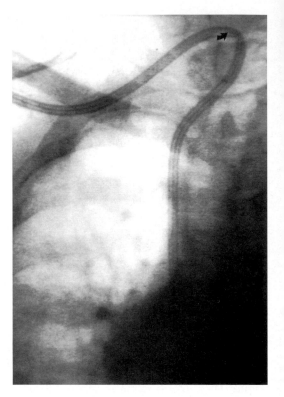

Figure 11–9 Catheter kink. The catheter is kinked at the transition between the subcutaneous tunnel and the venous entry site (*arrow*). Kinking is often caused by a venous puncture too high in the neck and poor tunneling causing an acute turn at the venous entry site.

1. Magnify the image to allow easier puncture of the vein using the catheter as a target.
2. Puncture the skin directly over the catheter with the needle at approximately 45 degrees.
3. Advance the needle, always staying superimposed over the catheter until the needle tip hits the catheter. Alternatively, ultrasound can be used to image the vein below the previous access site.
4. The guidewire then should advance into the vein.
5. Once the micropuncture dilator has been placed, the indwelling catheter can be removed, hemostasis obtained, and the new catheter placed in the usual fashion.

Catheter Misplacement

The most common cause of early catheter malfunction is misplacement of the catheter,[8] which is more likely to occur if the catheter was inserted without image guidance (Fig. 11–12). Migration of the catheter tip can occur soon after placement, however, especially in large patients (especially obese females) when using the subclavian approach (Fig. 11–13). It is not unusual for the catheter to be pulled back several centimeters when the patient sits up because the tunneled portion of the catheter is pulled down with the soft tissues of the chest. A catheter that was thought to be in a perfect position in the RA in the supine position can suddenly migrate to an inadequate position, possibly with the catheter tip against the vein wall. Furthermore, catheters placed in good position can become misplaced after

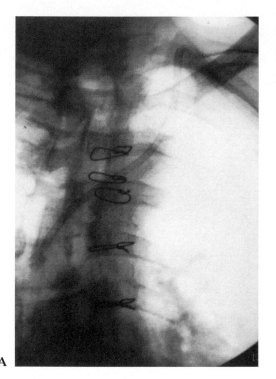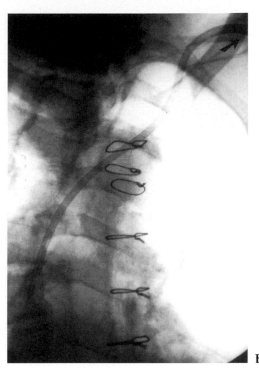

A   B

Figure 11–10 **(A)** The catheter is kinked because of the acute turn made by the tunnel. **(B)** The same venous entry was used, but a new tunnel was created resulting in a less acute angle at the venous entry site (*arrow*).

days or weeks. Sometimes, catheters located at the SVC–RA junction can migrate into the contralateral innominate vein, the azygous arch, or the jugular vein. In such cases of spontaneous migration of the catheter tip, it is best to replace the catheter, either de novo or over a guidewire with a longer one. If the catheter is simply repositioned, it will again migrate and become misplaced.

Nontunneled catheters are frequently placed by operators without image guidance; therefore, there is a high rate of misplacement. Misplacement is more common in patients who have had multiple previous central venous catheters and have central venous thrombosis or stenosis and distortion of the venous anatomy.[8] A catheter angiogram should be performed to evaluate venous patency. If the central veins are patent, the catheter can be repositioned by direct manipulation with a guidewire. Occasionally, a forceful injection of contrast or saline can reposition the catheter tip, although caution must be taken not to damage the catheter, especially small-caliber ones. Guidewire manipulation must be performed under strict sterile conditions. It is suggested that a new catheter be placed over the guidewire instead of advancing the indwelling catheter, which may introduce infection.

Replacement of a peripherally inserted central catheter (PICC) is done by withdrawal of the existing catheter, which is cut and replaced over a guidewire (from the kit of the new PICC). The wire is used to insert a peel-away sheath, and the PICC is placed in the usual fashion. When placement of a PICC into the central veins is difficult because of tortuosity or venous stenoses, a 0.018-inch glidewire can be advanced to facilitate placement and the catheter advanced over the wire.

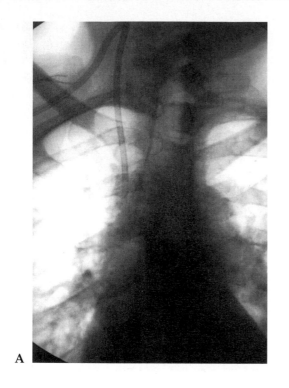

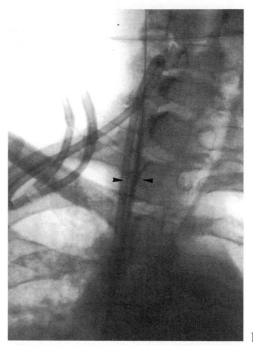

Figure 11–11 **(A)** The catheter is kinked because entry into the vein is too high in the neck. **(B)** The same jugular vein was punctured lower in the neck and a new sheath was placed (*arrowheads*). **(C)** The lower venous puncture was used to place a new catheter, and the old catheter was removed.

Misplaced tunneled catheters that are too short or too long need to be replaced over a guidewire for a catheter of the appropriate length (Fig. 11–14). Catheters of predetermined length can be replaced, based on the length of the existing catheter and making

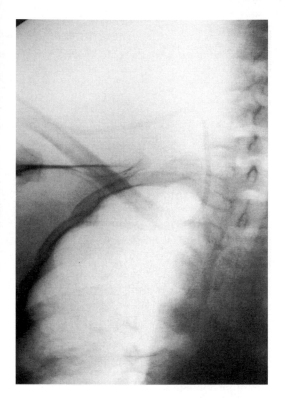

Figure 11–12 A right internal jugular vein catheter, which was placed without image guidance, was left with the tip in the right subclavian vein. This catheter could be repositioned by pulling it into the superior vena cava from a femoral approach.

the appropriate length adjustments (Figs. 11–14 and 11–15). Catheters that need to be trimmed (not predetermined length)

must be measured by placing a guidewire through the lumen and measuring the appropriate change needed in catheter length.

1. If the catheter is too short, for example, advance the wire through the catheter, and place the tip of the wire at the desired catheter tip position in the RA.
2. Place a clamp on the wire at the catheter hub.
3. Then pull the wire back until the tip of the wire is at the tip of the indwelling catheter.
4. Place another clamp on the wire at the hub of the catheter. The distance between the two clamps on the wire is the alteration needed in catheter length.
5. Remove the indwelling catheter over the guidewire and use the old catheter to measure the new catheter either adding or subtracting the needed length of catheter.
6. The new catheter then can be inserted over the guidewire.

Misplaced tunneled catheters of adequate length can be repositioned using several methods from a femoral approach with use of a pigtail catheter, a loop snare, or a tip-deflecting wire, or a combination of these devices. A pigtail catheter is advanced from a femoral vein

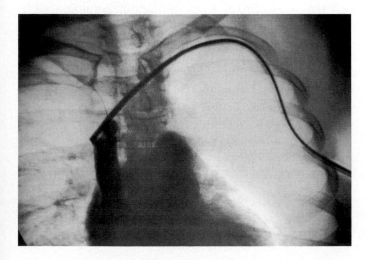

Figure 11–13 The left subclavian vein catheter was originally placed with the catheter tip in the distal superior vena cava (SVC). The catheter malfunctioned and was shown to have been pulled back; the tip is now against the SVC wall.

219

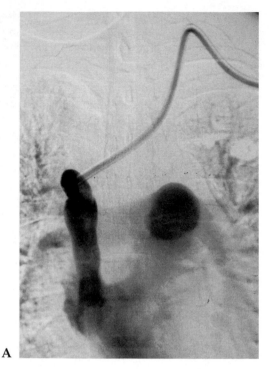
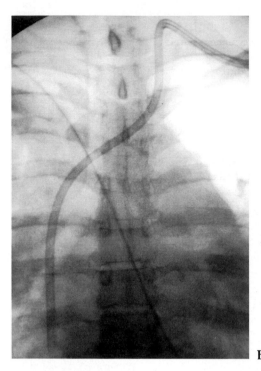

A   **B**

Figure 11–14   A recently placed dialysis catheter was malfunctioning. A catheter check showed the catheter was too short and the tip of the catheter was against the wall of the superior vena cava (SVC) **(A)**. Catheter exchange was performed over guide wires with placement of a longer catheter **(B)**.

approach to a position cephalad to the misplaced catheter. The pigtail catheter then is pulled down and rotated to encircle the malpositioned catheter and to pull it into the appropriate position. If the maneuver fails to reposition the catheter, more rigidity is provided by inserting a standard guidewire or tip-deflecting wire into the pigtail catheter. If this step does not work (which can happen with large-bore misplaced catheters or if the catheter tip is wedged in a small vein or thrombus), greater force can be applied by introducing a loop snare, snaring the guidewire and pulling both the guidewire and the snare loop at the same time. A misplaced catheter can be repositioned with an Amplatz gooseneck snare loop if the tip of the misplaced catheter is free within the vein (Fig. 11–16).

1. Place a femoral venous sheath and advance the guiding catheter over a guidewire into the vein where the tip of the misplaced catheter is located.
2. Remove the guidewire and advance the snare loop through the guiding catheter. The loop size should be chosen to open completely within the target vein.
3. Open the loop above the misplaced catheter tip.
4. Pull back the snare until the catheter is encircled.
5. Tighten the snare by advancing the guiding catheter over the snare wire until the snare is tightened.
6. Tension is maintained on the snare wire and guiding catheter, which are pulled into the RA, pulling the catheter tip into the proper position. Passage of a guidewire through the misplaced catheter may facilitate snaring.

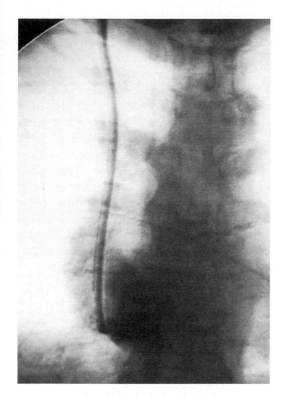

Figure 11–15 This dialysis catheter was too long, and the tip was against the wall of the right atrium. The catheter was exchanged for a shorter catheter.

Late Catheter Malfunction

Late catheter malfunction refers to catheters that initially worked well but eventually malfunctioned. The most common presentation is PWO. This may be a nuisance in smaller catheters meant primarily for infusion (portacaths, 9 F Hickman, Broviac, etc.) in that there is ability to infuse but inability to aspirate. On the other hand, large-bore catheters that require high flow for pheresis or hemodialysis can be rendered unusable by PWO. Causes of late catheter malfunction include catheter thrombosis, fibrin sheath formation, venous thrombosis, and, less commonly, catheter tip migration or catheter leakage.

Catheter Tip Migration

A catheter tip that was placed in the SVC can spontaneously become repositioned into the contralateral innominate vein, azygous vein, or jugular vein (Fig. 11–17). The catheter may malfunction because the tip is against the vein wall. Vein thrombosis is a frequent accompanying complication, especially if sclerosing materials such as total parenteral nutrition (TPN) or chemotherapeutic agents are being infused through the malpositioned catheter. Migration most commonly occurs when catheters are too short and is best treated by replacement with a longer catheter rather than repositioning the misplaced catheter.

Catheter Occlusion

Occlusion of the catheter is due most frequently to thrombus formation within the catheter. This complication possibly is due to inadequate blocking or flushing of the catheter with heparin when the catheter is not in use. Catheter thrombosis also may occur when infusions are allowed to run dry, allowing blood to back up into the catheter and thrombose. Infused blood products, if allowed to become stagnant in the catheter, also can thrombose. Other less common causes of catheter occlusion, suchas precipitation of medications and TPN, are discussed elsewhere (Chapter 12).

Thrombus within the catheter usually presents as an inability to infuse and aspirate rather than the classic PWO. Therapy for catheter occlusion is discussed in Chapter 12. The thrombolytic agent is injected and allowed to dwell in the catheter for 30 to 60 minutes to lyse the clot. The thrombolytic agent can be injected with a 5- or 10-mL syringe in a forceful to-and-fro action. Even if totally occluded, the soft Silastic or silicone catheter is compliant and will expand slightly with injection, allowing the thrombolytic agent to infiltrate the catheter around the thrombus and permeate the clot. Smaller syringes (1 or 3 mL) should not be used because the high pressure generated by these syringes can rupture the catheter. Historically, the agent used for thrombosed catheters was urokinase 5000 U (Opencath); and this is being reintroduced. Tissue plasminogen activator (tPA) 2 mg/mL or Retavase 0.5 U in 2 mL are now also available. After allowing the thrombolytic agent to dwell in the catheter for up to an hour, a large syringe (50–60 mL) is used to attempt to aspirate the thrombolytic agent and any residual clot. If aspiration is unsuccessful, flushing is attempted, again taking care not to rupture the catheter. If aspiration is still unsuccessful, the process of injecting a thrombolytic agent can be repeated several times.

Thrombolysis to open a malfunctioning catheter is easy and can be done in the dialysis unit, by nurses in the patient's room, in clinics, or at home by a visiting nurse. Thrombolytic agents are 81 to 95% successful at opening catheters,[2,4,9] but they do not provide long-term patency because the malfunction is frequently due to fibrin sheath around the catheter tip or venous thrombosis. If the thrombolytic therapy fails, radiologic evaluation and treatment are warranted.

Fibrin Sheath

Fibrin sheath formation is the most common cause of catheter malfunction. Venous catheters may lose functional patency when an encasing sleeve of fibrin acts like a ball valve, which allows infusion but prevents aspiration (i.e., PWO). This encasement of the catheter results in decreased flow, which precludes successful completion of hemodialysis.[10] This process reportedly complicates the use of nearly one half the large-bore hemodialysis catheters implanted.[9] Hoshal and colleagues[11] found fibrin accumulation around catheters as early as 24 hours and that all catheters were encased with fibrin sheath by 5 to 7 days. This study described the ubiquitous nature of fibrin sheath, found at autopsy in 100% of 55 patients with central venous catheters.

The fibrin sheath initially forms at sites of intimal damage, including the venous puncture sites and sites where catheters touched vessel walls. The sheath propagates from the sites of intimal injury to encase the entire catheter. The sheath usually is perforated along its course,

allowing infused fluids to enter the bloodstream at several points, but when negative pressure is applied to the catheter, the fibrin sheath prevents aspiration of blood in a one-way valve-like action. Histologically, the sheath consists of platelets and fibrin with a few red blood cells and polymorphonucleocytes. When catheters were removed, a "wind sock" of contrast-filled fibrin sheath (Fig. 11–18) was demonstrated in 40% of patients.[11,12] During catheter removal, part of the fibrin sheath often becomes detached and embolized to the pulmonary arteries. Fortunately, this rarely results in symptomatic pulmonary embolus (PE).

Treatment Options

Malfunctioning catheters with PWO or complete occlusion should be treated initially with low-dose thrombolysis as described. Function can be reestablished in as many as 74 to 95%.[2,4,9] In most cases, this therapy is ineffective and does not provide long-term patency. If low-dose thrombolytic agents do not reestablish catheter function or, if malfunction recurs, the patient should be managed by the catheter service. Traditionally, the treatment of a malfunctioning catheter consisted of catheter removal and placement of a new catheter at a different venous site.[4] Because venous access sites can become quickly depleted, however, a de novo catheter insertion is not optimal. The vascular and interventional radiologist now has several treatment options, including stripping, catheter exchange over a guidewire, exchange with angioplasty, disruption of the sheath with a tip-deflecting wire and thrombolysis. There is no agreement as to which method is better. We believe that the optimal therapy depends on the clinical circumstances; therefore, the venous catheter service should be familiar with all treatment options.

Catheter Stripping

Stripping removes the fibrin sheath from the catheter mechanically by tightening

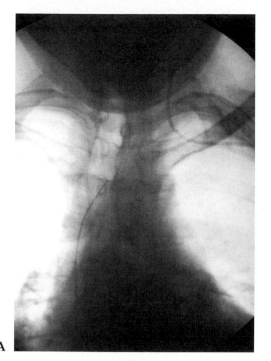
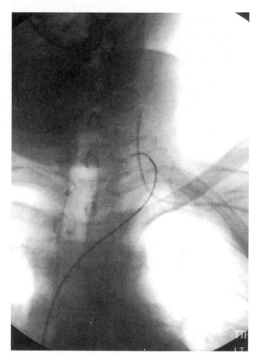

A   B

Figure 11–16 **(A)** A left subclavian vein catheter was placed without image guidance and was left with the tip in the left internal jugular (IJ) vein. A guidewire is seen passing through the right atrium and superior vena cava (SVC) from a femoral approach. **(B)** The catheter and guidewire have been advanced into the left IJ vein. (*Continued*) **(C)** The Amplatz gooseneck snare encircled the catheter and has been tightened. **(D)** The loop snare pulled the catheter into the SVC.

and pulling a snare down the shaft of the catheter. The fibrin sheath becomes dislodged and embolizes into the pulmonary arteries. This is a well-tolerated event, with sporadic cases reported of symptomatic PE. Contraindications include patients with known right-to-left shunt or with severe cardiopulmonary disease that would not tolerate a small PE.[13] The procedure should be performed only if the indwelling catheter is in adequate position with the catheter tip in the RA or at the junction of the SVC with the RA (otherwise, it would be best to exchange the catheter to place the new catheter in adequate position).

1. Using a femoral venous access, place a 6 F vascular sheath.
2. Advance a 6 F snare-guiding catheter into the RA or SVC.
3. Advance the Amplatz loop snare wire (Microvena, White Bear Lake, MN, U.S.A.) through the tip of the guiding catheter until the loop opens.
4. Snaring the catheter can be facilitated by inserting a guidewire through the catheter to be stripped and advancing the wire into the inferior vena cava, where snaring is easier.
5. Encircle the wire and use it as a monorail to advance the snare over the catheter as cephalad as possible in the innominate vein (Fig. 11–19A).
6. Tighten the snare (Fig. 11–19B) and slowly withdraw it off the catheter (Fig. 11–19C). The snare must be tight enough to strip fibrin but should not be tightened excessively because it could damage the catheter or make it difficult to pull the snare over the catheter.
7. Repeat this process 5 to 15 times.[13] If the guidewire is left in place in the catheter with the wire tip in the inferior vena

223

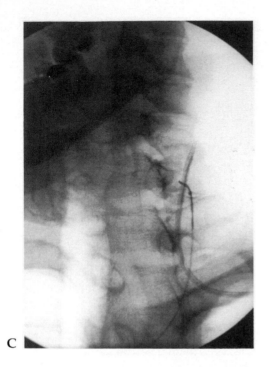

C

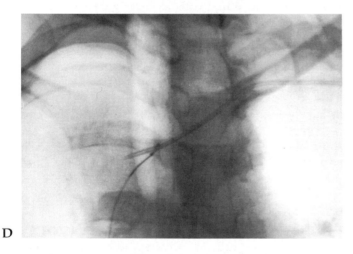

D

Figure 11–16 (*Continued*)

cava, the wire and catheter do not need to be resnared multiple times but only advanced over the wire and catheter into the innominate vein each time.

Results *Technical success,* defined as the ability to easily aspirate and inject both ports of the catheter with a 60-mL syringe, has been achieved in 95 to 100% of cases.[2,3,13–15] The duration of patency varies. Haskal and colleagues[14] reported technical success

in 22 procedures; however, 20 of 22 catheters had no improved flow (the beneficial effect was lost) after five hemodialysis sessions. Other studies, however, have reported greater patency following fibrin sheath stripping.[3,13,15] Brady and colleagues[13] reported a median duration of poststripping patency of 3 months, and 52 of 91 catheters were still functioning when they were removed. Likewise, Crain and associates[3] reported a patency of 45% at 3 months and

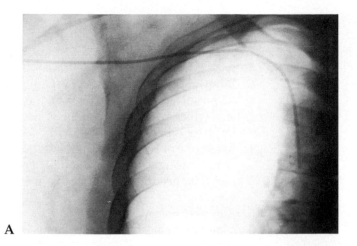

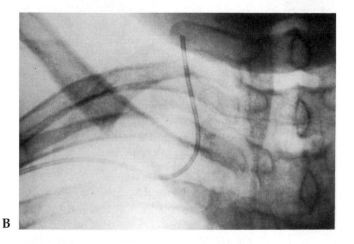

Figure 11–17 **(A)** A peripherally inserted central catheter (PICC) was placed in good position with the tip at the junction of the superior vena cava and the right atrium. One month later **(B)**, the PICC had "flipped" into the right internal jugular vein, which had thrombosed.

28% at 6 months with a median added patency of 2.8 months. Furthermore, repeated percutaneous fibrin sheath stripping procedures for recurrent functional occlusion can be performed and extended the patency to 83% at 3 months and to 72% at 6 months after the first procedure.[3] These investigators concluded that the ultimate result of percutaneous fibrin sheath stripping was a significant prolongation of catheter patency, from date of placement (catheter secondary patency) to 90% at 6 months and 81% at 1 year, which compares to the published patency of permacaths of 65 to 74% at 1 year.[9,16] That is, percutaneous fibrin sheath stripping can provide patency as good as placing a new catheter de novo. Similar results were achieved by Suhocki and colleagues.[2]

The disadvantages are the femoral puncture and its complications. The patient is required to lie flat in bedrest for 4 hours following the procedure, which is inconvenient for the patient and dialysis unit and can result in hospital costs approaching $1000.[6] Puncturing the femoral vein also risks formation of venous stenosis or deep vein thrombosis. Crain and coworkers[3] reported a femoral deep vein thrombosis following a catheter-stripping procedure, which is especially important in dialysis patients because the groin may be needed for future vascular access.

Catheter Exchange
The guidewire exchange procedure is another method to salvage malfunctioning, noninfected catheters and preserve venous

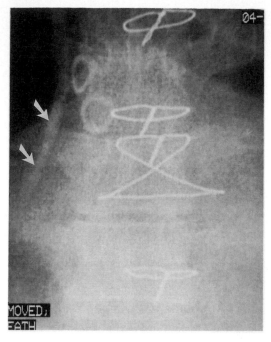

Figure 11–18 A "wind sock" of fibrin sheath. Contrast was injected through a catheter, revealing fibrin sheath encasing the catheter (not shown). Following catheter removal, the contrast-filled fibrin sheath remained in place (*arrows*) in the superior vena cava.

1. Prepare the skin site and the external portion of the catheter sterilely.
2. Anesthetize the exit site and the tunnel with lidocaine with epinephrine.
3. Bluntly dissect the cuff(s) by passing a hemostat along the catheter at the exit site, which results in the catheter becoming freely mobile.
4. Insert one or two hydrophilic stiff guidewires through the catheter (Fig. 11–20) and advance it or them into the inferior vena cava.
5. Remove the catheter.
6. Maintain hemostasis at the venous entry site.
7. An assistant places the new catheter on the two wires.
8. The wires are "pinned" and the catheter advanced through the tunnel and into the vein (Fig. 11–20C). Difficulty can be encountered as the blunt catheter enters the vein. The use of two guidewires makes this maneuver easier. Twisting and rotating the catheter may also facilitate entry into the vein.

When the catheter has been removed, the fibrin sheath detaches and embolizes to the lungs in most instances, but not always. It is not unusual for a "wind sock" fibrin sheath to remain. Therefore, just placing a new catheter into the residual sheath would cause the new catheter to malfunction. It is necessary to place the new catheter outside the culprit fibrin sheath either by advancing the catheter tip further into the RA or by exiting the fibrin sheath with the guidewire(s) before the new catheter is introduced.[6]

access sites. Multiple variations of this technique include guidewire exchange using the existing subcutaneous tract, with or without balloon dilatation, to macerate the residual fibrin sheath and cut-down at the venous entry site to exchange catheters with creation of a new subcutaneous tract.

Using the Existing Subcutaneous Tunnel This should be performed only when the existing subcutaneous tunnel is adequate. There should be no or minimal erythema at the skin exit site and no drainage from the tunnel. The length of the tunnel and angulation of the catheter at the venous entry site must be acceptable. If catheter exchange is performed through an inadequate subcutaneous tunnel, the new catheter will inherit the problems of the old catheter.

Exchange and Balloon Maceration Catheter exchange is fruitless if the new catheter is placed into the culprit fibrin sheath. Efforts can be taken to place the new catheter tip outside of the fibrin sheath, or the fibrin sheath can be fragmented and macerated with balloon dilatation using a large (10–14 mm) balloon.

The initial steps of catheter removal over a guidewire are the same as described for

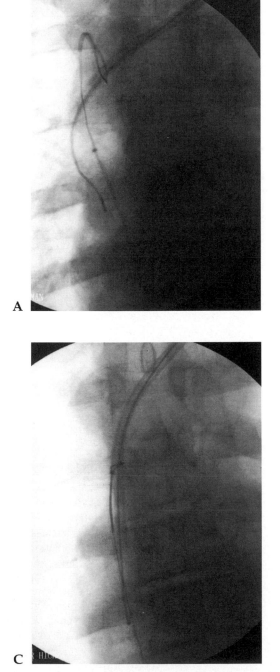

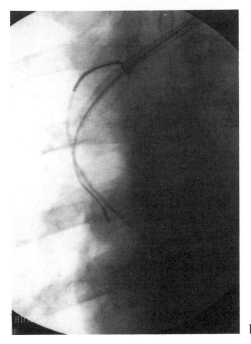

Figure 11–19 (A) The loop snare was advanced over the catheter as far cephalad as possible. Note the guidewire through the catheter to facilitate encircling the catheter. **(B)** The snare was tightened around the catheter. **(C)** While maintaining tension with the loop snare around the catheter, the snare is pulled off the catheter.

guidewire exchange of catheters (Fig. 11–21A). Instead of placing a new catheter over the guidewire, however, a long 12 or 13 F vascular sheath is advanced over the guidewire into the innominate vein (Fig. 11–21B).

The sheath should be large enough to tamponade bleeding from the venous entry site. The sheath may kink, but the balloon catheter still can be advanced because of the large diameter of the sheath. A large 10- to

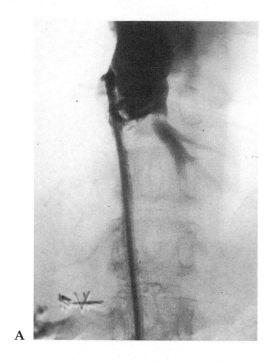

A

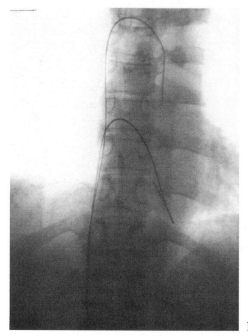

B

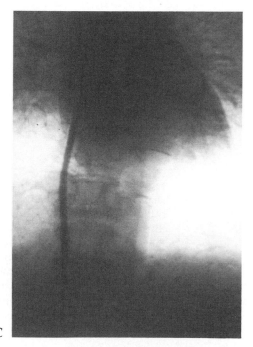

C

Figure 11–20 (A) Contrast injection through an inferior vena cava (IVC) catheter shows fibrin sheath at the catheter tip, which lies at the junction of the IVC and the right atrium. **(B)** Two stiff hydrophilic wires were advanced through the catheter, which was removed over the wires. **(C)** A new, longer catheter was advanced over the wires and positioned with the tip in the right atrium.

14-mm balloon is inflated to fragment the fibrin sheath, which should still surround the guidewire (Fig. 11–21C). Several short inflations are made throughout the RA and SVC. Care should be taken to avoid overdilating the innominate vein. A venogram can be done through the vascular sheath to assess results. A second wire can be inserted through the vascular sheath (Fig. 11–21D), the sheath removed, and a

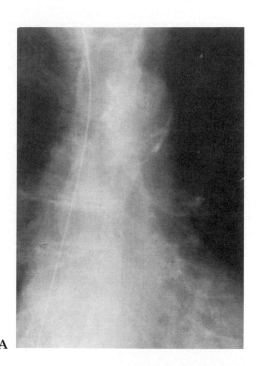

A

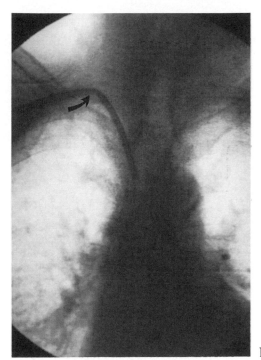

B

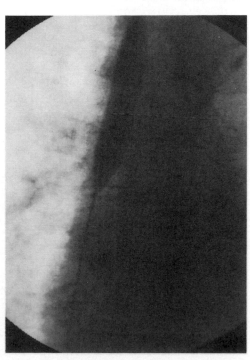

C

Fig. 11–21 A guidewire is placed through the existing catheter (A), which is removed. A long vascular sheath is advanced through the tunnel into the vein over the wire (B). Note that the sheath is kinked (*arrow*), but this does not prevent advancement of the balloon catheter. The balloon is inflated throughout the superior vena cava and right atrium (C). (*Continued*) A second wire can be advanced through the sheath to facilitate passage of the new catheter (D). The sheath is removed, and the new catheter (E) is placed over the wire(s).

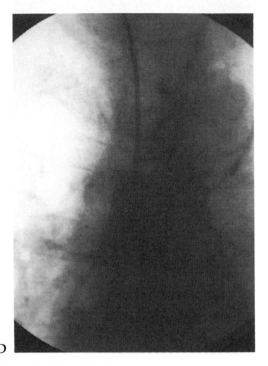

D

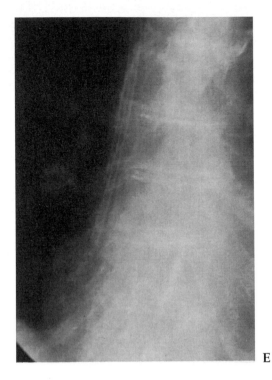

E

Figure 11–21 (*Continued*)

new permacath placed over the two wires (Fig. 11–21E).

Exchange via Cut-Down at the Venous Entry Site Catheter exchange can be performed over a guidewire with creation of a new subcutaneous tract. This technique is used when the existing subcutaneous tunnel is inadequate (because of inflammation, inadequate length, inadequate angulation, and so on), keeping the same venous entry site.

1. After routine preparation of the skin and catheter, anesthetize the tunnel, the skin exit site, and the venous entry site.
2. Make a skin incision at the venous entry site with a no. 10 or no. 15 blade. Usually, this incision corresponds to the scar of the incision made at the original catheter placement.
3. With blunt dissection using a forceps, identify the catheter in the subcutaneous tissue, grab it, and exteriorize it.

4. Clamp the catheter with the forceps at this site.
5. Using scissors, cut the catheter.
6. Advance a guidewire through the intravenous fragment of catheter, and remove the catheter.
7. Insert a peel-away sheath appropriate to the new catheter over the wire.
8. Then remove the remaining portion of catheter within the tunnel using blunt dissection to free the fixation cuff.
9. Make a new subcutaneous tunnel.
10. Place a new catheter.

Exchange via Cut-Down at the Venous Entry Site and Balloon Fragmentation
A new catheter never should be placed in the fibrin sheath "wind sock" of an old catheter. The described technique of cut-down, retrieval, and cutting the catheter can be performed, but instead of immediately placing the peel-away sheath over the guidewire, a 12 to 14 F short vascular sheath can be placed and balloon dilatation per-

formed through the sheath as previously described to fragment the residual fibrin sheath. The vascular sheath then is exchanged for a peel-away sheath, a new subcutaneous tunnel is created, and a new catheter is placed.

Results Only the method of guidewire exchange through the existing tunnel (without balloon inflations) has been well described in the literature.[6,17,18] Duszak and colleagues[6] found no difference in infection rates between de novo catheter placement and exchanged catheters, concluding that exchanging catheters through pre-existing tunnels carries no increased risk of infection if performed with the same sterile technique of the initial de novo catheter insertion. Catheters placed de novo in this study reportedly had 1.5 infections per 1000 catheter days compared with 1.1 infections per 1000 catheter days in the exchanged catheters. Likewise, function was not significantly different. The longevity of exchanged catheters in this report compared favorably with the reported primary patency following percutaneous fibrin sheath stripping. The primary patency was 51 and 37% at 3 and 6 months, respectively, compared with 45 and 28%, respectively, following percutaneous fibrin sheath stripping.[3] An advantage of the guidewire exchange technique is that a femoral venous puncture is not necessary (as in percutaneous fibrin sheath stripping), and therefore no bedrest is required following the procedure.

Thrombolytic Infusion
Thrombolysis is the least invasive means of restoring patency caused by fibrin sheath. No new venous puncture is required, and the venous access site is salvaged. The technique is atraumatic, requiring no dissection or creation of new subcutaneous tract. The drawback is the time needed for infusion and the cost of the thrombolytic agents. Numerous infusion regimens have been reported[4,9,19–22] using urokinase or streptokinase. Available thrombolytic agents are tPA or Retavase (alteplase). Urokinase is

about to be re-introduced. Protocols vary, but an accepted infusion is 0.5 mg tPA per port per hour (1.0 mg per hour) for 4 to 6 hours or 0.25 U of Retavase per port per hour for 4 to 6 hours. Urokinase can be infused at 100,000 units per hour per port, over 4 hours. These low doses allow lysis of the fibrin at the catheter without systemic fibrinolysis and the resultant bleeding complications. Larger doses may be used, or overnight infusions have been used. Dilution of the thrombolytic agent should be such that at least 5 mL per hour is infused through each lumen. For instance, tPA at 0.1 mg/mL could be infused at 10 mL per hour for a dose of 1 mg per hour. The larger volume of infusion is thought to allow greater distribution of the agent within the fibrin sheath.

Thrombolysis is 95% effective in salvage of functional patency.[20–22] There are, however, few reports of long-term patency following thrombolysis. Gray[23] reported a prospective, randomized trial that compared percutaneous fibrin sheath stripping with infusion of urokinase into malfunctioning catheters. The primary patency following percutaneous fibrin sheath stripping at 30 and 45 days was 50 and 33%, respectively. The primary patency of catheters following infusion of urokinase at 30 days and 45 days was 67 and 37%, respectively. No significant difference between the two methods was found.

Other Treatment Options
Knelson and colleagues[24] described the simple technique of placing a tip-deflecting wire into the catheter so that the curved tip just exited the tip of the catheter. The wire then is rotated in repeated 360-degree angles. This action reportedly removes the fibrin sheath from the tip of the catheter. Other researchers have reported advancing a ureteral brush through catheters to disrupt the fibrin sheath at the tip. Neither of these techniques has been evaluated in a large study to establish catheter patency following the procedures. Both techniques treat only the fibrin sheath at the catheter tip, implying

that recurrent occlusion from sheath "regrowth" can occur in a short period.

SUMMARY

The ubiquitous nature of fibrin sheath formation causing catheter malfunction has been well documented. Numerous techniques have been described to deal with this problem, but none has been shown to be superior. With all treatments described for fibrin sheath, the fibrin sheath will re-form and cause catheter malfunction. New techniques are constantly being developed, and evaluation of the efficacy of the various techniques is ongoing. Until the perfect treatment for catheter malfunction due to fibrin sheath is found, it is important to be aware of all treatment options. Different techniques will be useful depending on the clinical situation.

REFERENCES

1. Fan PY, Shwab SJ. Vascular access: concepts for the 1990's. *J Am Soc Nephrol.* 1992; 3:1–11.

2. Suhocki PV, Conlon PJ, Knelson MH, Harland R, Schwab SJ. Silastic cuffed catheters for hemodialysis access: thrombolytic and mechanical correction of malfunction. *Am J Kidney Dis.* 1996;28:379–386.

3. Crain MR, Mewissen MW, Ostrowski GJ, Paz-Fumagalli R, Beres RA, Wertz RA. Fibrin sleeve stripping for salvage of failing hemodialysis catheters: technique and initial results. *Radiology.* 1996;198:41–44.

4. Schwab SJ, Buller GL, McCann RL, Bollinger RR, Stickel DL. Prospective evaluation of a Dacron cuffed hemodialysis catheter for prolonged use. *Am J Kidney Dis.* 1988;11: 166–169.

5. Cimochowski GE, Worley E, Rutherford WE, Sartain J, Blondin J, Harter H. Superiority of the internal jugular over the subclavian access for temporary hemodialysis. *Nephron.* 1990;54:154–161.

6. Duszak R, Haskal ZJ, Thomas-Hawkins C, et al. Replacement of failing tunneled hemodialysis catheters through pre-existing subcutaneous tunnels: a comparison of catheter

function and infection rates for de novo placements and over-the-wire exchanges. *J Vasc Interv Radiol.* 1998;9:321–327.

7. Deitel M, McIntyre JA. Radiographic confirmation of central venous catheters. *Can J Surg.* 1971;14:42–52.

8. Boardman P, Hughes JP. Radiological evaluation and management of malfunctioning central venous catheters. *Clin Radiol.* 1998;53: 708–709.

9. Moss AH, Vasiliakis C, Holley JL, Foulks CJ, Pillai K, McDowell DE. Use of a silicone dual-lumen catheter with a Dacron cuff as a long-term vascular access for hemodialysis patients. *Am J Kidney Dis.* 1990;16:211–215.

10. Schneider TC, Krzywda E, Andris D, Quebbeman EJ. The malfunctioning silastic catheter: radiologic assessment and treatment. *JPEN J Parenter Enteral Nutr.* 1986;10:70–73.

11. Hoshal VL, Ause RG, Hoskins PA. Fibrin sleeve formation on indwelling subclavian central venous catheters. *Arch Surg.* 1971; 102:353–358.

12. Brismar B, Hardstedt C, Jacobson S. Diagnosis of thrombosis by catheter phlebography after prolonged central venous catheterization. *Ann Surg.* 1981;779–783.

13. Brady PS, Spence LD, Levitin A, Mickolich CT, Dolmatch BL. Efficacy of percutaneous fibrin sheath stripping in restoring patency of tunneled hemodialysis catheters. *AJR Am J Roentgenol.* 1999;173:1023–1027.

14. Haskal ZJ, Leen VH, Thomas-Hawkins C, Shlansky-Goldberg RD, Baum RA, Soulen MC. Transvenous removal of fibrin sheaths from tunneled hemodialysis catheters. *J Vasc Invest Radiol.* 1996;7:513–517.

15. Rockall AG, Harris A, Wetton CWN, Taube D, Gedroye W, Al-Kutoubi MA. Stripping of failing hemodialysis catheters using the Amplatz gooseneck snare. *Clin Radiol.* 1997; 52:616–620.

16. Gibson SP, Mosquera DL. Five years' experience with the Quinton Permacath for vascular access. *Nephrol Dial Transplant.* 1991; 6:269–274.

17. Carlisle EJ, Blake P, McCarthy F, Vas S, Vidall R. Septicemia in long-term jugular hemodialysis catheters: eradicating infection by changing the catheter over a guide wire. *Int J Artif Organs.* 1991;14: 150–153.

18. Shaffer D. Catheter-related sepsis complicating long-term tunneled central venous dialysis catheters: management by guidewire exchange. *Am J Kidney Dis.* 1995;25:593–596.

19. Vogt K, Tillmann U, Blumberg A. Successful fibrinolysis in permanent hemodialysis catheter obstruction. *Nephron.* 1987; 45:174–175.

20. Zajko AB, Reilly JJ Jr, Bron KM, Desai R, Steed DL. Low-dose streptokinase for occluded Hickman catheters. *AJR Am J Roentgenol.* 1983;141:1311–1312.

21. Haire WD, Lieberman RP, Lund GB, Edney J, Wieczorek BM. Obstructed central venous catheters: restoring function with a 12-hour infusion of low-dose urokinase. *Cancer.* 1990;66:2279–2285.

22. Haire WD, Lieberman RP. Thrombosed central venous catheters: restoring function with 6-hour urokinase infusion after failure of bolus urokinase. *JPEN J Parenter Enteral Nutr.* 1992;16:129–132.

23. Gray RJ, Levitin A, Buck D, et al. Percutaneous fibrous sheath stripping versus transcatheter urokinase infusion for malfunctioning well-positioned tunneled central venous dialysis catheters: a prospective, randomized trial. *J Vasc Interv Radiol.* 2000;11:1121–1129.

24. Knelson MH, Hudson ER, Suhocki PV, Payne CS, Sallee DS, Newman GE. Functional restoration of occluded central venous catheters: new interventional techniques. *J Vasc Interv Radiol.* 1995;6:623–627.

Chapter 12

Catheter Care

Philip C. Pieters
Melinda Pyle
Jaime Tisnado

This chapter discusses primarily the nursing tasks that need to be carried out long after the physician has placed a catheter. These issues are crucial to the long, effective life of the catheter and must be understood by all members of the venous access service.

Physicians placing central venous catheters must control wound care and dressing changes as needed, never assuming that catheter care and dressing changes will be handled appropriately by the admitting service (if other than the catheter service). If a catheter is not appropriately cared for, the risk of catheter-related infection increases. Even if orders for catheter care are written by the admitting service, these orders vary from one service to the next and can stray from the "state-of-the-art" techniques available for preserving the catheter. A perfectly placed and positioned catheter is useful only as long as it remains in place. If an infection occurs and the catheter must be removed, it does not matter how well it was placed initially. Therefore, the catheter service should write detailed postprocedure orders for catheter care and dressing changes.

DRESSING MATERIAL

Numerous studies have been conducted to identify and examine factors related to the incidence of infection in patients with central venous catheters. Most catheter-related infections (CRIs) appear to result from the migration of skin organisms at the insertion site into the subcutaneous tract, with eventual colonization of the catheter tip.[1] Another important contributor to colonization of the catheters is colonization of the catheter hub.[1-3] Less common mechanisms of CRI include hematogenous seeding of the catheter tip from a distal focus of infection and administration of contaminated infusate. According to guidelines of the Centers for Disease Control (CDC), an estimated 200,000 cases of nosocomial CRIs occur each year. CRI results in increased morbidity, mortality rates of 10 to 20%,[4] prolonged hospitalization (mean, 7 days),[5] and increased medical costs in excess of $3500 to $6000 per hospitalization[6,7] (1988 U.S. dollars).

Most CRIs begin as local infections of the catheter wound caused by organisms that colonize the patient's skin.[8] Several prospective studies reported coagulase-negative staphylococci, a predominant organism on human skin, as a common source of CRI.[1,2,9-13] These studies reported a correlation of heavy colonization of the insertion site with CRI. Furthermore, Maki and Ringer,[1] through a multivariate analysis, suggest that moisture under the dressing contributes to colonization and increased risk of CRI.[1] The CDC guidelines for the prevention of intravascular infections[14] state that because most intravenous (IV)-related infections result from inward progression of microorganisms contaminating the wound, control measures should prevent contamination of the site. Recommended measures include the use of sterile dressings, preparation of the site, and hand washing.

Transparent Adhesive Dressings versus Gauze Dressings: The Debate Continues

One of the most actively researched and controversial areas of catheter site care is the use of transparent adhesive dressings (TAD). Polyurethane transparent films became available for use as wound and catheter dressings in the late 1970s and offer many advantages, such as allowing continuous inspection of the site, securing the device, and allowing patients to bathe and shower. Concerns have been raised, however, regarding the potential increase in moisture under TAD[8] resulting in greater colonization and the possible increased risk of CRI.[10,15–20] Numerous studies have addressed these issues and are summarized in Table 12–1. A review of these studies indicates that the question of whether TAD increases risk of

CRI, compared with sterile gauze dressings, has not yet been answered.

Summary of the Literature: Dressings and Catheter-Related Infection

The difference in the CRI rate between TAD and gauze dressings remains controversial because contradictory results have been obtained. Some studies have suggested a trend of higher infection rates with TAD; however, statistical significance has not always been achieved because of small sample sizes in the individual studies. Other studies have concluded that there is no difference in infection rates for patients using the various dressing types, and some have suggested a higher infection rate with the use of sterile gauze and tape. Comparison of these studies is difficult because of differences in methods of wound care, methods of culturing, and definitions of infection. The question of which dressing prevents CRI more effectively has not been answered.

Further complicating the picture is the use of different types of TAD in the various studies. Assuming that collection of

Table 12–1 Studies of Transparent Adhesive Dressings (TAD) vs. Sterile Gauze and Tape (SGT)

Authors	Nehme and Trigger[21]
Year	1984
Study design	Prospective, randomized
Patient population	187 patients on TPN
Compared	Op Site dressings (T. J. Smith and Nephew LTD, UK) changed every 7 d vs. SGT changed every 2 d
Comments	Skin prep was the same for both groups
Results	No statistical significance in CRI between the groups (0.63% in SGT group and 0.34% in Op Site group)
Authors	Ricard et al.[22]
Year	1985

(Continued)

Table 12–1   *(Continued)*

Study design	Prospective, randomized
Patient Population	200 postop patients in the ICU
Compared	SGT
	Vs. Op Site film changed every 2 d
	Vs. Op Site film and Op Site spray changed every 2 d
	Vs. Op Site film and Betadine spray changed every 2 d
	Vs. Betadine ointment
Results	No statistical significance for colonization under the dressings between groups. No statistical significance for catheter-related sepsis between groups
Authors	Make and Ringer et al.[1]
Year	1987
Study design	Prospective, randomized
Patient population	1088 patients with *peripheral* catheters
Compared	Sterile gauze and tape changed every 2 d
	Vs. Tegaderm
	Vs. transparent dressing with iodophor antiseptic incorporated into the adhesive
Comment	Large sample size allows for generalization of findings for identifying risk factors of CRI
Results	No statistical significance for rate of catheter infection between the groups; CRI 4.6–6.1%
Authors	Petrosino et al.[15]
Year	1988
Study design	Prospective, randomized
Patient population	92 cancer patients with long-term catheters
Compared	SGT
	Vs. no dressing
	Vs. Op Site
	Vs. Tegaderm
Results	No statistical significance of CRI between the groups although the "trend" was toward a higher infection rate with the two transparent dressing groups. The "no dressing" group had the lowest infection rate

(Continued)

Table 12–1 *(Continued)*

Authors	Conly et al.[16]
Year	1989
Study design	Prospective, randomized
Patient population	79 patients
Compared	Sterile gauze with tape changed every 2 d vs. Op Site changed every 2 d (Smith and Nephew, Lachine, Quebec)
Results	Statistically significantly more colonization of catheter sites after 48 hours with TAD and statistically significantly more CRI in the TAD group

Authors	Eisenberg et al.[23]
Year	1990
Study design	Prospective, randomized
Patient population	193 patients, 252 catheters
Compared	SGT changed every day vs. Op Site changed every 7 d
Comments	Found decreased nursing time and decreased costs with TAD
Results	No statistical significance in CRI between groups

Authors	Shivnan et al.[24]
Year	1991
Study design	Prospective, randomized
Patient population	98 bone marrow transplant patients with long-term venous catheters
Compared	SGT changed every day vs. Tegaderm (3M Co., St. Paul, MN, U.S.A.) changed every 4 d
Comments	1. Found increased skin irritation with tape and gauze
	2. Statistically significant increased patient satisfaction with TAD
	3. Difference in nursing time was highly significant between the groups: TAD group required 172.7 min nursing time/30 d and the SGT group required 377 min nursing time/30 d
	4. Higher costs of supplies for the SGT group: $87.08/30 d compared with the TAD group, which cost an average of $27.06/30 d
Results	No statistical significance in CRI between groups. There was 1% CRI in both groups.

(Continued)

Table 12–1   *(Continued)*

Authors	Maki et al.[25]
Year	1994
Study design	Randomized, prospective
Patient population	442 patients with pulmonary catheter
Compared	SGT replaced every 2 d vs. Tegaderm replaced every 5 d vs. Op Site 3000 replaced every 5 d
Results	No statistical significance in catheter colonization or sepsis between the groups. There was, however, greater colonization of the skin under the dressings of the TAD group
Authors	Brandt et al.[26]
Year	1996
Study design	Randomized, prospective
Patient population	101 cancer patients with long-term tunneled catheters
Compared	SGT changed every day vs. Op Site 3000 changed every 7 d
Comments	Cost of supplies greater for the SGT group averaging $23.10/week compared to the cost of the Op Site 3000 group, which averaged $8.98/wk
Results	No statistical significance when all categories of CRI considered between the groups
Authors	Treston-Aurand et al.[5]
Year	1997
Study design	Retrospecive, nonrandomized
Patient population	3931 patients with various central venous catheters
Compared	SGT changed every day vs. Tegaderm changed every 2 d vs. Op Site 3000
Comments	Greater staff satisfaction with TAD
Results	Statistically significant more CRI with SGT

moisture under a dressing facilitates colonization of microflora, which, in turn, increases the risk of CRI, it is reasonable to assume that the differences in moisture transmission of dressings would influence the risk of CRI. The permeability of the TAD in these studies varies dramatically. Tegaderm is relatively impermeable to water vapor (moisture vapor transmission rate = 80), Op Site is semipermeable, and Op Site 3000 is highly permeable (moisture vapor transmission rate = 2930).[25,26] Using the highly permeable TAD, recent studies suggest lower CRI rates with TAD that are more comparable to CRI rates of sterile gauze dressings.

Patient Satisfaction

Studies that have compared patient satisfaction among dressings have shown greater patient satisfaction with TAD because fewer dressing changes are required, and because patients do not need to be as vigilant about not getting the dressings wet (they can take showers).

Personnel Satisfaction

Studies that evaluated staff acceptance have shown significantly greater satisfaction with TAD.

Costs

Although the cost of a single TAD is greater than a single dressing of sterile gauze and tape, TAD need be changed only every 4 to 7 days instead of the daily changes required for gauze dressings. Studies have shown overall cost savings for supplies with TAD.[5,24] In addition, cost savings are realized with TAD because of decreased nursing time.[24,26]

Recommendations

Greater patient satisfaction, greater staff satisfaction, and less overall cost while maintaining at least the same quality of care in terms of CRI make TAD a viable (if not preferred) alternative to sterile gauze dressings. Regardless of which alternative one chooses as the primary method of dressing catheters, it is vitally important to realize that viable options exist. Patients' preference or events such as skin irritation may dictate changing or alternating dressing types.

Perhaps of greater importance than the type of dressing used is the establishment of appropriate catheter care by the nursing staff. One study demonstrated the benefits of a nursing educational program on the CDC recommendations for control of CRI. Statistically significant reduction of inappropriate catheter care and a reduction in the rate of skin colonization have been shown. Because maintenance of catheters by inexperienced staff may increase the risk of catheter colonization,[27] many institutions have established infusion therapy teams. Available data suggest that personnel trained in the maintenance of IV access devices can provide a service that effectively reduces catheter-related infections and costs.

DRESSING CHANGE

Techniques

The materials needed are as follows:

- Nonsterile gloves
- Sterile gloves
- Povidone–iodine swab sticks
- Alcohol pads and swab sticks
- Sterile barrier
- Sterile gauze or transparent dressing
- Tape

The steps involved in changing a dressing are as follows:

1. Wash hands.
2. Set up sterile field with supplies.
3. Don nonsterile gloves.
4. Carefully remove old dressings.
5. Inspect the exit site, surrounding skin, and tunnel for skin integrity, erythema, drainage, tenderness, swelling, bruising, or bleeding.
6. Remove nonsterile gloves.
7. Don sterile gloves.
8. Clean the exit site and surrounding skin with an alcohol pad. Repeat twice. Start at the skin exit site and work outward in a circular fashion without returning to the skin already cleaned.
9. Hold the catheter with an alcohol swab at the skin exit site. Wipe the catheter with another alcohol swab from the proximal to the distal ends.
10. Lay the catheter on a sterile towel.
11. Clean the exit site and surrounding skin with povidone–iodine swab sticks. Again, start at the exit site, working in a circular fashion outward for 3 to 4

inches. Repeat twice. Allow to air dry. Avoid getting iodine on the catheter.

12. Protective skin barrier may be applied to the skin underlying the dressing. Apply dressing over the catheter exit site and form an occlusive seal by pinching the adhesive portion around the catheter.

13. Loop the catheter, if length allows, and secure to skin with tape.

14. Remove gloves and wash hands.

15. Label dressing with date and time of change.

Documentation

Nursing personnel should enter the following information in the chart:

- Date and time of dressing change
- Appearance of skin exit site, surrounding skin, and tunnel
- Presence of any tenderness, erythema, drainage, hematoma, or bleeding
- Appearance of sutures, if present
- Type of dressing used
- Replacement of IV fluids

REPLACEMENT OF ADMINISTRATION SETS AND INTRAVENOUS FLUIDS

Contamination of infused fluids and administration sets is a less common cause of CRI. The CDC's "Recommendation for the Prevention of Nosocomial Intravascular Device-Related Infections" recommends the following guidelines:

Administration Sets

Administration sets include the spike of the tubing entering the fluid container to the hub of the vascular device. Replacement of the administration set involves the following steps:

1. Replace IV tubing, including piggyback tubing and stopcocks, at 72-hour intervals. No recommendation has been made for the frequency of replacement of IV tubing used for intermittent infusions.

2. Replace the tubing used to administer blood, blood products, or lipid emulsions within 24 hours of initiating the infusion.

Parenteral Fluids

No recommendation has been made for the starting time of IV fluids, including non–lipid-containing parenteral nutrition.

1. Complete infusions of lipid-containing parenteral nutrition fluids (e.g., 3-in-1 solutions) within 24 hours.

2. When lipid emulsions are given alone, complete the infusion within 12 hours of hanging the emulsion.

MANAGEMENT OF CUTANEOUS REACTIONS

Patients needing long-term central venous catheters are frequently debilitated and have increased skin sensitivity from chemotherapy, antibiotics, or radiation. Bone marrow transplant patients with graft-versus-host disease also may have increased skin sensitivity. Skin irritation, rash, and breakdown may occur with the dressings. Localized skin reactions are a challenge and can be difficult to treat. Progression of skin reactions may result in skin breakdown and infection, and eventually the catheter must be removed. Early recognition and management of cutaneous reactions are important and illustrate the importance of inspection of the catheter exit site and surrounding skin by the nurse. Instituting alternative dressing techniques at the onset of obvious cutaneous reactions may avert infection of the line and progression of skin breakdown.

Bagnall-Reeb and Ruccione's[28] criteria for cutaneous involvement are outlined in Table 12–2. When these signs and symptoms are found, the central venous access service should be notified and alternative care procedures instituted. If moderate ery-

Table 12–2 Skin Assessment Criteria

Mild erythema

Urticaria

Superficial redness of epidermis

+ / − patchy cutaneous peeling

Moderate erythema

Exanthematous eruptions

Urticaria

Scattered epidermal abrasion

Cutaneous excoriation

Purpuric eruptions

Urticaria

>50% epidermal abrasion under catheter dressing

(Reprinted from *Oncol Nurs Forum*, 17, Bagnall-Reeb HA, Ruccione K, Management of cutaneous reactions and mechanical complications of central venous access devices in pediatric patients with cancer: algorithms for decision making; 677–681, 1990, with permission from the Oncology Nursing Society.)

thema is present, the site should be cultured and catheter care changed to an application of 50% solution of peroxide–sterile water, povidone–iodine. Neosporin ointment (Burroughs Wellcome Co., Research Triangle Park, NC, U.S.A.) should be applied at the catheter exit site and a Cover Roll applied.

Patients with excoriation at the exit site should have a culture taken and alternative catheter care instituted. The site should be cleansed with a 50% solution of peroxide–sterile water and 1% Silvadene ointment (Marian Laboratories, Inc., Kansas City, MO, U.S.A.) applied. A Duoderm wafer (Conva Tec, Skillman, NJ, U.S.A.) cut to fit around the catheter and covering a radius of 4 to 6 cm from the catheter is recommended to be used as a dressing.[28] The wafer can be secured with transparent adhesive dressing. Brandt and colleagues[26] used strips of Duoderm to anchor sterile gauze dressing at the periphery of the gauze.

DRAWING BLOOD FROM CENTRAL VENOUS CATHETERS

Recommendations for drawing blood from catheters are from the National Institutes of Health Clinical Center, *Clinical Pathology and Transfusion Medicine Guide*, 9th edition, August 1995. Blood should not be drawn from peripherally inserted central catheters (PICCs) smaller than 4 French (F), vacutainers should not be used when drawing blood from PICCs, and syringes smaller than 10 mL should not be used to flush PICCs.

Materials

- Double stopcock with male Luer lock
- 10-cc syringe or vacutainer holder with Luer lock adapter
- Collection tubes
- Alcohol swabs

- Luer lock syringe with saline to flush catheter after blood drawing (10 mL for adults, 5 mL for children)
- Luer lock syringe with heparin flush
- Nonsterile gloves

Steps

1. Wash hands.
2. Assemble double stopcock system with vacutainer or syringe closest to the male end of the stopcock, and turn the valve off in the direction of the vacutainer or syringe.
3. Attach the saline flush to the next port and turn off the valve to the female end of the stopcock.
4. Attach syringe with heparin flush to the female end of the stopcock.
5. Don nonsterile gloves.
6. Clean cap of catheter with alcohol pad.
7. Attach male end of double stopcock to the catheter.
8. Turn off all infusions.
9. Turn first stopcock valve off in the direction of the heparin syringe.
10. Open catheter clamp.
11. Discard 10 mL of blood from the catheter by inserting "discard tube" in vacutainer or by filling 10-cc syringe.
12. Insert specimen tubes into vacutainer holder or withdraw appropriate amount of blood in syringe.
13. Turn stopcock valve off in the direction of the syringe every time a syringe is removed.
14. Turn stopcock valve off in direction of vacutainer or syringe.
15. Inject appropriate amount of saline.
16. Turn second stopcock off in the direction of saline syringe.
17. Flush catheter with heparin (described in next section).

HEPARIN FLUSH OF CATHETERS

Heparinized saline solutions are used to maintain the patency of venous access devices. Indwelling central venous catheters, including Hickman, Broviac, and open-ended portacaths, should be routinely flushed with heparin. Groshong catheters may not require routine flushing with heparin.

Materials

- Nonsterile gloves
- Alcohol pads
- Luer lock syringe with saline to flush catheter after blood drawing
- Luer lock syringe with either 100 U/mL heparin or 1000 U/mL heparin
- Infusion caps

Steps

1. Wash hands and don nonsterile gloves.
2. Clean infusion cap with alcohol pad.
3. For dialysis and apheresis catheters, withdraw 5 mL of blood from each port and discard it (because it contains heparin).
4. Attach syringe with saline.
5. Unclamp catheter.
6. Aspirate to check for free-flowing blood, and flush with saline (10 mL for adults, 5 mL for children).
7. Attach syringe of heparin. Fill catheter with appropriate amount of solution (see below), closing the catheter clamp while flushing, before the syringe completely empties (positive-pressure techniques).
8. Remove gloves and wash hands.

The "appropriate amount" of heparin flush depends on the volume of the catheter lumens. Usually, these volumes are marked on the catheters and range from 1.5 to 3.0 mL, depending on the length of the catheter. The exact volume of the lumen of nondialysis Hickman, Broviac, PICC, and Hohn catheters, as well as portacaths, is unknown because they are cut to the desired length when inserted. It is recommended that 2.5 mL be injected into Hickman and Broviac catheters, 3.0 mL into portacaths, and 2.0 mL into PICCs of heparin 100 U/mL.

In general, all catheters must be flushed with heparin after every use. When not in use, portacaths should be flushed with heparin at least monthly. PICC, Hickman, and Broviac catheters need to be flushed daily or every other day.

RESTORING PATENCY OF OCCLUDED CENTRAL VENOUS CATHETERS

Catheter occlusion is the most common noninfectious complication of long-term central venous catheters. Preventing or minimizing the risk of occlusion is the best way to avoid interruptions in crucial or lifesaving therapy. Therefore, when catheter occlusion occurs, patency must be reestablished so that therapies can resume.

Catheter occlusion results from different causes, and it is crucial to establish the exact cause before initiating maneuvers that may be fruitless and time consuming if misdirected. Inspecting the catheter may eliminate some causes (kinking at the clamp, impinging sutures), including a chest radiograph (check the tip position and kinking in the subcutaneous tunnel) and examination of the patient for evidence of venous occlusion (swelling, distended collateral veins). When these causes of dysfunction are ruled out and the catheter cannot be aspirated or flushed, it is likely occluded.

Occlusion of catheters may be due to a variety of causes, such as thrombosis, lipid deposits, or precipitation of medications or minerals. It is important to check what has been infused through the catheter to make a reasonable assumption as to the cause of the occlusion. Thrombosis is by far the most common reason and may result from the slow infusion of blood products, formation of a fibrin sheath at the catheter tip, blood backing up into the catheter lumen, or blood being left in the lumen and not adequately flushed. Injection of a thrombolytic agent into the clotted catheter has been found to be effective in opening the lumen.[29,33]

Urokinase has been the most commonly used agent and is being re-introduced. Urokinase activates the natural fibrinolytic system by accelerating conversion of plasminogen into plasmin, an active proteolytic enzyme that lyses fresh fibrin and clot mesh. The dose of Abbokinase is 5000 U of urokinase per milliliter, 1 or 2 of which should be injected into the clotted lumen.[29–32] If the catheter does not irrigate or aspirate, the urokinase should be instilled with a gentle push–pull action. Alternatively, 1 to 2 mg of tissue plasminogen activator (tPA) (1 mg/mL) (Alteplase, Genetech) may be used for the same purpose. Most institutions fractionate and freeze small aliquots of tPA (2–5 mg) and thaw the individual dose when needed.

A Silastic catheter is soft and elastic, and a slow injection of the thrombolytic agent will expand the lumen around the thrombus so that the agent will come into direct contact with the clot. The agent should be allowed to dwell in the catheter for 30 to 60 minutes. Then a 60-mL syringe is used to aspirate the agent and any residual thrombus. If this does not open the lumen, the process can be repeated up to four times in a 24-hour period.[29–32]

Aggregation of lipid particles should be suspected in a patient receiving total parenteral nutrition (TPN), especially with dextrose, amino acids, and lipids mixed in one container. The aggregation of lipid particles causes occlusion with a waxy lipid material.[34–37] If this agent is the cause of catheter occlusion, patency can be reestablished with a lipid solvent, such as ethyl alcohol. One to two milliliters of a 70% solution of ethyl alcohol (prepared by mixing 3.5 mL of 98% ethyl alcohol and 1.5 mL sterile water) is injected in the same manner as described above for urokinase and tPA. It is allowed to dwell for 1 to 2 hours[29] and then is aspirated with a 60-mL syringe. Ethyl alcohol is 80% successful at reestablishing patency in catheters occluded with lipid.[37]

Another potential cause of catheter occlusion is precipitation of incompatible medications or poorly soluble medications. Medications that have been reported to precipitate and cause catheter occlusion include etopside crystals, calcium phosphate in TPN, phenytoin, heparin, and a number of antibiotics. The mixture of heparin and incompatible antibiotics is especially prone to precipitation. The first step is to determine what infusate precipitated. Then the goal is to lower the pH if an acidic material precipitated or to raise the pH if a basic material precipitated.

Acidic medications and minerals that precipitate include calcium phosphate, etopside crystals, amikacin, piperacillin, and vancomycin.[29,38,39] Occlusions by precipitation of these substances are successfully treated with the injection of hydrochloric acid in the catheter lumen.[29,38,39] The pharmacy should prepare a solution of 0.1 N HC1, and 1 mL should be injected slowly with a gentle repeated push-and-pull action with a 3- to 5-mL syringe.[29] The hydrochloric acid should be allowed to dwell for 60 minutes and then aspirated and discarded. Often, the precipitate forms in the proximal portion of the catheter, and blood clot forms in the distal portion of the catheter; so a dose of thrombolytic agent may be needed following removal of the precipitate with HC1.

If the occlusion is secondary to basic medications, including phenytoin, ticarcillin/clavulanic acid, oxacillin, and heparin, increasing the pH within the catheter lumen may improve the solubility and clear the occlusion.[40] Sodium bicarbonate, with a pH of 7.0 to 8.5, may be injected in much the same manner as described already.

Frequently, it is difficult to establish the cause of occlusion, and it is reasonable to treat for possible thrombosis initially with a thrombolytic agent. If these efforts are unsuccessful and the patient is receiving the 3-in-1 mixture of TPN, a trial of injecting 70% ethyl alcohol should be used in an attempt to treat occlusion possibly secondary to lipid aggregation. If the patient is not receiving TPN and lipid aggregation is unlikely, the next step would be to change the acid/base of the catheter, depending on which medication is likely to have precipitated. The decision of whether to increase or decrease pH is often difficult, and if one is tried and unsuccessful, the pH should be changed in the other direction.

REPAIR OF TORN AND BROKEN CATHETERS

A tear or a hole in tunneled catheters can result from various causes, including injection with too great pressure, such as when an occluded catheter is flushed to "blow out" the clot, or as a result of catheter "fatigue" from clamping, twisting, or kinking of the catheter. It is important to salvage these catheters, the lifeline of many patients, and avoid unnecessary catheter removal and catheter placement. Repair kits for each of the catheters used should be kept on hand. In each instance, the instructions for use are enclosed and should be followed closely. Repair requires the following steps:

1. Sterilize the catheter with alcohol/betadine and lay it on a sterile field.
2. Don sterile gloves.
3. Clamp the catheter below the tear.
4. Cut the catheter just below the tear.
5. Slide the metal cannula of the kit into the lumen of the catheter and into the new catheter hub.
6. Apply adhesive at the junction of the catheter pieces.
7. Slide the plastic sleeve over the junction and fill the sleeve with adhesive.
8. Unclamp.
9. Aspirate from both lumen and flush with saline and then heparinized saline.
10. If the catheter is occluded, thrombolytic treatment should be given.

Catheter repair need not be done urgently. A temporary repair has been described[28] that should allow safekeeping of the catheter overnight. A temporary repair involves clamping and cutting the catheter in the same manner as already described and then placing a blunt-ended 16- or 18-gauge needle into the open lumen. The catheter over the needle is sutured tightly to create a seal, then flushed, and the needle hub capped.

BASIC CATHETER CARE

Patients frequently inquire about the basic aspects of catheter care. Questions such as "Can I take a shower?" and "Can I work out?" are important to the patient's life. It is important that the radiologist not act surprised by such questions and provide a reasonable answer. Otherwise, the patient may lose confidence in the doctor if he or she does not know the answer. Simple answers and reasonable advice are expected. The following are a few frequently asked questions and some helpful answers:

Question Can I work out?

Answer Physical exertion results in increased venous return and increased venous pressures, thereby increasing the risk of hematoma formation due to leakage of blood around the catheter, at least in the immediate postprocedure period. It is prudent to avoid physical exertion for 24 to 48 hours and vigorous physical activity for 3 or 4 days after catheter placement. Keeping the dressing clean and dry is also a consideration. Perspiration may gather under the dressing and can loosen adhesives holding the dressing in place. The dressing should therefore be changed after every workout. Exercise activities and heavy housework may increase the risk of getting the catheter caught on something and accidentally pulling it out. Always take extra care to ensure that the catheter is especially well secured when performing physical activities. An Ace bandage around a PICC in the arm may be a good idea. Catheters that exit from the anterior chest wall can be fairly well secured with a tight T-shirt that will hold the catheter firmly against the body. Too much tape over the catheter is not recommended because

the tape may become loosened with perspiration.

Question Can I go swimming?

Answer No. There is no way to keep the skin site clean and dry during swimming. If the patient is insistent on swimming after placement of a catheter, then a subcutaneous device is a better choice. After the wounds are healed, swimming does not increase the risk of infection with a subcutaneous port.

Question Can I play golf?

Answers Yes. All suggestions pertaining to working out apply. That is, the catheter needs to be secured such that it does not get caught on something and pulled out. If the dressings get wet from perspiration, they should be changed. Using a golf cart instead of walking the course may decrease the amount of perspiration and keep the dressing dry.

Question Can I take a shower?

Answer Any catheter that exits the skin (or any wound not yet healed) must be kept dry. Therefore, a bath is better than a shower, being careful to keep the dressings dry. The catheter should not be submerged in water. A well-wrung washcloth can be used to clean the skin surrounding the dressings, trying not to drip any soap or water on the dressings. If showering, a plastic wrap can be placed over the entrance area to keep the dressings dry. The plastic wrap should be removed immediately after the shower. Plastic adhesive dressings (PADs) should protect the site from becoming wet, but the seal around the catheter is incomplete and water gets through. Every effort should be made to keep the area dry even if a PAD is used. One should not take a bath or shower that is exceedingly hot and causes perspiration. If a dressing becomes wet or loose during a bath or shower, it must be changed immediately.

245

Question Can I still have sex?

Answer Yes. All suggestions pertaining to working out apply; however, securing the catheter may be somewhat difficult.

Question Could the catheter get pulled out when I roll over in my sleep?

Answer This is possible and happens, although infrequently. Securing the catheter is more difficult at bedtime because most people like to wear loose clothing to bed. Taping the catheter is a possible solution, but frequent use of tapes irritates the skin. Changing the position of the tape on the skin each time it is applied may lessen this risk. A tight shirt may hold the catheter against the chest and not allow too much catheter movement. Tank tops and sleeveless shirts should be avoided.

OTHER RECOMMENDATIONS

When IV tubing is connected to a catheter, the tubing can be secured to the clothing or gown with a safety pin, wrapping a small piece of tape around the tubing and pinning the tape to the clothing. IV lines tend to get pulled and tripped over, and it is best if the pulling is applied to the patients clothing rather than to the catheter in the subcutaneous tunnel. Care must be exercised not to puncture the catheter when pushing the pin through the tape.

HELPFUL HINTS
The tape is easily applied and removed by using the following technique:

1. **Use 1-inch silk tape.**
2. **Cut pieces 2 to 3 inches long.**
3. **Create multilayered tape by placing a piece of tape, sticky side down, on a smooth, clean surface and placing several more pieces of the same length on top.**
4. **Pull the multilayered tape off the counter, turn it over, and fold both ends ($\sim\frac{1}{4}$ inch) over.**

5. **Tape the tubing with the folded, nonsticky ends facing each other.**

Do not apply deodorant to the dressings and skin exit site. Deodorants irritate, sting, and burn an open wound and decrease adherence of dressings. Maintain good hygiene. Dirt and grime may be transferred to the dressing and increase the risk of CRI. One hand may be used to scratch or touch a contaminated region of the body and then will touch the dressing or catheter. When changing clothes, be conscious of the catheter location. When removing a shirt, if possible, secure the catheter with the ipsilateral hand and use the contralateral hand to pull off the shirt. No matter how, always keep the catheter in the forefront of your thoughts.

REFERENCES

1. Maki D, Ringer M. Evaluation of dressing regimens for prevention of infection with peripheral intravenous catheters. *JAMA.* 1987;258:2396–2403.
2. Moro M, Vigano E, Lepri A. Risk factors for central venous catheter-related infections in surgical and intensive care units. *Infect Control Hosp Epidemiol.* 1994;15:253–254.
3. Murphy LM, Lipman JO. Central venous catheter care in parenteral nutrition: a review. *JPEN J Parenter Enteral Nutr.* 1987;11:190–201.
4. Lau CE. Transparent and gauze dressings and their effect on infection rates of central venous catheters: a review of past and current literature. *J Intraven Nurs.* 1996;19:240–245.
5. Treston-Aurand J, Olmsted RN, Allen-Bridson K, Craig CP. Impact of dressing materials on central venous catheter infection rates. *J. Intraven Nurs.* 1997;20:201–206.
6. CDC Public Health Focus. Surveillance, prevention and control of nosocomial infections. *MMWR Morb Mortal Wkly Rep.* 1992;41:783–787.
7. Putterman C. Central venous catheter-related sepsis: a clinical review. *Resuscitation.* 1990;20:1–16.
8. Maki D. Infections due to infusion therapy. In: Bennett JV, Brachman PS, eds. *Hospital*

Infections. Boston, MA: Little, Brown; 1992: 849–898.

9. Mermel L, McCormick R, Springman S, et al. The pathogenesis and epidemiology of catheter-related infection with pulmonary artery Swan-Ganz catheters: a prospective study utilizing molecular subtyping. *Am J Med.* 1991;91(suppl 3B):197S–205S.

10. Richet H, Hubert B, Nitemberg G, et al. Prospective multicenter study of vascular-catheter-related complications and risk factors for positive central-catheter cultures in intensive care unit patients. *J Clin Microbiol.* 1990;28:2520–2525.

11. Graham D, Keldermans M, Klemm L, et al. Infectious complications among patients receiving home intravenous therapy with peripheral, central, or peripherally placed central venous catheters. *Am J Med.* 1991; 91(suppl 3B):95S–100S.

12. Snydman DR, Gorbea HF, Pober BR, Majka JA, Murray SA, Perry LK. Predictive value of surveillance skin cultures in total-parenteral-nutrition-related infections. *Lancet.* 1982;2: 1385–1388.

13. Flower RH, Schewenzer KJ, Kopel RF, Fisch MJ, Tucker SI, Farr BM. Efficacy of an attachable subcutaneous cuff for the prevention of intravascular catheter-related infection. A randomized controlled trial. *JAMA.* 1989;261:878–883.

14. Centers of Disease Control. Guidelines for prevention of intravascular infections. *Infect Control.* 1981;3:61–72.

15. Petrosino B, Becker H, Christian B. Infection rates in central venous catheter dressings. *Oncol Nurs Forum.* 1988;15:709–715

16. Conly JM, Grieves K, Peters B. A prospective, randomized study comparing transparent dry gauze dressings for central venous catheters. *J Infect Dis.* 1989;159:310–319.

17. Dickerson N, Horton P, Smith S. Clinically significant central venous catheter infections in a community hospital: association with type of dressing. *J Infect Dis.* 1989;160:720–721.

18. Hoffman KK, Weber DJ, Samsa GP, et al. Transparent polyurethane film as an intravenous catheter dressing: a meta-analysis of the infection risks. *JAMA.* 1992;267:2072–2076.

19. Craven DE, Lichtenberg DA, Kunches LM, et al. A randomized study comparing a transparent polyurethane dressing to a dry gauze dressing for peripheral intravenous catheter sites. *Infect Control.* 1985;6:361–366.

20. Powell C, Regan C, Fabri PJ, Ruberg RL. Evaluation of Opsite catheter dressings for parenteral nutrition: a prospective randomized study. *JPEN J Parenter Enteral Nutr.* 1982;6:43–46.

21. Nehme AE, Trigger JA. Catheter dressing in central parenteral nutrition: a prospective randomized comparative study. *Nutr Support Serv.* 1984;4:42–50.

22. Ricard P, Martin R, Marcoux A. Protection of indwelling vascular catheters: incidence of bacterial contamination and catheter-related sepsis. *Crit Care Med.* 1985;13:541–543.

23. Eisenberg P, Howard P, Gianino M. Improved long-term maintenance of central venous catheters, with a new dressing technique. *J Intraven Nurs.* 1990;13:279–284.

24. Shivnan JL, McGuire D, Freedman S, et al. A comparison of transparent adherent and dry sterile gauze dressings for long-term central catheters in patients undergoing bone marrow transplant. *Oncol Nurs Forum.* 1991;18: 1349–1356.

25. Maki DG, Stolz SS, Wheeler S, Mermel LA. A prospective, randomized trial of gauze and two polyurethane dressings for site care of pulmonary artery catheters: implications for catheter management. *Crit Care Med.* 1994; 22:1729–1736.

26. Brandt B, DePalma J, Irwin M, Shogan J, Lucke JF. Comparison of central venous catheter dressings in bone marrow transplant recipients. 1996;23:829–836.

27. Parras F, Ena J, Bouza E, et al. Impact of an educational program for the prevention of colonization of intravascular catheters. *Infect Control Hosp Epidemiol.* 1994;15: 239–242.

28. Bagnall-Reeb HA, Ruccione K. Management of cutaneous reactions and mechanical complications of central venous access devices in pediatric patients with cancer: algorithms for decision making. *Oncol Nurs Forum.* 1990;17: 677–681.

29. Holcombe BJ, Forloines-Lynn S, Garmhausen LW. Restoring patency of long-term central venous access devices. *J Intraven Nurs.* 1992; 15:36–41.

30. Winthrop AL, Wesson DE. Urokinase in the treatment of occluded central venous catheters in children. *J Pediatr Surg.* 1984; 19:536–538.

31. Gale GB, O'Connor DM, Chu JY, et al. Restoring patency of thrombosed catheters

with cryopreserved urokinase. *JPEN J Parenter Enteral Nutr.* 1984;8:298–299.

32. Lawson M, Bottino JC, Hurtubise MR, et al. The use of urokinase to restore the patency of occluded central venous catheters. *Am J Intraven Ther Clin Nutr.* 1982;9:29–32.

33. Brown LH, Wantroba I, Simonson G. Reestablishing patency in an occluded central venous access device. *Crit Care Nurs.* 1989; 9:114–121.

34. Freund HR, Rimon B, Muggia-Sullam M, et al. The "all-in-one" system for TPN causes increased rates of catheter blockade. *JPEN J Parenter Enteral Nutr.* 1986;10:543.

35. Fleming CR, Barham SS, Ellefson RD, et al. Analytical assessment of Broviac catheter occlusion. *JPEN J Parenter Enteral Nutr.* 1985; 9:314–316.

36. Rubin M, Bilik R, Aserin A, et al. Catheter obstruction: analysis of filter content of total nutrient admixture. *JPEN J Parenter Enteral Nutr.* 1989;13:641–643.

37. Pennington CR, Pithie AD. Ethanol locks in the management of catheter occlusion. *JPEN J Parenter Enteral Nutr.* 1987;11:507–508.

38. Duffy LF, Kerzner B, Gebus V, et al. Treatment of central venous catheter occlusions with hydrochloric acid. *J Pediatr.* 1989;114: 1002–1004.

39. Testerman EJ. Restoring patency of central venous catheters obstructed by mineral precipitation using hydrochloric acid. *JVAN.* 1991;1:22.

40. Goodwin ML. Using sodium bicarbonate to clear a medication precipitate from a central venous catheter. *JVAN.* 1991;1:23.

Chapter *13*

Complications of Central Venous Access

Jaime Tisnado
Philip C. Pieters

The use of central venous catheterization is becoming more widespread. The indications for its use are expanding every day. It is estimated that more than three million central catheters are placed in this county each year. The annual cost is estimated at 230 million dollars. Chronic central venous catheters account for 15%, ports 29%, hemodialysis catheters 13%, and short-term catheters 26%.[1] Therefore, the demands for insertion of central venous catheters are increasing every day.

Most central venous catheters are placed by interventional radiologists in the interventional radiology suite or by surgeons in the operating room. Despite advances in methods and techniques and improvements in equipment, it is inevitable that complications related to central venous catheter placement increase as more procedures are being performed. Central venous catheters are being placed by some operators who are not familiar with the techniques and methods of placing them. This situation sometimes occurs when expert personnel are not available or when a busy department has too many patients needing central venous access at the same time so that not enough experienced operators are available to insert the catheters.

Central venous catheters are placed for therapeutic and diagnostic indications, such as long-term systemic chemotherapy, administration of blood products, hemodialysis, plasmapheresis, total parenteral nutrition (TPN), stem cell harvesting, intravenous (IV) fluid administration, administration of IV medications, repeated blood samplings for laboratory tests, and to monitor response to treatment.[2] The indications for placement of central catheters are expanding continuously. It is natural that, despite the use of careful techniques and adequate equipment, complications related to the procedure can eventually develop.

Advances in radiologic equipment and the routine use of fluoroscopy and ultrasound guidance during placement of central venous catheters in the vascular interventional radiology suite have allowed interventional radiologists to perform the procedures with fewer complications and lower costs.[3,4] In a recent study of the costs of radiologic versus surgical placement of central venous catheters, the cost of the former was half that of the latter.[5,6] In many aspects, the rate of complications of procedures done in the operating room, without fluoroscopy or ultrasound, is much higher.[3,4,7] On the other hand, the rate of some delayed complications is similar, regardless of who inserts the catheters or where they are inserted. In addition, the rate of complications is directly related to the expertise of the operators placing those devices, regardless of their subspecialty.

Interventional radiologists frequently are called to solve problems originating from central catheter placement by operators with no experience in catheterization techniques; therefore, the vascular interventional radiologist must be ready to solve most of these problems.

It is important that personnel who place and care for catheters know and be familiar with the types of complications, the mechanisms of occurrence, and the prevention and management of complications. Emphasis on preventing complications is an ideal goal. Although prevention of complications should be the primary goal, it is impractical to think we can change the course of some events that are likely to occur in patients with long-term central venous catheters, who are thereby maintained and kept alive for a long time. The longer a central venous catheter is in place, the greater the risk that complications will develop.

We can therefore expect complications to occur sooner or later and must be prepared to manage these problems. Health workers responsible for central venous catheter maintenance must be familiar with the topic so they can notify the vascular interventional radiologists or surgeons in a timely manner because these persons eventually will take care of the problems. A combined approach with different operators would be ideal, particularly to maintain the functionality of hemodialysis catheters.[8]

As we shall see, it is much better to tackle a problem early, as soon as it is suspected, because it is easier to correct it, and the success of maintaining the access is higher. As a general principle, the central access should be maintained as long as possible, with every effort made to keep the catheters functioning. This is particularly important in patients who will have central catheters, perhaps for the remainder of their lives, such as patients on chronic hemodialysis. We must consider that many of these patients, particularly those on hemodialysis, have depleted most of their venous accesses, and their central venous catheters could be one of the last resources for hemodialysis. Therefore, we must make every effort to keep the access functional. We emphasize here that many catheters sooner or later will require revision.[9]

Sometimes it is better to be overconcerned about central venous catheter function. Health care personnel should not hesitate to contact the vascular interventional radiologist as soon as suspicion of catheter malfunctioning is raised, even if the problem seems "trivial." The interventional radiologist must be ready and available at all times for consultation and should not question the call. We must realize that the degree of knowledge and expertise of the health workers are variable and sometimes limited.

On the other hand, health care personnel can take numerous steps to avoid or prevent complications and to improve the longevity of the catheters. Some such ideas are mentioned during the discussion of the different complications.[10] We foster a "team approach" to central venous catheter maintenance that involves numerous individuals.[8,11] The interventional radiologist must be involved in the care of the patients through the entire "life" of the catheter and port.[1] Patients also must be educated and participate in the care of their access. Better patient education will result in lower rates of complications and improved patency. The rate of complications, however, remains low (3% in some series).[12]

TYPES OF COMPLICATIONS

For the sake of discussion, most authorities classify the complications in two large, broad categories.

Acute, Immediate, Early, and Procedural

These complications occur within 30 days of the procedure[2] and include failure of placement, pneumothorax, hemothorax, hemopneumothorax, hemorrhage, misplacement of catheters, arterial injury, air embolism, thoracic duct injury, spasm of veins, injury to veins, injury to cardiac chambers, arrhythmias, injury to neural structures, inferior vena cava (IVC) filter dislodgement or extrusion, among others. Concerning peripherally inserted central catheters (PICCs), early complications are those occurring within less than 3 days after insertion.[13] Some of these complications are rare, and others may be very unusual indeed and are listed here for completeness only. It is obvious that the better the technique and experience of the operators and the equipment used, the less likely it is that complications will occur.

Chronic, Delayed, Late, and Postprocedural

These complications occur later (after 30 days of the procedure) as a consequence of the long-term presence of the central venous catheter.[2] The longer the catheter is in place, the more likely a complication will develop. With advances in catheter care, patients can be maintained with their accesses for many years and therefore are likely to develop complications. Concerning PICCs, late complications are those occurring more than 3 days after insertion.[13]

This group of complications includes infection, thrombosis, venous stenosis or occlusion, injury to vessels, migration of the catheter, fracture of the catheter, peripheral or central embolization of catheter fragments, malposition of catheter tip, erosion of skin and subcutaneous tissues, fibrous sheath deposition, hemorrhage, and others. In separate sections, we briefly describe most complications, the radiologic findings, and ways to prevent them, and we present some information about their management and treatment. Most of the information is derived from our own experience of many years with thousands of central venous catheterizations and also from a review of the works of other authors.

Acute Complications

Failure to Place a Central Catheter

Although not a true complication, here we include failure to place a central catheter as a complication. In our experience, inability to gain access is rare and almost nonexistent. Success rates of almost 100% are reported in the radiologic literature.[2,14–16] Failures of placement of PICCs are almost nonexistent as well.[13]

We preferentially place central venous catheters in the internal jugular veins. If these veins are not available, the next access sites are the subclavian veins, the external jugular veins, and then the common femoral veins. If all these veins are occluded, the IVC by translumbar approach is the next step; finally, the hepatic veins by percutaneous puncture of the liver are used. Other less conventional accesses will be mentioned here as well. Most failures of catheter placement are by physicians and health workers with limited experience in catheterization techniques. The clinical literature reports failure rates of 4 to 33% during central venous catheter placement, except during bedside PICC placement, where high rates of success have been obtained.[17–19]

Vascular interventional radiologists have a very low or negligible failure rate because they access the veins with ultrasound or venographic "road mapping" guidance.[20] With real-time ultrasound, the success rate of catheter placement approaches 100%, provided the central veins (internal jugular or subclavian) are patent. When the upper-body central veins are depleted, ultrasound and venography can be used to access the femoral veins, and when these veins are depleted, the IVC or the hepatic veins can be punctured with imaging guidance. Thereafter, other less common sites of access, such as azygous and hemiazygous, intercostal, external jugular, or collateral veins can be used. Ultrasound and venography, in addition to facilitating puncture of the venous structures, prevent inadvertent puncture of adjacent arteries and other structures because the arteries usually course parallel to the veins.

Occasionally, computed tomography (CT) guidance can be used for IVC or hepatic vein access. We have placed catheters in the IVC under CT guidance. Thereafter, the patients were transported to the interventional radiology suite for final placement of the catheter. Many patients have completely depleted their veins for access. Sometimes, in some of these patients, the lumen of a chronically occluded vein can be recanalized, and a careful manipulation of wires and catheters may permit access into the superior vena cava (SVC) and right atrium (RA). The small lumen of the vein may not allow a large-bore catheter to be inserted into the RA, however. In some of these cases, fibrinolytic therapy with recombinant tissue plasminogen activator (tPA) alteplase (Activase), urokinase, or recombinant reteplase (Retavase) may be successful in recanalizing the vein and can be followed by angioplasty and stenting of the vein for central venous access. Angioplasty of venous stenoses to facilitate placement of central venous catheters must be encouraged and done as liberally as possible. There is no reason to struggle during catheterization of stenotic central veins, when the lesion can be dealt easily, quickly, and effectively with balloon dilatation and stenting, if needed.

In conclusion, vascular interventional radiologists know the central venous anatomy and have the materials and equipment needed for central venous catheterization. In experienced hands, the rates of failure of catheter placement are negligible: less than 1%. Vascular and interventional radiologists use creativity and intuition to place central venous catheters in patients with limited accesses, even after other less experienced operators may have failed. Furthermore, vascular interventional radiologists can perform various procedures, such as thrombolysis, percutaneous transluminal angioplasty (PTA), stenting, and stent-grafting of occluded or stenotic veins before placement of a central venous catheter, in situations when accesses are limited or almost completely depleted.[20]

Several options are available for catheter placement when conventional sites and placement are depleted. There are isolated reports of placement of catheters in unusual places, such as collateral veins, azygous system, external jugular veins, and others. Certainly, a close discussion between patients, referring physicians, and vascular interventional radiologists is necessary to determine the type of catheter and how long it will be needed. Sometimes, if a central catheter is needed for short-term therapy only, a peripheral IV insertion may be sufficient. So the message is that although central venous catheters are important and necessary, many times they are not needed if a simple IV access will do the job.

Inadvertent Removal of the Catheter

A problem that occurs occasionally is the inadvertent or accidental removal of a catheter. Sometimes the catheter falls out by itself, but this usually occurs because the patient removes the catheter for some reason; some uncooperative patients may do this. Although not a complication per se, it is mentioned here because it requires placement of a new catheter. Sometimes clinicians remove catheters, without consulting the interventional radiologist, when they think the catheter might be malfunctioning but in reality it is functioning well. Of course, this practice must be discouraged.[9,21]

Pneumothorax

Pneumothorax is now a rare complication of venous access caused by transgression of the pleural space, usually during the venous puncture.[22] In a recent report, the incidence was 0.1% (one case in 880 procedures).[14] In the past, this complication was more frequent because the subclavian veins were preferentially used for initial access. The subclavian veins are the preferred initial access for clinicians and other operators. Vascular interventional radiologists prefer the internal jugular veins for access, and therefore the rate of pneumothorax is low, reported to be between 0 and 1.7%.[1,21] We try to spare or avoid the subclavian veins for central access, particularly in patients undergoing hemodialysis, for reasons that are described later.

Furthermore, even in the event that the subclavian veins are used for access, the puncture of the subclavian veins is done under digital venography "road mapping" or ultrasound guidance, and therefore the rate of pneumothorax has significantly decreased to almost nonexistent. Puncture of the subclavian veins should be performed under direct vision of the vein. We prefer to puncture the subclavian veins lateral to the intersection of the first rib and the clavicle to avoid pneumothorax and the "pinch-off" syndrome and catheter fracture and embolization (described in foregoing paragraphs). The likelihood of pneumothorax during an internal jugular puncture is almost nil or nonexistent.

The reported rate of pneumothorax during subclavian vein puncture approaches 1 to 6%, depending on the techniques used.[17,23] The higher rate is likely during "blind" punctures by operators unfamiliar with the technique. In our experience, the rate of pneumothorax is less than 0.1%. It has been reported that pneumothorax may account for 30% of complications during "blind" punctures.[17]

On occasion, air is aspirated during venipuncture. If the patient complains of some tracheal irritation and cough during the puncture, it is likely that the trachea has been punctured. In this case, the contaminated needle should be discarded before a new puncture of the vein is attempted.

The diagnosis of pneumothorax can be made with fluoroscopy but more appropriately with "conventional" upright chest radiographs in frontal and lateral views on inspiration and expiration. CT has been used to depict small pneumothoraces not visualized with conventional radiographs. If a small pneumothorax is suspected, it is clinically not significant and follow-up chest radiographs are adequate (Fig. 13–1).

Treatment Management of a pneumothorax varies, depending on the specific circumstances and particularly on the degree of lung collapse. If there is a small pneumothorax (less than 15%) and the patient is asymptomatic, treatment is conservative and includes observation and serial chest radiographs. A repeat chest radiograph may be obtained in 6 to 8 hours before discharge.

If the pneumothorax is asymptomatic, but the amount is more than 15%, a chest catheter or tube needs to be placed. The chest tube can be inserted in the interventional radiology suite by interventional radiologists. A catheter with a Heimlich valve is used for small pneumothoraces. If the pneumothorax is large, the patient will need to have a chest tube placed by the surgeon or by the interventional radiologist (if he or she is knowledgeable about the technique). We prefer that a surgeon place the tube and manage the complications.

Hemothorax

Bleeding into the thoracic cavity is a serious complication and usually is a result of injury to a vessel (vein or artery) during puncture and transgression of the thoracic cavity. Another rare cause of hemothorax is injury to vessels during catheter removal in the unexpected situation in which the tip of the catheter is adherent to the vessel wall, causing a tear of the vessel wall during withdrawal.

The degree of bleeding varies. Minor bleeding usually causes no significant sequela; however, serious bleeding requires immediate treatment. Serious hemothorax is usually due to puncture and laceration of a large artery, such as the subclavian, internal mammary, or carotid, which are in close apposition to the veins being punctured. Tears to the central veins also can result in serious hemothoraces. Fortunately, this complication is rare, especially when the access is done under ultrasound or fluoroscopic venographic guidance. The subclavian venous approach may be more likely to result in major vessel injury. During subclavian vein punctures, lateral to the junction of the first rib with the clavicle, the risk of pneumothorax and hemothorax is very low.

Isolated reports of injuries to the aorta, brachiocephalic arteries, and even the pulmonary arteries during central venous catheter placement have resulted in serious

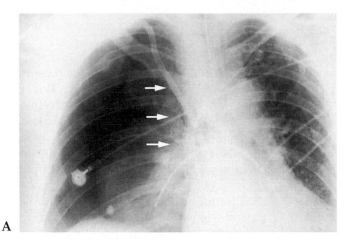

A

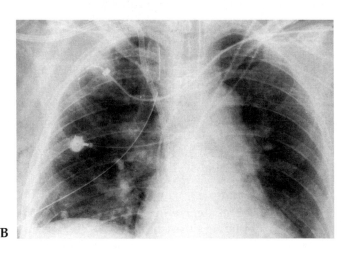

B

Figure 13–1 **(A)** Large pneumothorax (*arrows*) after central catheter placement by internal jugular vein puncture. **(B)** A chest tube was placed. The patient recovered uneventfully.

hemothoraces requiring emergency intervention. Injuries to the arteries resulting in hemothorax are not uncommon when inexperienced house officers try to place central venous catheters in the emergency room or bedside without ultrasound or fluoroscopic guidance.

Prevention It is most important that the veins be punctured under ultrasound or fluoroscopic guidance. Also, personnel unfamiliar with imaging guidance should not try "blind" approaches in seriously ill, uncooperative, intoxicated patients, particularly in the emergency department.

Treatment Consists of maintaining the patient's hemodynamic stability and insertion of a chest tube for drainage of the blood

and, perhaps, repair of the injured vessel, if possible. With the advent of stent grafts, this complication can be managed in the interventional radiology suite. If an arteriovenous fistula (AVF) is present, transcatheter embolization is preferable to surgery. Fortunately, this event is rare.

Air Embolism
Air embolism is a serious and potentially fatal complication, but it is fortunately rare. An incidence of 1.4% was reported in a recent article.[14] A mortality rate of 50% is associated with this complication. Air can be introduced (sucked in) into the veins through needles, catheters, sheaths, and peel-away sheaths during the procedure.[22] Obviously, air can enter the veins during the many different steps of central

venous catheter placement. The negative intrathoracic pressure, particularly during inspiration, will allow air to be sucked into the veins if there is an opening (communication) between the atmosphere and the bloodstream during insertion (or removal) of needles or catheters in the RA or central veins.[1,17,24]

It has been estimated that a large amount of air can enter the bloodstream rapidly via needles or catheters used for central venous access. One or two deep breaths may be enough to introduce sufficient air to result in a fatal embolism. Some uncooperative patients may cough, take deep inspirations, or perform a Mueller maneuver during catheter insertion, thereby decreasing the intrathoracic pressure, facilitating aspiration of air into the venous system. Some patients are deeply sedated during the procedure and may not be able to cooperate. It is important to cover open needles and catheters and to be as expeditious as possible during the steps of catheter insertion, including during wire insertion into the needle after the vein has been punctured or dilatation of the tract for catheter or peel-away sheath insertion.

One of the most dangerous steps for air embolism is during removal of the dilator from the peel-away sheath and insertion of a large-diameter [12–14 French (F)] tunneled catheter. It is important to ask the patients to take a deep breath, stop breathing, perform the Valsalva maneuver (if possible), or hum during final insertion of the catheter into the peel-away sheath.

These maneuvers are intended to increase the intrathoracic pressure, with resultant increasing bleeding from the sheath but decreasing the risk of air embolism. If the patient is under general anesthesia, we suspend the respiration, if possible. Pinching the peel-away sheath immediately after removal of the dilator is also recommended if the catheter cannot be inserted immediately into the peel-away sheath to obliterate the large lumen that is a direct communication between the atmosphere and the central venous system or RA. Obviously, if

the peel-away sheath is crushed or pinched, it must be restored to normal shape quickly; otherwise, it may be difficult to insert the soft Silastic catheters through the sheath.

One important concept is the possibility of air embolism during removal of catheters. In many institutions, removal of catheters is delegated to nursing or ancillary personnel. If they are not aware of this potential problem or if they are not careful enough, a catastrophic air embolism could result. This is mentioned in another section.

Pressure changes in the intrathoracic cavity are responsible for air embolism during catheter insertion or removal. During inspiration, the intrathoracic pressure drops below atmospheric pressure. During expiration, the reverse is true. There are also changes in pressures in the central veins. The pressure decreases during inspiration and increases during expiration. During inspiration, therefore, air can easily be sucked into the veins in the same manner as air enters the lungs.[24]

Moreover, because a fibrin sheath usually develops around indwelling catheters, a fibrin tract may be formed from the skin entry site to the central vein. Therefore, as soon as a catheter is withdrawn, air could easily enter into the venous system if one is not careful to obliterate the entry site, tunnel, pathway, or tract into the vein. Air into the right heart gets trapped in the pulmonary outflow tract and right-sided heart failure, shock, and death may ensue.[24]

Prevention Increasing intrathoracic pressure during removal of the catheter to prevent air from entering the venous system can be done by stopping respiration, taking a deep breath, and bearing down (Valsalva) or humming. Placing the patient in Trendelenburg position during catheter insertion is also effective but not practical in most angiographic suites.[1]

Treatment

1. Observe the patient carefully. Monitor vital signs closely.

2. Give oxygen 100% by mask. A loud churning sound may be auscultated over the chest in the presence of serious air embolism.
3. Place the patient in the left lateral Trendelenburg position to trap air in the RA.
4. Aspirate air from the RA via the catheter just placed, or place another catheter in the RA to aspirate air. Some investigators advocate percutaneous puncture of the RA with a needle and aspiration of trapped air.[17,24]

Thoracic Duct Injury

This is a rare complication that may occur when the left internal jugular or left subclavian vein approach is used. The thoracic duct ascends in the left hemothorax and curves anteriorly to drain into the left subclavian vein. The thoracic duct may be enlarged in cirrhotic patients, making this complication more likely. Care must be taken during left subclavian vein puncture in cirrhotic persons and in patients with chronic lymphatic obstruction because enlargement of the thoracic duct may be present. This injury is suspected when the patient develops a left chylothorax after access.

Prevention A lateral puncture during left subclavian vein access lateral to the junction of the left clavicle and the left first rib should prevent thoracic duct injury. Imaging guidance should decrease the number of unsuccessful punctures and decrease the risk of this complication as well.

Treatment Treatment is to remove the catheter, apply pressure, and observe the patient. No other sequela is expected. Surgery is rarely indicated.

Catheter Misplacement

The ideal location for central venous catheters is at the junction of the SVC and RA.[25] We prefer to place the catheter a little more into the RA, where the blood pool is more abundant, particularly for hemodialysis

and pheresis catheters. The same can be said for PICCs and portacaths.

The incidence of catheter misplacement by vascular interventional radiologists is very low (less than 1%) because most, if not all, catheters are placed under ultrasound or venographic guidance for access and fluoroscopy for definitive placement of the tip of the catheter. We usually leave the catheter in its final location after a "survey" is taken by the vascular interventional radiology team, including technologists, nurses, and others. We look at the monitor and agree on the final position of the catheter. If any discrepancy or question exists concerning location of the tip of the catheter, an injection of contrast material is made and digital subtraction angiography (DSA) or "one-shot" pictures are taken. If the catheter is in an anomalous position, we immediately investigate and try to determine why the catheter is lodged there. On occasion, anomalies of the venous system, such as double SVC, left SVC, absence of jugular veins, and so on may be the cause.

We do not terminate the procedure until we are sure that the catheter is in the correct position and is working properly. Blood must be aspirated easily from all ports of all catheters. By rotating the C-arm in different obliquities, we make sure that a catheter taking an unusual course is not lodged in an unusual or anomalous vein (such as azygos, small veins, contralateral central veins). If any question exists, contrast material must be injected to ascertain the position of the tip of the catheter.

When dealing with obese patients, particularly women with large breasts, we tape the breasts down caudally, toward the lower chest and waist, and then make sure that a longer catheter (about 5 cm longer) is used.[25] This is because of the migration of the catheters when the patients sit or stand and walk.[26,27] Sometimes we obtain chest radiographs in the supine and upright positions to evaluate changes in catheter tip position; however, some do not obtain chest radiographs.[28] If the catheter is too short in the SVC in the supine position, when the patient is supine or when the patient stands, the catheter can migrate cephalad and abut the vessel wall (either the SVC or central veins) and become nonfunctional. On occasion, we ask the patients to sit up and we check the position of the tip of the catheter with fluoroscopy for changes in position from supine to erect and correct any misplacement before the patient leaves the room.[25]

If the catheter is too low or too long into the RA, it may impair the functioning of the cardiac valves with resultant arrhythmias. On occasion, if the catheter is too long, it may prolapse across the tricuspid valve into the right ventricle with resultant arrhythmias as well. Furthermore, complications from a long or misplaced catheter are not uncommon. Endocardial damage, vegetations, thrombosis, damage to valves, inflammation, infection, endocarditis, and other problems have been described related to the abnormal position of the misplaced catheters.

Inadvertent malposition of catheters in an artery is possible but very unlikely when using ultrasound or fluoroscopic guidance. Furthermore, if one punctures an artery rather than a vein, a pulsatile flow of bright red blood will be obvious and unmistakable. Less-experienced operators doing "blind" punctures may experience this complication. In addition, because the arteries and veins are in close apposition to each other, and because large-bore catheters may need to be inserted, there is a possibility of creating an AVF. This could happen during puncture of the internal jugular vein (with the carotid arteries) or subclavian veins (with the subclavian arteries) and common femoral veins (with the common femoral arteries), among others. Arterial occlusion, thrombosis, embolism, pseudoaneurysm, and arteriovenous fistula are rare but possible complications of placement of central catheters.

One common malposition during "blind" insertion of a subclavian catheter is when the tip of the catheter becomes lodged in the ipsilateral internal jugular vein as the catheter goes cephalad rather than caudad into the SVC. In addition, the catheter could be placed across the midline into the contralateral subclavian vein, internal jugular vein, azygous, hemiazygous, or accessory hemiazygous veins. Sometimes the catheters are lodged in small peripheral veins and small thoracic veins. In these cases, the catheters eventually will malfunction because of venous thrombosis causing persistent inability to withdraw blood. Malpositioned catheters frequently become malfunctional or nonfunctional, and thrombotic complications may ensue. Misplacement of catheters is one of the most common etiologic factors of catheter or venous thrombosis (Figs. 13–2 and 13–3).

Rare reports of perforation of the pleura and insertion of the catheter into the pleural cavity have been published. Extravascular insertion in other sites may occur, such as in the neck, mediastinum, chest, and so on.

Treatment The malpositioned catheter must be repositioned using a variety of maneuvers and techniques. If the problem is found immediately during or after placement and the patient is still on the angiographic table, the catheter can be repositioned by advancing one or two guidewires (preferable hydrophilic) through one or both lumens of the catheter and trying to reposition the tip.

When a catheter is found malpositioned sometime after placement, it may be repositioned via a common femoral vein approach using the gooseneck loop snare technique. This procedure is rather simple and is described in another section. Briefly, a sheath is inserted into a common femoral vein. An Amplatz gooseneck loop snare or a Dotter basket is advanced into the RA or SVC. The catheter tip is snared with the loop or snare, the loop or snare is closed, and the catheter repositioned. This technique works if the tip of the catheter is free and not attached to the vessel wall. Otherwise, one can use a tip-deflecting wire to release the tip of the catheter from the wall of the vessel and once one end of the catheter is free,

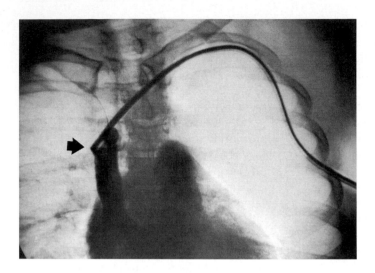

Figure 13–2 Malpositioned left subclavian catheter. The tip is in the superior vena cava (*arrow*). Fibrin deposits are noted.

a gooseneck loop snare, a basket, or a Curry loop can be used to snare the catheter and reposition in the correct location. This procedure is simple and efficacious, it can be done in a few minutes, and it is used when other techniques fail, especially when dealing with a malpositioned portacath. Finally, if a catheter cannot be repositioned, it must be exchanged for a new one using conventional catheter exchange methods.

Vascular Injuries

Arteries and veins (and lymphatics) can be injured during central venous catheter placement. Clinically significant arterial puncture occurred in 12 of 880 procedures (1.4%) in a recent study.[14] Fortunately, these mishaps are uncommon. Some of these problems are described with the different complications, either acute (procedural) or chronic (postprocedural). Possible problems include the following:

- Injury to the carotid artery during internal jugular vein puncture. One carotid puncture occurred in 82 placements in a recent series.[29] Pseudo-aneurysms resulting from inadvertent catheterization of the carotid artery with large-diameter catheters have been described. AVFs are possible but rare occurrences.

- Injury to the subclavian artery and branches may occur during subclavian vein access. The close apposition between the artery and the vein makes the artery vulnerable to injury during attempts at venous puncture (Fig. 13–4).
- Injuries to the abdominal aorta and branches are very unlikely but could occur during IVC catheter placement by a translumbar approach.
- Injuries to the femoral arteries are more common during arteriographic studies but also sometimes occur during venous catheterization.
- Trauma to the upper-extremity arteries (brachial artery) is rare but possible during PICC line placement.[13]
- Arteriovenous fistulas are rare complications but can be a major problem for management. Fortunately, these lesions are so rare that we have no experience in this specific problem. If a large AVF occurs during central venous catheterization, embolization or placement of stent grafts should solve the problem.
- The thoracic aorta and brachiocephalic arteries and branches may be injured during internal jugular vein or subclavian venous puncture if a low puncture is made or a needle that is too long is used. We therefore favor the use of

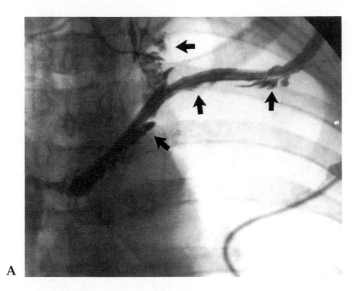

A

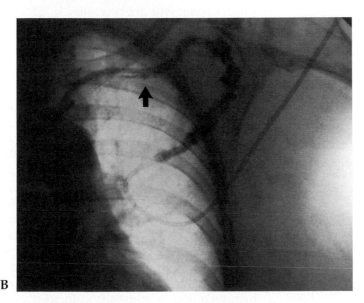

B

Figure 13–3 (A, B) Misplaced catheter in the left innominate vein. Extensive thrombosis has developed.

"short" (4–5 cm long), small-gauge (22-gauge) needles and micropuncture sets for venous puncture. In cases of inadvertent arterial puncture, the needle is withdrawn and manual pressure is applied for a few minutes for hemostasis, which usually is sufficient.[14]

Prevention One of the most important factors in preventing these rare complications is the use of ultrasound and fluoroscopic venography "road mapping" guidance for puncture. "Blind" punctures are discouraged and are no longer considered acceptable in this era of technologic advances and sophistication in angiographic equipment.[21,30]

Small, portable, inexpensive, practical ultrasound units are available on the market for puncturing central and peripheral veins. These units are a must in any vascular interventional radiology service. It has been clearly demonstrated that the incidence of complications is significantly lower when

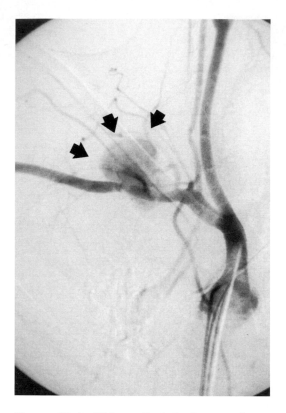

Figure 13–4 This patient had several unsuccessful attempts at right subclavian venous puncture and developed a pulsatile mass in the supraclavicular region. A large pseudoaneurysm from the right subclavian artery is noted.

the punctures are made with guidance. As mentioned, the success rate of venous puncture with ultrasound and fluoroscopy is very high (almost 100%), and the incidence of complications is very low, decreasing proportionally to the sophistication of the equipment and the experience of the operator.

One of the best ways to prevent bleeding is to make sure that the patient has coagulation abnormalities corrected before the procedures are done. The platelet level should be greater than $50,000/mm^3$ and the international normalized ratio (INR) less than 1.5. Platelets and fresh frozen plasma must be given to correct coagulopathies.[1]

Treatment Arterial injuries are treated either by surgical exploration or by angio-

graphic intervention, such as embolization, stenting, and stent graft placement. Ultrasound compression may be used to control some acute pseudoaneurysms or AVFs in small vessels. Manual compression may be sufficient, in some instances, to control bleeding, pseudoaneurysm, and AVF development. If the conservative or vascular interventional radiologic treatment does not work, surgical exploration may be necessary. Thrombin injection into a pseudoaneurysm is another option.

Neural Injury
This complication is rare but possible. Damage to the phrenic and vagus nerves has been reported in isolated cases.[23] No further comments are necessary.

Arrhythmias
Arrhythmias during central venous catheterization are expected problems because the catheters and wires undoubtedly will be in contact with the walls of the right-sided heart chambers. No matter how careful an operator may be during central venous access, irritation of the right side of the heart is likely, with resultant arrhythmias.

Diverse types of alterations in cardiac rhythm are observed: ventricular ectopies, ventricular tachycardia, and atrial disturbances are the most common problems. Supraventricular tachycardia is an uncommon event. Most of those arrhythmias are expected during blind punctures and manipulations of wires and catheters.[17]

Vascular and interventional radiologists should not encounter arrhythmias as often as other operators, who place catheters blindly, because the wires can be more easily manipulated under fluoroscopic observation. Furthermore, because patients are monitored by electrocardiogram, pulse oximeter and blood pressure measurements, and a nurse is always present to watch the monitors, any disturbance in rhythm should be corrected immediately by changing the position of the catheters or guidewires or advancing the devices. We always try to advance the wires through the right side of the heart into the IVC and all the manipulations necessary for central venous catheter placement are done over a securely placed stiff guidewire in the IVC.

Prevention Careful technique is of paramount importance. Advancement of wires and catheters under fluoroscopic observation is critical. DSA can be used if questions arise as to the position of the catheter. Manipulation of dilators and catheters should be done over stiff guidewires advanced into the IVC, avoiding placing wires into the right ventricle or pulmonary outflow tract. The ancillary personnel must be fully trained in critical care and advanced life support. Also, personnel must be familiar with the pharmacologic effects of antiarrhythmic and other drugs.[1]

Treatment Wires and catheters should be quickly removed from sites where they may be irritating the right side of the heart chambers. Vagal stimulation by massage of the carotid body region, if the patient develops supraventricular tachycardia, may be an option. Injection of 6 mg intravenously of adenosine or IV injection of 50 mg of lidocaine is indicated in cases of continuous arrhythmias.[1,17]

Other Miscellaneous Complications
Injury to nerves is uncommon and not a cause of major concern. Nerve injury is rare during PICC line placement.[13,31] IVC filter dislodgement or extrusion rarely occurs during central catheter placement. A basic principle is to review the chart and examine the chest and abdomen with fluoroscopy before any central catheter is placed. If an IVC filter is found, attempts must be made to avoid placing catheters and guidewires through the filter.[1,17] The placement of catheters and guidewires through filters is relatively safe, however, so long as it is done under fluoroscopic observation.

The Vena Tech filter, because of its configuration, seems to be more prone to guidewire entrapment, especially if a hydrophilic wire is used. The wire can get caught between the struts and legs of the filter, and the filter could be completely or partially extruded and misplaced in the central veins. We have seen this problem in few patients with portions of filters lodged in the neck. On occasion, we have been called to remove a wire caught in a filter. We carefully dislodge the wire from the filter struts with the aid of other catheters or balloon catheters or guidewires. Of importance is preventing the insertion of wires and catheters through IVC filters placed recently because the filters may not be lodged yet well in the IVC wall, and filter migration is likely.

Chronic Complications

Venous Occlusion and Thrombosis
Catheter-related or catheter-induced central venous thrombosis is one of the most frequent delayed complications of central venous catheterization. This topic includes several related processes, all the direct result of the presence of a long-term central venous catheter. For the sake of discussion, these thrombotic problems are arbitrarily divided into three categories: (1) thrombosis and occlusion of the catheters, (2) thrombosis or occlusion of the veins, and (3) fibrin sheath deposition and formation around the catheter.

The overall incidence of these complications is high (up to 70%), but the numbers vary considerably due to the lack of standardization of how to report and categorize complications or problems. Furthermore, the variation is related to the methods of diagnostic evaluation. Some authors' reports are based on the clinical situation and include every malfunctioning catheter, assuming that the malfunction is due to thrombosis of the catheter lumen. Others consider thrombosis only when the vein is occluded. Some do not consider fibrin sheath deposition as a thrombotic complication. In addition, the incidence is different if the diagnosis is made with ultrasound or venography.

In general, the incidence of catheter-related thrombosis depends on many factors, such as the duration of the catheter in place, material and composition of the catheter, position of the catheter and its tip, nature and composition of the infusion, expertise in catheter care, and whether or not an associated infection may be present because there is a direct link between thrombosis and infection. Other considerations are the presence of malignancy and hypercoagulable states. From the aforementioned discussion, it is obvious that prevention and correction of associated etiologic factors have important roles in the maintenance of central venous catheters and avoidance of thrombotic complications.

Catheter Thrombosis

Catheter thrombosis is one of the most common presentations.[32] Aspiration of blood is diminished or absent. Usually, with catheter thrombosis, one is unable either to aspirate blood or to inject fluids. The length, position of the tip, and any kinking or twisting of the catheter can be evaluated radiographically. If no problems are noted radiographically, it is assumed that thrombosis of the catheter or venous thrombosis may be present, and treatment is established.[1,33]

Prevention One of the most important factors for the prevention of catheter thrombosis is adherence to strict recommendations for catheter flushing. Sufficient heparin must be injected in the lumens of the catheters to keep them patent. Some recommend a low-dose oral Coumadin (warfarin) maintenance at a dose of 1 mg per day to prevent catheter thrombosis and to avoid systemic anticoagulation with its attendant problems. This regimen has been successful in preventing thrombotic complications of central venous catheterization in some patients, but it is not widely accepted or routinely used by most operators. Maintenance of the catheter under strict sterile conditions to prevent infections is also important to prevent thrombosis because it

is recognized that infection plays a very important factor in the development of catheter-related thrombosis. Positioning of the catheter tip is an essential factor; the ideal position for the tip of the catheter is in the SVC–RA junction.[11]

Treatment Intraluminal thrombolysis is one of the methods to reestablish patency of the lumen of thrombosed catheters. The approach has been to instill 5000 U of urokinase in the catheter lumens and allow to dwell for about 30 to 60 minutes. This can be repeated twice, if needed, to establish patency. This treatment is highly successful, but the recurrence can be high. In some cases, a systemic IV infusion of 40,000 U of urokinase per hour for 12 to 24 hours was recommended.[17,34] If there was recurrence of catheter thrombosis, radiologic evaluation and further therapy were needed.

Other fibrinolytic agents are also available: recombinant tissue plasminogen activator (tPA) alteplase recombinant (trade name Activase) and reteplase recombinant (trade name Retavase). The dose of alteplase recombinant is 2 mg diluted in 1 to 2 mL of saline solution and instilled to dwell in each of the catheter lumens as described for the urokinase protocol. The dose of reteplase recombinant is 2 U diluted in 1 to 2 mL of saline in each of the catheter lumens. These protocols for "catheter clearance" can be done on the floor by house officers or by ancillary personnel. This method is usually successful in restoring patency due to blood clots in the catheter, but it is not effective if the occlusion is due to fibrin sheath deposition and other materials. Successful results have been obtained in 94% of cases.

Alternatively, the insertion of guide-wires in the lumens of the catheters may be sufficient to restore patency of thrombosed catheters. This will clear the catheter lumens of clots, fibrin deposits, sludge, and other debris from precipitated and crystallized medications.[35] We prefer hydrophilic guidewires for this purpose. Lately we have been using ureteral biopsy brushes to restore patency of catheters

(Cook Urological, Spencer, IN, U.S.A.). The brush is inserted into the catheter to clean the lumens with to-and-fro and rotation motions of the brush. Further, we insert the brush beyond the tip of the catheter and release the vein from clots, debris, and fibrin deposits with brushings.

If all these maneuvers fail, catheter exchange may be the best option, using the conventional exchange techniques, making sure that any alterations in catheter position, which may have precipitated the thrombosis in the first place, are corrected (i.e., tip must be in ideal location, no twisting or kinking of the catheter, repuncture of the vein if a too-high puncture existed, and so on). Also, the vein must be patent and free from clots, scars, fibrin deposits, or a fibrin sheath.

Fibrin Sheathing
Sooner or later, fibrin deposition occurs around all central venous catheters, regardless of the time they have been in, regardless of technique for insertion and maintenance, and regardless of the material from which the catheter is made. The nature of the infused solution is important. TPN increases the likelihood of fibrin deposition. The catheter material is also important. Polyvinyl chloride catheters are the most fibrogenic (fibrin sheath deposition), then polyethylene, polyurethane, and silicone (Silastic) in decreasing order of thrombogenicity and fibrin sheath production.

Because the fibrin sheath deposition is outside the lumen of the catheter, passing wires or brushes through the lumens will not solve the problem, as there is fibrin all around the catheter. The fibrin sheath is a major cause of catheter malfunction because it will encircle the shaft and tip and eventually will occlude the tip in a "one-way valve" manner (i.e., it is possible to inject fluid in the vein, but it is not possible to aspirate blood).[36] To assess the presence and extension of fibrin sheathing, contrast material must be injected through the catheter. Contrast material tracking back

around the shaft of the catheter will be noted (Fig. 13–5).

Studies have reported that fibrin sheath deposits can be present as early as 24 hours after catheter insertion, and a full sheath can develop in a week or so.[36] It is interesting to mention that although most investigators consider "fibrin" to be the material present, experimental work has demonstrated that the sleeve around the catheter is not fibrin but rather cellular collagen tissue covered by endothelium. Smooth-muscle cells migrating from the injured vein wall are responsible for fibrin deposition.[36]

Treatment Several methods can be used to manage this common problem. A wire can be used to clean the lumens of the catheters, but this usually does not work well and is a temporary measure. Lately, we have been using a ureteral brush inserted in the lumens of the catheter to release the fibrin deposits with to-and-fro and rotating movements. Sometimes we insert two wires, one in each lumen of the catheter, and withdraw the catheter almost to the entry site in the vein, making sure that the catheter does not come out of the vein to prevent bleeding. Manual compression at the entrance of the catheter in the vein avoids bleeding. Thereafter, we withdraw the wires into the SVC, innominate vein, and entrance into the RA, and with to-and-fro movements, we try to break, fragment, macerate, and dislodge the fibrin sheath. Alternatively, one wire can be left in the IVC to make sure that the access is not lost and one wire can be used for fibrin sheath destruction. We prefer small "J" (3-mm) wires for these purposes.

Another method to fragment the fibrin is to keep one wire in the IVC and use the other wire to insert an angioplasty balloon catheter with a 10- to 12-mm × 4-cm balloon. The balloon can be inflated and deflated several times over the fibrin sheath deposits in the SVC, RA, innominate, or subclavian veins. Also, the balloon can be inflated mildly and withdrawn through the fibrin sheath (as doing Fogarty embolectomy).

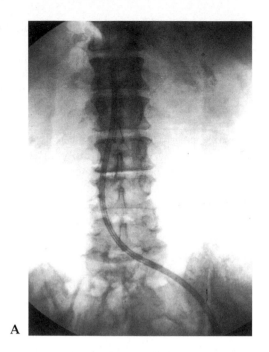 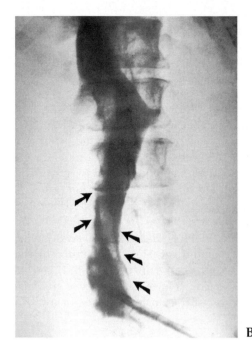

Figure 13–5 **(A)** This patient had placement of a catheter in the inferior vena cava from a left common femoral vein approach. **(B)** On removal of the catheter, a large, thick fibrin sheath is noted.

Catheter stripping is another method, albeit more cumbersome. An Amplatz gooseneck Nitinol loop snare is inserted through an introducer catheter via a femoral vein sheath. The introducer catheter is advanced into the RA, and the loop snare is advanced through the catheter tip. The snare is opened in the RA and SVC, and the catheter tip floating in the RA and SVC is snared. The loop snare is closed tight enough to encircle the catheter, but not too tightly, so the snare can be withdrawn and slide from the catheter as one assistant holds the external portion (outside the patient) of the catheter (hub). This maneuver is performed repeatedly. The catheter is flushed with saline, and contrast material is injected two or three times to assess results. This technique is similar to cleaning the stick to check the oil of an automobile.

Finally, the best method to correct this complication is to exchange the catheter for a new one using the different techniques for catheter exchange. Care must be taken to ensure that the tip of the catheter is placed in

an ideal location and to correct the initial problem (whatever it was) to avoid recurrence of the fibrin sheath, if possible. We believe catheter exchange is a more long-lasting procedure and the same venous access can be preserved. On occasion, a new catheter needs to be inserted in a different site. This, of course, will contribute to depleting venous access sites, although the site used last, the one with the fibrin sheath, can be left to rest, the fibrin sheath may recanalize spontaneously, and the access site may be available for future use.

Venous Thrombosis
This frequent complication is caused by numerous etiologic factors, including the following: (1) malignancy, which may produce a hypercoagulable state favoring thrombosis; (2) the presence of a large-bore catheter in a narrowed vein, which may compromise the flow and make the blood flow stagnant enough for thrombosis to develop; (3) venous irritation caused by the catheter resulting in intimal injury, which in

turn promotes platelet adherence and aggregation; and (4) the toxic and irritative effects of infusions, such as TPN, chemotherapeutic agents, and so on. All these factors contribute to the development of venous thrombosis. These etiologies follow the well-known dictum of the triad of Virchow: venous stasis, endothelial damage, and hypercoagulability.

The presence of a fibrin sheath contributes to venous thrombosis by forming a nidus for red thrombus and a medium on which bacteria and fungi may grow. It is well known that infection and thrombosis are related to each other because infection plays an important role in the development of deep venous thrombosis (DVT). Endothelial injury during catheter placement and constant trauma caused by the catheter during cardiac contractions, respirations, and motion of the patient is also a factor. Injury to the endothelial layer exposes the underlying thrombogenic layers, allowing platelet adherence and aggregation, which can initiate the clotting cascade (Figs. 13–6 and 13–7).

Catheter position is an important factor as well. The site of venous access may be important because studies have shown that there is an increased incidence of thrombosis when a left internal jugular vein or a left subclavian venous approach instead of a right one is used. These studies infer that a right internal jugular vein access is preferable. Also, the position of the tip of the catheter is important. The position of the catheter tip abutting against the lateral wall of the SVC is thought to be a factor for thrombus development because of irritation and erosion of the intima. Catheter tips placed in the SVC and proximally in the innominate and subclavian veins and in the intrahepatic IVC (when an IVC approach is used) will result in a higher incidence of venous thrombosis.

Infusion of hyperosmolar or caustic materials results in injury to the endothelium, which may cause thrombosis (by loss of the nonthrombogenic lining). Therefore, if these infusants are given into a

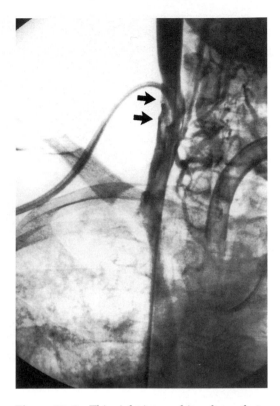

Figure 13–6 This right internal jugular catheter was inserted too high in the vein. A large loop of catheter is seen. Thrombus formation at the venous entry site is noted.

relatively low-flow vein, there is more contact with the endothelium before the caustic material is diluted and taken away with the blood flow. On the other hand, if infused into the high-flow and turbulent RA, the caustic fluids are immediately diluted and contact with the endothelium is minimized; therefore, there is less injury to the endothelium and less likelihood of thrombosis.

The ideal position for the tip of the catheter is at the junction of the SVC with the RA or more centrally into the RA. We prefer to place catheters into the RA, where the flow is better and the chances of thrombosis or fibrin development may be less because of the large pool of blood.

In summary, the duration of the central venous catheterization, the material and composition of the catheter, the location of

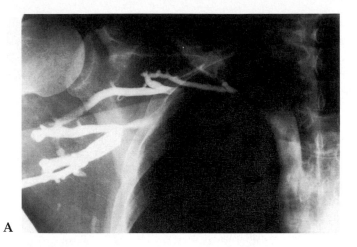

A

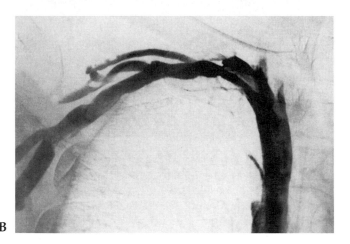

B

Figure 13–7 (A) This patient had a peripherally central catheter line inserted in the right basilic vein. Thereafter, he developed swelling of the right upper extremity. Venogram shows extensive thrombosis of the axillary and subclavian veins. **(B)** Thrombolytic therapy with urokinase successfully relieved symptoms. The catheter was removed as soon as the diagnosis was made.

the tip, the site of access, the presence of catheter-related infections, and the nature of the fluids being infused all play an important role in the development of DVT.

Clinically, patients with catheter-related DVT may present with swelling of one or both upper extremities or SVC syndrome (if the SVC is occluded) with neck and face swelling or lower-extremity swelling, when dealing with femoral catheters. Most patients, however, are asymptomatic.[1] The presence of edema in patients with indwelling central venous catheters should immediately suggest catheter-related DVT. Ultrasound or venography must be obtained as soon as thrombosis is suspected.[37–39]

The reported incidence of catheter-related venous thrombosis is high and may reach 70% with a median of 20%.[35,39–41] Surprisingly, many patients may be asymptomatic (40%), and only about 30% may present with the classic symptoms and signs of DVT. The incidence of thrombotic complications with PICCs is low.[18] Thrombophlebitis may occur in 1 to 10% of patients with PICCs and local cellulitis in 2% of patients with PICCs.[13]

Treatment Low-dose urokinase, at the rate of 40,000 to 100,000 U per hour, via infusion catheter in the thrombosed vein is used for fibrinolytic therapy of extensive DVT. The classic treatment of not catheter-related venous thrombosis has been systemic anticoagulation. When the venous thrombosis is due to complication of central venous catheters, an aggressive approach with fibrinolytic therapy is warranted.

Other options include using recombinant tPA alteplase recombinant (Activase) at a dose of 1 mg per hour via multiport infusion catheters. The dose for reteplase recombinant (Retavase) is 1 U per hour with or without a bolus of 2 to 5 U. The patients are sent to the intensive care unit (ICU) and observed carefully. Systemic heparin is administered at the rate of about 400 to 500 U per hour only, not at the usual systemic dose of 800 to 1000 U per hour, to prevent or minimize serious bleeding complications during tPA recombinant and reteplase recombinant treatment, which are believed to be due to systemic fibrinolytic state.

During initial fibrinolytic therapy, the central venous catheter can remain in place and need not be removed until the results from fibrinolytic therapy are evaluated. The main objective of the therapy, in addition to recanalize the thrombosed vein, is to maintain the central venous access, particularly in patients with limited accesses. If the low-dose fibrinolytic therapy with the agents described does not result in recanalization of the occluded vein and relief of the clinical condition of the patient, the catheter must be removed and a new access used for central catheter placement. The catheter tip must be sent for culture to make sure that infection is ruled out as a factor. The success rate of thrombolysis in catheter-related DVT is 73 to 95%.[40,41]

Surgical thrombectomy is rarely indicated at this time. If an infection is suspected, the catheter must be removed and antibiotics administered in addition to fibrinolytic therapy. A course of 7 to 10 days of IV antibiotics is warranted.

Following a successful thrombolysis, the positioning of the catheter must be reevaluated. Did the position of the catheter tip cause or contribute to the venous thrombosis? If so, the catheter must be exchanged or repositioned to decrease the likelihood of rethrombosis. If the tip is too high in the SVC, the catheter must be repositioned or exchanged and placed in the ideal position to prevent further venous thrombosis.

One important consideration here is the risk of pulmonary embolism resulting from catheter-related thrombosis of upper-extremity and central veins. There is a general belief that venous thrombosis of the upper extremities rarely results in pulmonary embolism. This concept, however, may not be true when dealing with catheter-related venous thrombosis of the upper extremities because the capacious central veins can be occluded with a large amount of clot. Recent studies have indicated that in up to 35% of patients with catheter-related venous thrombosis, pulmonary embolism may originate from the upper-extremity veins.[1,17,42] Therefore, if a patient with no evidence of lower-extremity or pelvic venous thrombosis presents with clinical symptoms of pulmonary embolism, this possibility still must be considered if the patient has a central venous catheter.

One regimen proposed to prevent catheter-related venous thrombosis is low-dose Coumadin administration at 1 mg per day. This has proven to diminish the incidence of thrombosis in patients with long-standing central venous catheters.[39]

Venous Stenosis

This is a frequent complication of central venous catheterization. Sooner or later, the central veins will become stenotic as a result of trauma during placement, fibrin deposits, scar tissue, bleeding, organized thrombosis, and other factors. Stenoses are found more frequently at the entrance of the internal jugular vein into the subclavian vein, at the midportion of the subclavian vein, and at the SVC. The degree of stenosis varies, and the hemodynamic compromise caused by the presence of a large-bore catheter in a stenotic vein may result in complete thrombosis.

The problem is more frequent during subclavian vein access, for which the reported incidence of stenosis may reach 50%.[30,38] We avoid, if possible, subclavian venous access and prefer exclusively the internal jugular vein access, especially in patients on chronic hemodialysis.[37] The presence of a stenosis in the subclavian vein may preclude the placement of an AVF in the arm or render the fistula nonfunctional if the stenosis is not suspected and corrected, either before or after placement of the AVF.

Furthermore, if a subclavian vein stenosis is present and an AVF fistula is placed in the ipsilateral arm, the increased blood flow will result in progressive swelling of the upper extremity that may be so symptomatic that it may require closure of the fistula or render the AVF nonfunctional. Therefore, we try to preserve the subclavian veins, if possible, and do not use those veins for central venous catheterization. Unfortunately, many house officers and clinicians prefer the subclavian vein because they are accustomed to puncturing the vein blindly. Avoidance of this practice will result in saving veins for future use. As a general rule, we do not place catheters in the subclavian veins unless they are the only options for venous access.[37]

The management of venous stenosis is relatively simple but not necessarily effective over the long term. The stenosis can be dilated with percutaneous transluminal angioplasty. Large balloons are necessary to dilate central veins, such as subclavian, internal jugular, innominate, and SVC (10–20 mm) according to the diameter of the normal vessel. High-pressure balloons are usually needed. We prefer balloon catheters that can be inflated to 18 to 20 atmospheres (Fig. 13–8). Unfortunately, these high-pressure-rated balloons are available only in diameters of 12 mm or smaller. Larger-diameter balloons (15–20 mm) do not tolerate inflations more than 10 atmospheres, which may not be adequate to dilate thick and hard venous stenoses. For this reason, we frequently use two balloons inserted from the same femoral venous approach (using a large sheath to accommodate two catheters) or from two different venous approaches (i.e., two femoral veins,

a femoral vein and an AVF, a femoral vein and a basilic vein, and so on). This is similar to the "kissing balloon" technique for arterial dilatations (Fig. 13–9).

Whatever access is chosen, the use of two balloons of the same or different diameters will dilate the vessel to the ideal diameter (e.g., for SVC of 20-mm diameter, we could use two 10-mm balloons or one 8-mm and one 12-mm balloons). Those balloons will withstand the high pressure necessary to dilate the veins. Stenting of the central veins remains controversial. Stenting of venous stenoses should be avoided as long as acceptable results are obtained with angioplasty because of the poor long-term patency of stented central veins. Recurrence of stenosis is common 3 to 6 months after PTA, but the vein can be redilated. Only if angioplasty fails and the stenosis persists (or becomes worse) should the vein be stented. At this time, stenting of central veins should be an intervention of last resort. A patency rate of 28 to 40% at 1 year after central venous stenoses stenting is expected.[37]

For venous stenting, we prefer the Smart stent or the Wallstent because of its radial force and flexibility. We do not use Palmaz stents in curved, tortuous central veins, although they are useful for localized stenosis of the SVC. Wallstents and Smart stents are flexible, thus allowing placement in curved and tortuous veins. We prefer using one or more long (68–94 mm) stents. We make sure that if more than one stent is used, they overlap each other for a long segment. Otherwise, migration into the RA, right ventricle, or pulmonary arteries is likely, with serious consequences requiring retrieval. We have retrieved many of these stents with Amplatz gooseneck loop snares, Dotter retrieval baskets, Curry loops, forceps, and so on (Figs. 13–10 and 13–11).

Catheter Migration
This late complication refers to migration of a catheter or its tip to an abnormal position after it was placed in a correct position.

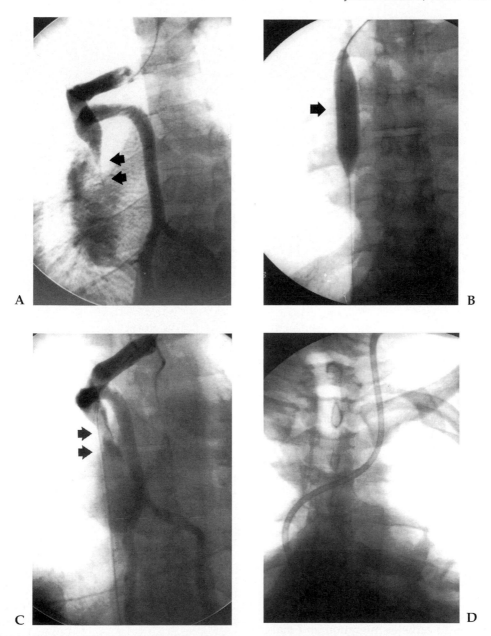

Figure 13–8 This patient, on chronic hemodialysis for many years, had placement of central catheters in numerous occasions at different entry sites. Eventually, she developed superior vena cava (SVC) syndrome. **(A)** Superior vena cavogram after accessing the left internal jugular vein shows marked stenosis and almost complete occlusion of the SVC. The entire venous drainage of the head and neck is made into the azygous system. **(B)** Dilatation of the SVC was done with progressively larger balloons, up to 20 mm. **(C)** After percutaneous transluminal angioplasty (PTA), there is significant reconstitution of luminal diameter of the SVC. The drainage into the azygous has markedly decreased. **(D)** A 14 French dialysis catheter was inserted. The patient underwent hemodialysis uneventfully. The SVC syndrome disappeared immediately after PTA. The patient felt dramatically better while she was still on the angiographic table.

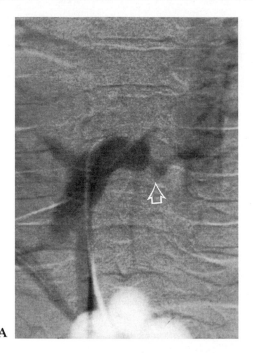
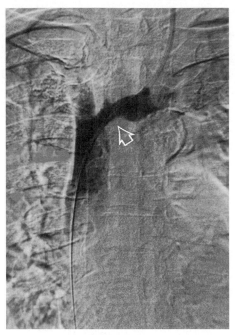

A   B

Figure 13–9 **(A)** Chronic occlusion of both innominate veins as a result of numerous central venous catheterizations. **(B)** Recanalization of the left innominate vein was accomplished with percutaneous transluminal angioplasty (PTA) by a combined approach via right common femoral vein and left internal jugular vein. A dialysis catheter was inserted through the left internal jugular vein, and the patient continued on chronic hemodialysis.

The following are some of the factors contributing to migration:

- Excessive coughing or vomiting
- Large, oversized tunnels or pockets that allow the catheter to migrate, become malpositioned, and, therefore, malfunctioning
- Poor securing of the catheter or port to the subcutaneous tissues that progresses to catheter migration and malposition
- Too-vigorous flushing and testing of the catheter that produces a jet-and-whip effect to the catheter tip
- Too-vigorous exercise and hyperextension of the neck, shoulders, and upper extremities

A catheter in a precarious position will become malpositioned in these circumstances. Sometimes the catheter becomes lodged in a small tributary vein and the infusion of caustic of other infusates irritates the vein with resulting thrombosis. Correctly placed catheters in the SVC may migrate into the azygous vein, contralateral innominate vein, or ipsilateral subclavian vein.

The anatomic constitution of the patient also plays an important role in catheter migration. In obese women, the catheter may be in a correct position checked by fluoroscopy during the placement with the patient supine. When the patient stands up and the chest, neck, and breast soft tissues drop, however, the catheter tip may migrate about 5 cm or more. The migrated tip may abut the lateral wall of the SVC and become malfunctional. We occasionally obtain chest radiographs to assess catheter migration. Some researchers have said that the routine use of chest radiographs is not warranted, and we agree.[28]

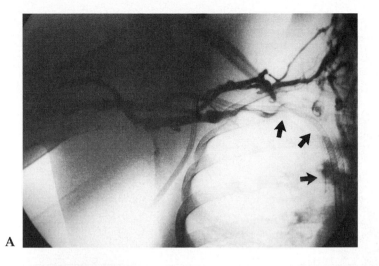

A

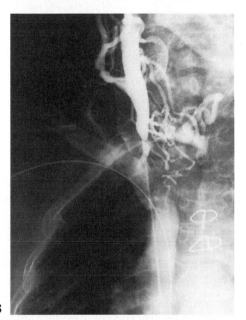

B

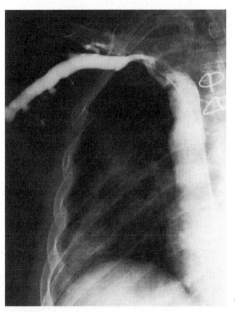

C

Figure 13–10 This patient developed recurrent chronic thrombosis of all the central veins, including both internal jugular, both subclavian, and both innominate veins. She underwent repeated episodes of fibrinolytic therapy, venous angioplasty, and stenting of the central veins. **(A)** A Wallstent is noted in the right subclavian and innominate veins. A dialysis catheter was inserted by a right subclavian venous approach. Although the central veins are chronically occluded, even after repeated recanalizations, the catheter remains functional. As long as the access is maintained, the patient can undergo dialysis. **(B–E)** Another patient with similar problems had complete recanalization and stenting of the right internal jugular, innominate, and subclavian veins (*Continued*).

Prevention Placing the catheters in a correct position in the first place is the best preventive measure to avoid migration. The catheter should be longer than usual (about 3–5 cm) in obese women. When dealing with ports, one should ensure that the pocket is made as small and tight as possible and that the port is sutured to the

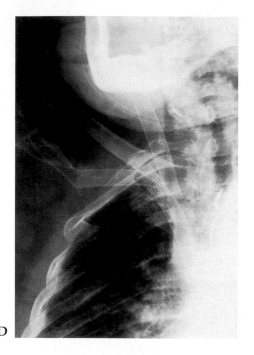

D

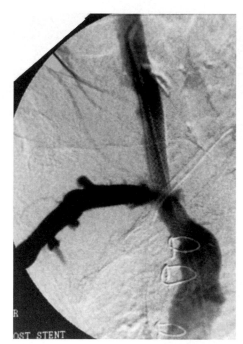

E

Figure 13–10 (*Continued*)

deep fascia. The pocket should be more cephalad than usual, in the anterior chest wall in obese women. It is important to make a low puncture in the neck for internal jugular venous catheters so that no redundancy or kinking or looping of the catheter exists. If a large loop is formed in the base of the neck because of a high puncture, migration of the tip of the catheter is likely.

A special situation is the misplacement and migration of IVC catheters inserted by a translumbar approach. Migration into the retroperitoneal space, subcutaneous tissues, iliac veins, and other locations is possible.[43]

Treatment Forceful injection of saline solution or contrast material creates a jet-and-whip effect on the tip of the catheter and may be repositioned in a correct place. Hydrophilic guidewires can be inserted through the catheter to reposition it. Because one of the most common factors in catheter malposition is insertion of catheters that are too long or too short, catheter length

must be correct to prevent misplacement or migration and the catheter should be trimmed during initial placement. If the catheter is not of adequate length after repositioning, it will likely "migrate" again and should be replaced or exchanged with a catheter of adequate length.

Catheter "retrieval" is another effective method:

1. Puncture the femoral vein.
2. Insert a sheath and an Amplatz gooseneck loop snare or retrieval basket to snare the misplaced catheter and reposition it. We prefer the gooseneck loop snares (15–25 mm diameter), inserted via a 6 F introducer catheter into the RA and into the vein where the misplaced catheter is lodged.
3. Snare the catheter with the loop.
4. Withdraw the loop over the introducer catheter to encircle the catheter.
5. Then withdraw both the loop and the introducer catheter to reposition the misplaced catheter in a correct position.

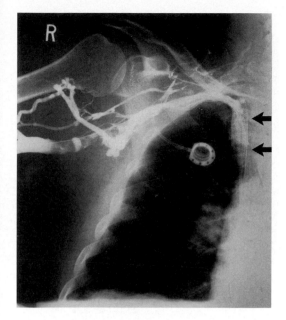

Figure 13–11 This patient received chemotherapy for a long time, resulting in chronic occlusion and recurrent thrombosis of the central veins. A portacath had been inserted in the right subclavian vein, the only patent vein at that time. She developed recurrent massive acute deep venous thrombosis (DVT) of the right axillary, subclavian, and innominate veins and the superior vena cava (SVC). Fibrinolytic therapy and stenting of the subclavian vein and SVC were done, which allowed the central catheter to be maintained for chemotherapy and relieved the symptoms of SVC syndrome.

A disadvantage of this technique is that a new puncture is needed. Different retrieval devices (routinely available in most vascular and interventional radiology laboratories) are needed as well.

Catheter Rupture, Fracture, Migration, and Embolization

Catheter fracture due to "pinch-off" effect used to be a relatively common complication of subclavian venous catheter insertion, but it is less common now that the etiology and prevention are well known. Central venous catheters are frequently placed by surgeons and other house officers who prefer the subclavian approach over the internal jugular venous approach be-

cause of their training and because they are not current with the new interventional techniques. These blind venous punctures often are made medial to the intersection of the first rib and clavicle, and the catheter gets compressed and entrapped between the subclavius muscle and the costoclavicular ligament.[1]

The radiologist may be the first to detect the "pinch-off" syndrome on chest radiographs and should alert the surgeons or the interventional radiologists about a possible catheter breakage and embolization. Four grades or steps of pinch-off are recognized: (1) no compression; (2) catheter slightly kinked but lumen not affected; (3) lumen compromised; (4) catheter fracture, migration, and embolization of the distal fragment into the RA, right ventricle, or SVC.

If the pinch-off syndrome is found in follow-up chest radiographs and the catheter is not fragmented or separated, some researchers advocate a conservative approach, not removing the catheter. A monthly chest radiograph is obtained for 6 months because it is believed that the average time for a catheter to become fractured and separated is more than 6 months. Because the complication of fragmentation and embolization is potentially lethal, we recommend immediate removal of the catheter when the problem is detected on chest radiographs (Fig. 13–12).

When rupture and embolization occur, retrieval of the fragment is done with the conventional retrieval techniques using an Amplatz gooseneck, a Nitinol loop snare, or a Dotter retrieval basket. Forceps, Curry loops, and other devices are less commonly used. The steps are as follows:

1. Puncture a common femoral vein.
2. Insert a sheath.
3. Advance a nontapered catheter introducer into the RA.
4. Insert the loop snare in the introducer catheter and advance it through the tip of the catheter until the loop opens in the RA, right ventricle, or IVC (wherever the embolized fragment is lodged).

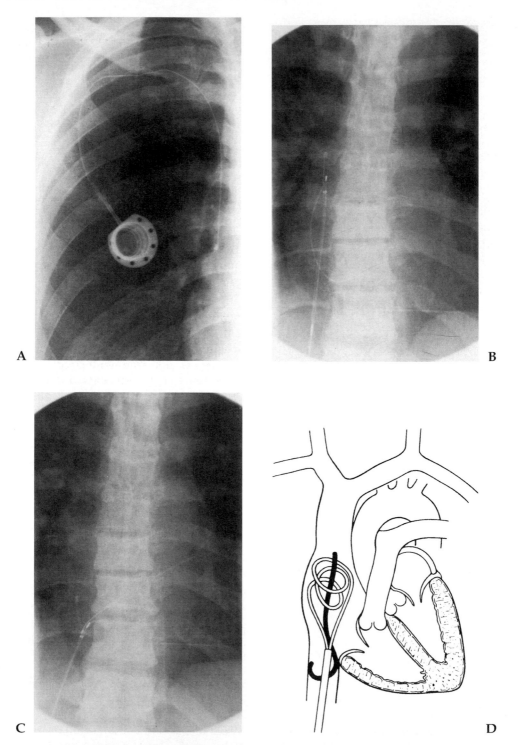

Figure 13–12 **(A)** Chest radiograph shows kinking of the subclavian venous catheter. This is the second stage of the "pinch-off" syndrome. Thereafter, the catheter ruptured and embolized into the right atrium **(B, C)**. The fragment was retrieved **(D)** using a Dotter basket.

5. Snare the fragment with the loop.
6. Close the loop by pulling the loop over the catheter.
7. Remove both the loop and the catheter together carefully under fluoroscopic observation with an assistant.
8. If no free end of the embolized fragment is accessible, a pigtail catheter or a deflecting-tip wire can be used to pull the fragment free from the vessel wall so that a free end is available for retrieval.

The success rate of retrieval is almost 100% in experienced hands.

Embolized catheters and guidewires and other foreign bodies in the vascular system are serious complications of catheterization techniques. A mortality rate of 40% was reported if the fragments were not removed.[17] A high morbidity rate of 70% also was reported that resulted from misplaced catheters, wires, and foreign bodies. Therefore, we firmly believe that embolized catheters, guidewires, and other foreign bodies must be removed as soon as possible.

This potentially serious complication is almost exclusively the result of nonguided ("blind") subclavian punctures. Therefore, we strongly recommend not inserting subclavian venous catheters blindly, without ultrasound or venographic guidance. The subclavian venous puncture should be done lateral to the junction of the clavicle and first rib. This can be accomplished easily using venography "road mapping" puncture or ultrasound, making sure that the puncture is lateral to the bony structures, entering the subclavian vein lateral to the costoclavicular space. In this manner, the vein wall protects the catheter from repeated trauma.[17] This step will also decrease the risk of pneumothorax, as already described.

Infection

Infection is one of the most common complications of central venous catheterization. The incidence is 30 to 50%, depending on the type of report and who is reporting.[22,33] A rate of 1.4 infections per 1000 catheter days has been estimated.[39] Catheter-related infections are manifested in three manners, categories, or types: (1) exit-site infection; (2) tunnel, pocket infection; and (3) catheter-related sepsis.

Most catheter-related infections are due to invasion of the exit site and ascent through the tract into the venous system of skin germs. Therefore, one of the most important factors in preventing infection is to maintain a strict sterile technique during central venous accesses. A procedure-related infection occurs 5 to 30 days after placement of the device; however, most authorities consider the period to be within 2 weeks of placement.[44] Concerning the etiologic factors, the most common germs are *Staphylococcus epidermidis* and *Staphylococcus aureus*. The incidence of infection by *S. epidermidis* is 25 to 50%, by *S. aureus* 25%, and by *Candida albicans* 5 to 10%.[44] Other more virulent germs are *Enterobacter proteus*, *Escherichia coli*, *Pseudomonas* species, and *Serratia* organisms.[1,35,44,45] Other routes of contamination are the hematogenous one, contamination by the infusates, and contamination during manipulation or exchange.

In general, prevention is the best way to avoid or decrease the incidence of infectious complications because there is always a risk of contamination during the initial placement of the central venous catheter. The methods and techniques for these purposes are described in other sections.

Some institutions are installing an operating room environment in the vascular interventional radiology suite. A positive-pressure ventilation is ideal.[17] The incidence of infections increases with the traffic of people. Therefore, control of personnel traffic is important.

It is also important to follow strict rules for catheter maintenance. Education of home care personnel must be encouraged. Personnel of hemodialysis units must be educated about this problem. There has been an explosive creation of dialysis centers, and many people working there do not have expertise in infection control.[10] The incidence of infectious complications decreases if capable nursing teams are available.[10,39]

Some factors to be considered when one deals with infection are the type of catheter and the number of lumens. The more lumens, the more risk of infection.[46] Bone marrow transplant patients are at a high risk of infection by bacteria, fungi, and opportunistic germs. In addition, these patients receive chemotherapy and radiation therapy, making them more vulnerable to infection.[30] Septic patients sooner or later will have a contaminated catheter. It is important to remember that PICC lines have a very low rate of infectious complications.[19]

Exit-Site Infection This type of infection usually manifests by redness (erythema) and swelling for 1 to 2 cm around the entrance site. The catheter does not need to be removed. The incidence of this complication is 20 to 40%, and the success of therapy with antibiotics and local care is more than 90%.[21,47] To minimize the incidence of infectious complications of central venous catheters for hemodialysis, the catheter maintenance should be done by specially trained staff.[48]

Tunnel or Pocket Infection Tunnel or pocket infection presents with pus in the tunnel or port site or pocket. This infection does not respond to antibiotics and requires removal of the catheter or port. Antibiotics must be administered, either orally or preferably IV.

Catheter-Related Sepsis is septicemia in the absence of exit-site or tunnel or port infections and when other sources of infection have been ruled out. The blood cultures from the catheter tip are positive, and usually there is a 10-fold increase in the number of colonies compared with cultures from peripheral blood.[1]

Catheter-related sepsis usually presents with bacteremia, fever, and elevated white cell count. If an obvious source of sepsis or infection is not found, it may be assumed that the patient has sepsis related to the presence of the central venous catheter; therefore, the catheter must be removed, a course of IV antibiotics administered, and the catheter tip cultured. In general, sepsis responds to antibiotic therapy.

Treatment Some infections do not respond well to antibiotics: *Candida albicans*, *Pseudomonas* organisms, and other nosocomial infections. The catheters and ports must be removed and multidrug therapy instituted.[1] Also, patients who are human immunodeficiency virus (HIV)-positive have an increased incidence of infectious complications.[49]

The routine use of prophylactic antibiotics is controversial. Some use it, but some do not.[17,50,51] It is generally agreed that prophylactic antibiotics should be used during subcutaneous port placement. Some advise against prophylaxis because of reports of increased bacterial colonization of catheters after prophylactic antibiotics.[17,50]

During placement of catheters, cefazolin can be used preprocedure and nothing after the procedure. On the other hand, during placement of ports, cefazolin can be used preprocedure and dicloxacillin for 5 to 7 days after the procedure.

Port Disruption, Leakage, and Skin Erosion

Some uncommon complications of ports are mentioned here. Difficulty in accessing or aspirating the port, ulceration at the port site, hematoma at the port site (pocket), port leakage, catheter disruption, septum disruption, and so on are uncommon problems associated with ports.[44]

Port-site skin ulceration and dehiscence are usually due to improper access with leakage of caustic or toxic substances or chemotherapeutic agents and lack of enough subcutaneous fat and tissue as a result of placing the port too superficially, rendering the covering skin too thin. Therefore, repeated punctures of the same skin site for access eventually can result in ulceration. If a port is placed too deep in the subcutaneous tissues, especially in an obese person, particularly obese women with large, pendulous breasts, it can be hard to palpate and difficult to access. In these cases, fluid infusates may leak in the subcutaneous tissues and cause pain and necrosis.[44]

In cases of skin ulceration or dehiscence, the port must be removed and placed in another site (another pocket). If it is too superficial, the port must be replaced more deeply. If it is too deep, it must be placed more superficially. Insertion of the port must be such that it lies against bony structures for easy access but not too deep in the subcutaneous tissues that it cannot be felt and accessed. If a port is needed in a morbidly obese person, an arm port may be preferable because arm ports are easy to insert and access.

Port leakage is usually due to defects in the port, too-vigorous infusion, or too-vigorous flushing when the catheter is occluded or flushing at high pressure with a small syringe. It also may be due to poor catheter–port connection, separation, or rupture. The port must be removed and a new one inserted in the same or different pocket and tunnel.[32,44] Septum dehiscence is a rare event that is due to repeated trauma to the septum by needle punctures. Eventually, the septum may be damaged if too-large or -blunt needles are used[35,44] (Fig. 13–13).

Ports also can migrate or rotate around their longitudinal or transverse axis so that they are upside down or backward. Some of these problems can be avoided by making sure that the pocket is small and tight enough to accommodate the port only. Ports must be sutured and anchored to the deep fascia and subcutaneous tissues. The skin

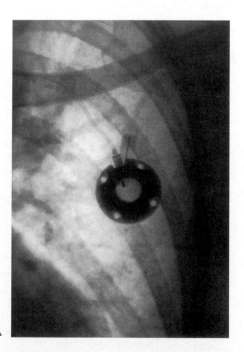

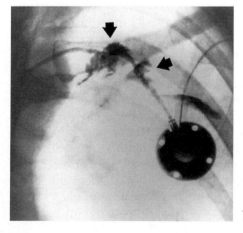

Figure 13–13 **(A)** Portacath in the left anterior chest wall inserted by surgeons. **(B)** The patient complained of severe burning and chest pain during infusion. Contrast was injected in the port. There is massive extravasation in the subcutaneous tissues as a result of catheter leak. The port and catheter were removed, and a new port was inserted by the interventional radiologist by right internal jugular vein puncture.

over the port must be closed carefully in layers, and the bleeding site(s) must be controlled before closing the pocket.[35]

Disruption of the port–catheter junction may be serious if it is not recognized. It will result in leakage of infusate with significant risk of tissue damage. The port must be removed unless the catheter can be reattached to the port or if the disrupted catheter can be replaced. Catheter disruption also may occur if the catheter is injured, perforated, or severed during access with the needle, particularly in patients in whom the port is not well palpated or identified in the subcutaneous tissues. If the catheter becomes separated from the port, peripheral or central embolization into the RA, right ventricle, or pulmonary arteries may occur, necessitating percutaneous retrieval with Amplatz gooseneck loop snares, Curry loop snares, Dotter retrieval baskets, or forceps.

An interesting, albeit rare, complication of ports is the "twiddle syndrome," which involves patients constantly fiddling with the port and eventually inverting the port. Also, trauma has been reported as a cause of port inversion.[44]

Catheter Removal Distress Syndrome

In this rare, poorly documented complication, patients develop neurologic paresis, coma, respiratory failure, and shock on complete removal of central catheters. Such problems can be potentially life threatening. This problem is mentioned here but it is not a well-recognized complication.[52]

SUMMARY

The vascular interventional radiologist places central venous catheters, such as PICC lines, subcutaneous ports, tunneled catheters, and temporary catheters using ultrasound and fluoroscopic guidance. Even using correct and current techniques, equipment, and supplies, complications related to the procedure cannot be avoided. The vascular interventional radiologist knows and is ready to manage these complications.

Prevention of complications must be the goal of every operator. Every effort must be made to keep a central venous access functional because sites of venous access become depleted as patients live longer and their primary problems are being managed. The vascular interventional radiologist must be familiar with the different methods, devices, and techniques for management of complications.

The vascular and interventional radiologist places catheters as soon as a request is made. There is no need to wait for operating room or other delays, and the results are significant cost savings, improved safety, decreased procedural time, improved precision, and increased convenience.[15,33,53] As long as vascular and interventional radiologists provide excellent patient care, educate ancillary personnel, and conduct research for developing better tools and methods, they will be an integral part of the team dealing with central venous access.

REFERENCES

1. Namyslowski J, Patel NH. Central venous access: a new task for interventional radiologists. *Cardiovasc Intervent Radiol.* 1999;22:355–368.
2. Lewis CA, Allen TE, Burke DR, et al. Quality improvement guidelines for central venous access. *J Vasc Interv Radiol.* 1997;8:475–479.
3. Patel NH. Alternate approaches to central venous access. *Semin Interv Radiol.* 1998;15:325–333.
4. Foley MJ. Venous access devices: low-cost convenience. *Diag Imag.* 1993;87–94.
5. Noh M, Kaufman JA, Rhea JT, et al. Cost comparison of radiologic versus surgical placement of long-term hemodialysis catheters. *AJR Am J Roentgenol.* 1999;172:673–675.
6. Robertson LJ, Mauro MA, Jaques PF. Radiologic placement of Hickman catheters. *Radiology.* 1989;170:1007–1009.
7. Mody MK, Shetty PC, Kastan DJ, et al. Implanted chest ports placed by interventional radiologist: immediate and delayed complications in 350 cases. SCVIR 1997 Annual Meeting Syllabus, 1997:218.

8. Gelbfish GA. Surgery versus percutaneous treatment of thrombosed dialysis access grafts: is there a best method? *J Vasc Interv Radiol.* 1998;9:875–877.

9. Jaques PF. Maintenance of long-term dialysis catheters. *Technol Vasc Interv Radiol.* 1998; 1:148–153.

10. Mauro MA. Introduction to techniques in vascular and interventional radiology. *Technol Vasc Interv Radiol.* 1998;1:115.

11. Paplham PD. Post-procedural care of central venous catheters. *Semin Interv Radiol.* 1998; 15:297–303.

12. Johnson EM, Saltzman DA, Suh G, et al. Complications and risks of central venous catheter placement in children. *Surgery.* 1998; 124:911–916.

13. Angle JF, Hagspiel KD, Spinosa DJ, et al. Peripherally inserted central catheters. *Appl Radiol.* 1998;31–39.

14. Docktor BL, Sadler DJ, Gray RR, et al. Radiologic placement of tunneled central catheters. *AJR Am J Roentgenol.* 1999;173:457–460.

15. Morris SL, Jaques PF, Mauro MA. Radiology-assisted placement of implantable subcutaneous infusion ports for long-term venous access. *Radiology.* 1992;184:149–151.

16. Sandhu J. Peripheral devices. *Technol Vasc Interv Radiol.* 1998;1:140–147.

17. Owens CA, Yaghmai B, Warner D. Complications of central venous catheterization. *Semin Interv Radiol.* 1998;15:341–355.

18. Andrews JC, Marx MV, Williams DM, et al. The upper arm approach for placement of peripherally inserted central catheters forprotracted venous access. *AJR Am J Roentgenol.* 1992;158:427–429.

19. Yaghmai B, Owens CA, Warner D. Peripherally inserted central catheters. *Semin Interv Radiol.*1998;15:305–314.

20. Trerotola SO. Interventional radiology in the management of dialysis access sites. RSNA Categorical Course in Vascular Imaging Syllabus, 1998:323–332.

21. Fan CM. Tunneled catheters. *Semin Interv Radiol.* 1998;15:273–286.

22. Mauro MA, Jaques PF. Radiologic placement of long-term central venous catheters: a review. *J Vasc Interv Radiol.* 1993;4:127–137.

23. Fernando C, Juravsky L, Yedlicka J, et al. Subclavian central venous catheter insertion: angiointerventional technique. *Semin Intervent Radiol.* 1991;8:78–81.

24. Thielen JB, Nyquist J. Air embolism during removal of subclavian catheters. *J Interv Vasc Nurs.* 1991;14:114–118.

25. Funaki B, Szymski GX, Leef JA, et al. Radiologic placement of tunneled central venous catheters: techniques and pitfalls. *Appl Radiol.* 1998;8–13.

26. Kowalski CM, Kaufman JA, Rivitz SM, et al. Migration of central venous catheters: implications for initial catheter tip positioning. *J Vasc Interv Radiol.* 1997;8:443–447.

27. Nazarian GK, Bjarnason H, Dietz C Jr, et al. Changes in tunneled catheter tip position when a patient is upright. *J Vasc Interv Radiol.* 1997;8:437–441.

28. Lucey B, Varghese JC, Haslam P, et al. Routine chest radiographs after central line insertion: mandatory postprocedural evaluation or unnecessary waste of resources? *Cardiovasc Intervent Radiol.*1999;22:381–384.

29. Caridi JG, Grundy LS, Ross EA, et al. Interventional radiology placement of twin Tesio catheters for dialysis access. *J Vasc Interv Radiol.* 1999;10:78–83.

30. Deutsch LS. Venous access develops into core technology. *Diagn Imag.* 1996;35-42.

31. Boardman P, Hughes JP. Radiological evaluation and management of malfunctioning central venous catheters. *Clin Radiol.* 1998;53: 10–16.

32. Lokich JJ, Bothe A Jr, Benotti P, et al. Complications and management of implanted venous access catheters. *J Clin Oncol.* 1985;3:710–717.

33. Mauro MA. Interventional radiologic placement of central venous catheters. *Hosp Physician.* 1996;55–59.

34. Haskal ZJ, Cohn MC. Management of hemodialysis catheters. *Appl Radiol.* 1999;14–24.

35. Mauro MA. Delayed complications of venous access. *Technol Vasc Interv Radiol.* 1998;1:158-167.

36. Xiang DZ, Verbeken EK, Van Lommel ATL, et al. Composition and formation of the sleeve enveloping a central venous catheter. *J Vasc Surg.* 1998;28:260–271.

37. Saker MB, Chrisman HB, Matsumoto AH. Dialysis access preservation. *Appl Radiol.* 1999;27–32.

38. Lund GB. Hemodialysis access catheters. *Semin Intervent Radiol.* 1998;15:287–295.

39. Denny DF Jr. Placement and management of long-term central venous access catheters

and ports. *AJR Am J Roentgenol.* 1993;161: 385–393.

40. Semba CP, Dake MD. Thrombolysis in venous and pulmonary occlusive disease. RSNA Categorical Course in Vascular Imaging Syllabus, 1998:177-182.

41. Seigel EL, Jew AC, Delcore R, et al. Thrombolytic therapy for catheter-related thrombosis. *Am J Surg.* 1993;166:716–719.

42. Prandoni P, Polistena P, Bernardi E, et al. Upper extremity deep vein thrombosis. *Arch Intern Med.* 1997;157:57–62.

43. Rajan DK, Croteau DL, Sturza SG, et al. Translumbar placement of inferior vena cava catheters. *Radiographics.* 1998;18:1155–1167.

44. Ahmad I, Ray CE Jr. Radiologic placement of venous access ports. *Semin Intervent Radiol.* 1998;15:259–272.

45. Haskal ZJ. Temporary access for hemodialysis and problem solving to maintain it.SCVIR Annual Meeting Syllabus, 1997: 113–120.

46. Millner MR, Kerns SR, Hawkins Jr IF, et al. Tesio twin dialysis catheter system: a new catheter for hemodialysis. *AJR Am J Roentgenol.* 1995;164:1519–1520.

47. Moss AH, Vasilakis C, Holley JL, et al. Use of silicone dual-lumen catheter with a Dacron cuff as a long-term vascular access for hemodialysis patients. *Am J Kidney Dis.* 1990; 16:211–215.

48. Kaufman JA, Greenfield AJ. Selection of venous access devices. In: *New Developments in Central Venous Access* [newsletter]. Glenview, IL: Physicians & Scientists Publications, Winter 1998–1999.

49. Whigham CJ, Goodman CJ, Fisher RG, et al. Infectious complications of 393 peripherally implantable venous access devices in HIV-positive and HIV-negative patients. *J Vasc Interv Radiol.* 1999;10:71–77.

50. Trerotola SO, Johnson MS, Moresco KP, et al. Antibiotic prophylaxis [letter to the editor]. *J Vasc Interv Radiol.* 1999;10:235–237.

51. Sawhney R. Arm ports provide long-term central venous access. *Diagn Imag.* 1998; 59–61.

52. Kim DK, Gottesman MH, Forero A, et al. The CVC removal distress syndrome: an unappreciated complication of central venous catheter removal. *Am Surg.* 1998;64:344–347.

53. McBride KD, Fisher R, Warnock N, et al. A comparative analysis of radiological and surgical placement of central venous catheters. *Cardiovasc Intervent Radiol.* 1997;20: 17–22.

Chapter 14

Central Venous Access Catheter Infections: An Overview

Robert D. Lyon
Allen Meglin

Long-term central venous access devices represent a major advance in medical care, allowing continuous access to the circulatory system for ongoing intravenous infusional therapy and therapeutic interventions such as plasmapheresis and hemodialysis. As with any invasive therapy, complications occur. The goal of this chapter is to provide an overview of infectious complications of these devices. Although much of what is published in the medical literature on this subject involves studies of nontunneled, acute-use devices, most of the principles regarding the pathogenesis, treatment, and prevention of catheter-related infection apply to long-term devices as well and are worth reviewing in this context.

The placement of any venous access device involves disruption of the normally protective integument, allowing the potential access of microorganisms into the body. Catheter-related infection results in a spectrum of difficulties, ranging from minor inconvenience, to device removal, to life-threatening sepsis.

Device removal as a result of infection can be a particularly serious outcome in vein-depleted patients, who then must suffer the placement of additional temporary or long-term devices to complete therapy. Indeed, the prevention of catheter infection becomes one of the primary goals of both the providers and recipients of central venous access devices.

DEFINITIONS OF INFECTION

One of the difficulties in comparing results in the medical literature regarding infectious complications is that there is an inconsistency in the definitions used for the various forms of catheter-related infections. For the purpose of this chapter, the following definitions will be used:

Colonization refers to the presence of pathogens in quantities in excess of generally accepted thresholds by either quantitative or semiquantitative culture techniques. *Contamination* refers to the presence of pathogens in quantities below these thresholds. *Device-related infection* requires the presence of clinical symptoms of infection in addition to device contamination. *Exit-site infection* refers to evidence of infection confined to the skin wound or the catheter tunnel within 2 cm of the skin wound. *Tunnel infection* refers to evidence of infection anywhere in the path of the subcutaneous catheter tract greater than 2 cm from the skin wound to the venous entry site. *Pocket infection* refers to evidence of infection confined to the subcutaneous pocket of an implanted venous access port. *Catheter-related bacteremia* is defined as the presence of the same organism colonizing the device that is present in the bloodstream. *Catheter-related sepsis* is present when clinical sepsis occurs in the presence of a proven catheter-related bacteremia.

MECHANISMS OF INFECTION

Several theories exist regarding the mechanism of venous access device infection. A clinically evident infection begins with colonization by pathogens of the device or its surrounding tissue. Most investigators believe that the primary source of infecting flora is commensal organisms living on the skin at the device entry site.[1] This is practically substantiated by the observation that most catheter-related infections are caused by staphylococcal species such as *S. epidermidis*, which is a prolific human skin commensal. One pathway of bacterial contamination may begin with the migration of organisms through the wound at the catheter entry site. The extent of the resulting invasion depends on multiple factors, including the health of the host and the vigor of the host's immune response, the virulence of the organism, and the integrity of the soft tissues at the access site. Colonization may be confined to the area of the entry site, or organisms may ascend along the catheter surface to cause a more widespread contamination of the subcutaneous tunnel or the reservoir pocket of an implanted port. Ultimately, this may result in the spread of organisms to the vessel and the onset of bacteremia.

Another well-investigated source of device colonization is contamination of the device hub.[2,3] The pathway of infection in this case is colonization of the lumen of the catheter by organisms introduced to the hub during catheter manipulation. This infection may progress to bacteremia as a result of ascending colonization of the catheter lumen. Similarly, the reservoir of an implanted venous access device may harbor thrombus as a result of insufficient flushing following aspiration of blood or transfusion of blood products. This may become colonized and thus become a source of ascending endoluminal bacterial contamination. A parallel concern with the endoluminal route of catheter infection is the resulting colonization of the fibrin sheath that ubiquitously forms around the catheter inside the vessel. In theory, colonization of this entity can lead to ongoing bacteremia and risk for sepsis.

Contamination of the infusate is another possible cause of catheter-related infection. Several instances of epidemic sepsis as a result of contaminated intravenous solutions were widely reported in the United States in the 1970s. These infections are usually caused by gram-negative organisms that grow well in nutrient infusates such as lipid emulsions used for total parenteral nutrition. Fortunately, this is a rare cause of infection today, but clusters of infections caused by unusual organisms, especially in patients with low-risk factors for catheter-related infection, should be regarded with suspicion for infusate contamination.

Last, catheter infection may result from an internal source of organisms contaminating the device by hematogenous spread. In this case, the fibrin sheath or thrombus at the catheter becomes colonized by bacteremia resulting from the breakdown of mucosal surfaces from a variety of causes, such as mucositis resulting from chemotherapy, tumor invasion of the bowel or bronchus, or the denuded skin surface of burn patients.

PATHOGENESIS

The remarkable feature of catheter infection is that rather ordinary organisms are most frequently responsible for catheter-related infection. The most common organisms are those usually found on the normal skin surface, the skin commensals such as coagulase-negative and coagulase-positive staphylococcal species, diphtheroids, and certain streptococcal species. Most yeast infections appear to result from hematogenous spread from another site.[1] Bacteremia caused by gram-negative organisms should implicate the gut or viscera as sources because contamination of a venous access device by these organisms by the usual routes of colonization is unusual in the absence of infusate contamination.

Interactions between pathogens, blood proteins, and the surface of the catheter are thought to play a role in bacterial colonization of venous access devices. Following placement, the intravascular portion of the device becomes rapidly coated with certain proteinaceous components of blood, including fibronectin, fibrin, and other associated substances.[4] These elements form a continuous surface over the catheter, referred to as the *fibrin sheath*. Besides being implicated in catheter malfunction, the constituents of the fibrin sheath can act as a "scaffolding" that allows bacterial attachment. It also may cause changes in the local immunologic milieu that protect attached pathogens from antibiotic eradication.[5] Individual organisms have their own qualities that promote affinity to the catheter surface. *S. epidermidis* produces glycoproteins that create a "slime" that aid in its adherence to the catheter surface.[6] Both *S. epidermidis* and *S. aureus* attachment appears to benefit from interaction with proteins adherent to the catheter surface, including constituents of thrombus.[7] This fact has been implicated in the difficulty of in situ treatment of *S. aureus* catheter infections.[5]

DIAGNOSIS

Signs and Symptoms

The contamination of a venous access device may merely result in colonization with no clinical evidence of infection. There are clinical mimics of infection that should be recognized. Mild erythema at the entry site of a catheter is a frequent occurrence and may not be the result of infection. Irritation from cleansing agents, tape, or other types of catheter dressings can cause redness and discomfort. Superficial phlebitis also can result in a syndrome of erythema, warmth, and pain that may involve the catheter entry site and the catheter tunnel and can be mistaken for infection. Extravasation of infusate from access needles incorrectly placed in the reservoir can result in a spectrum of clinical findings that could be mistaken for infection, ranging from local swelling to skin exfoliation.

In general, as infection progresses, a discharge of some type can be expressed from the entry site. This is a more sensitive indicator of infection compared with other causes of the clinical syndrome of pain, warmth, and redness. The discharge may be frankly purulent, but it can also be serous in quality. The presence of any type of discharge should raise the level of suspicion for catheter-related infection. Tunnel and pocket infections may demonstrate fluctuance and tenderness indicating drainage, and device removal may be necessary. Fever is not an uncommon symptom of catheter-related infection, but usually it is more often associated with bacteremia or sepsis. Fever associated with localized infection is a clear indicator of severity. Fever alone as a presenting symptom of local infection would be unusual without other associated clinical signs.

Bacteremic patients are also more likely to exhibit leukocytosis than patients with localized extravascular infections. Others symptoms of catheter-related sepsis are typical and include malaise, anorexia, chills and night sweats, and, in advanced cases, hypotension and cardiovascular collapse. Immunocompromised patients are of particular concern because they more often present with symptoms of florid sepsis than do patients with intact immune systems capable of more subtle responses to bacteremia.

A rare, but dreaded, presentation of catheter-related infection is suppurative thrombophlebitis, which can occur in both superficial and deep veins. In this syndrome, a catheter-related thrombus becomes colonized and the patient exhibits signs typical of occlusive deep venous thrombosis, such as arm swelling, but also exhibits other manifestations of infection. Since the advent of long-term central venous catheterization for venosclerosing infusates, superficial suppurative thrombophlebitis is rare.

Laboratory

The precise role of cultures in the management of suspected catheter-related infection has been the subject of numerous clinical and laboratory investigations. A sick patient with a venous access device who becomes febrile presents a management dilemma because catheter-related sepsis has no distinguishing clinical features from sepsis resulting from another focus of infection. Prompt catheter removal is an effective way of proving or disproving suspected catheter-related sepsis, but it necessitates removal of the venous access device and placement of another catheter to provide antibiotic therapy and for ongoing treatment of the patient's underlying condition. On the other hand, making a decision about catheter removal by simply verifying growth of the same organism in both catheter and peripheral blood aspirates is a nonspecific practice of little clinical value. Quantitative bacterial and fungal cultures have been advocated to pinpoint the role of a venous access device in a particular case of sepsis.

Where there is suspicion of systemic or vascular infection, peripheral blood cultures are very important when bacteremia is present. The fate of the venous access device depends on several considerations. If determination of the source of infection is unclear, the results of semiquantitative cultures of the catheter tip must be evaluated. Maki and associates compared 388 peripheral and central catheter tip cultures with peripheral blood cultures. They found that the presence of 15 or more colonies on the tip culture plate was associated with a 16% incidence of bacteremia in patients with mostly peripheral catheters; however, all cases of clinical sepsis and asymptomatic bacteremia were associated with colony counts above this threshold. No cases of bacteremia were associated with growth of less than 15 colonies.[8] The test is useful in that a low colony count "exonerates" the catheter as the source and focuses the search for the source of infection elsewhere. Unfortunately, the technique requires catheter removal.

Several studies describe the value of obtaining and comparing simultaneous quantitative blood cultures from a peripheral vein and the venous access device in cases of suspected catheter-related sepsis.[9–12] This test evaluates for an increase in the number of organisms in the catheter aspirate versus the peripheral aspirate. Step-ups in counts from the catheter blood culture of five to ten times the counts from the peripheral culture were found to correlate well with the diagnosis of catheter-related infection as evidenced by patient improvement following catheter removal and antibiotic therapy.[9,10,13] This method has the advantage of in situ evaluation for catheter-related infection. Unfortunately, these tests are complicated and expensive; however, quantitative cultures are useful in certain situations, such as when the cost or difficulty of line replacement is unacceptably high or for the evaluation of implanted venous access devices.

Another technique that does not require catheter removal was described in a study that compared semiquantitative cultures of catheter tips with semiquantitative cultures of the skin at the insertion site and the interior of the catheter hub with peripheral blood cultures in patients suspected of having catheter-related sepsis.[14] The positive predictive value of positive superficial cultures was 66%, but the negative predictive value of negative cultures was 96.7%, making this method of detection potentially useful in the triage of patients with venous access devices and unexplained fever.

MANAGEMENT

The most important factor in decision making for suspected catheter-related infection is the condition of the patient and the severity of the signs and symptoms of infection. Few would hesitate to remove a device in a patient with clear signs of sepsis and serial positive blood cultures for a typical organism, despite appropriate antibiotic therapy. These patients generally require hospitalization, intravenous antibiotics, and close observation. Likewise, purulent tunnel or pocket infections or pocket infections that present with wound dehiscence have little hope of eradication and device preservation with antibiotic therapy alone. Antibiotic therapy, device removal, and wound packing or surgical drainage is the best option in these situations.

On the other hand, tunnel or pocket infections presenting with mild signs of infection and serous or minimal purulent exudate often respond well to a short course of intravenous antibiotics, followed by 2 weeks of oral antibiotics based on the results of the culture. In these situations, salvage of the device becomes a priority, especially in patients who have limited accesses as a result of previous cannulations. There are no precise guidelines for which strategy to pursue, however, and the decision to remove a catheter should made on a case-by-case basis.

Treatment of bacteremia in immunocompetent patients with intravenous antibiotics and close observation, rather than catheter removal, may be considered in certain cases,[10,12,15,16] including infections caused by coagulase-negative staphylococcal species, streptococcal species, and other skin diphtheroids, because negative outcomes of sepsis from these organisms are uncommon. Treatment is followed by serial peripheral blood cultures, and catheter removal may be necessary for persistent bacteremia. Special caution is needed when dealing with infections by *S. aureus, Candida* and other fungal species, and *Pseudomonas* species. Serious complications from incompletely treated infections and hematogenous seeding of distant organs may occur. *S. aureus* is a particularly tenacious organism because of its tendency to become adherent to proteins of the fibrin sheath, which decreases the effectiveness of antibiotic therapy. Infection secondary to resistant staphylococcal species is an indication for catheter removal. *Pseudomonas* infections in patients with colonized venous access devices are rarely, if ever, eradicated by antibiotic therapy alone, and fear of *Pseudomonas* sepsis dictates device removal.

INFECTION PREVENTION

Device Choice and Placement

Multiple studies have shown a reduced rate of infections with tunneled catheters and implanted venous access devices compared with nontunneled central venous access devices.[17] Peripherally inserted central venous catheters have rates of bacteremia comparable to tunneled, cuffed central venous catheters.[18] There is evidence of an increased risk of bacteremia for multiple lumen nontunneled central lines,[19] but no similar data are available regarding a similar risk for multiple-lumen tunneled or implanted devices. Silver-impregnated antibiotic cuffs have been studied as a method of reducing infection by reducing the risk of ascending bacterial colonization of the subcutaneous tunnel before complete fibrous attachment of the Dacron catheter cuff. These studies have described decreased rates of local infection and catheter-related sepsis for acute-use, nontunneled catheters.[20,21] Other studies, however, have not shown the same benefit for tunneled catheters.[22,23]

Certain patients may be considered at increased risk for infection from tunneled or implanted devices. These include severely malnourished patients, whose incision for a reservoir pocket may not heal adequately, patients with specific antibody deficiencies, and patients with resistant bacteremia from endocarditis or other difficult-to-eradicate sources of blood-borne infections. In general, an implanted port is not a good choice for a patient receiving a continuous infusion, such as total parenteral nutrition or continuous chemotherapy. The transcutaneous access needle into the device reservoir for more than several days eliminates one of the advantages of an implanted device, namely, the need for frequent flushing and dressing changes, and should be avoided.

There are reports of using novel antiseptic or antibiotic-impregnated catheters to decrease the incidence of infection. A randomized, controlled trial showed that nontunneled devices coated with a combination of chlorhexidine and silver sulfadiazine were significantly less likely to become colonized and caused a lower rate of sepsis than noncoated devices.[24] These results were not duplicated by others.[25,26] Minocycline and rifampin in combination also have been studied as a catheter coating in a randomized study of nontunneled catheters in the critical care setting. A statistically significant decrease in both catheter colonization and catheter-related sepsis was reported.[27] No reports of randomized trials of these coatings on extended-use devices are available. Indeed, at least one investigator raises the concern of the possibility that these coatings may support the selection of resistant strains of organisms.[5]

Skin preparation for device placement is a matter of preference. Most operators follow preexisting guidelines for surgical preparation with iodine-based solutions for skin disinfection. There is evidence that chlorhexidine-based cleansers are better than iodine-based solutions or alcohol,[28] but their use has not been universally adopted because of the increased cost. Caution must be used when preparing the skin for jugular access not to splash chlorhexidine agents into the eyes because permanent corneal damage has resulted from prolonged contact with the eye.

Most operators give antibiotics during placement for tunneled or implanted devices. No randomized trials have addressed the use of procedural antibiotics specifically for the placement of venous access devices. There are reports, however, on the use of antibiotics for other vascular procedures that are worth considering when deciding whether to include antibiotic prophylaxis as a part of the implantation procedure. A randomized trial for arterial reconstructive surgery showed a reduction of the infection rate from 6.8% with placebo to 0.9% with cefazolin given intravenously immediately before the procedure.[29] Almost identical results were reported recently in another randomized trial evaluating intravenous vancomycin versus placebo in the placement of upper-extremity polyfluoroethylene grafts for hemodialysis.[30] A recent metanalysis of randomized studies examining the impact of antibiotics on the risk of pacemaker-related infections showed a statistically significant reduction in the risk of pocket or tunnel infections.[31]

A typical protocol would be the intravenous administration of a first-generation cephalosporin, such as cephalexin, immediately before device placement, followed by several days of oral antibiotic therapy with an agent such as dicloxacillin. Vancomycin can be a substitute in penicillin-allergic patients, but because of its cost and its special role in the treatment of resistant gram-positive infections, it should not be given as a first-line agent for prophylaxis. Antibiotic choice is directed primarily at gram-positive organisms, and common skin commensals will be sensitive to those antibiotics described.

No antibiotic regimen will substitute for scrupulous adherence to sterile technique during placement, including maintenance of cleanliness of the operative suite. Fluoroscopic suites used for placement of tunneled or implanted venous access devices must be maintained with the cleanliness expected in the operating room.

Device Care

Care of a venous access device after placement is the single greatest determinant of risk for catheter-related infection. Most clinical series on venous access devices have reported low rates of periprocedural infection (i.e., infection occurring within several days of placement). Despite the fact that the Centers for Disease Control defines any infection occurring within 1 year of placement as placement related,[32] mismanagement of dressing care and maintenance unfairly involves accountability of the operator who placed the device. Careless technique during infusion can lead to hub or reservoir contamination and colonization with risk of clinical infection. Studies have demonstrated significantly reduced rates of catheter-related infection in centers where dedicated, well-trained practitioners (primarily nurses) are in charge of catheter access and site management.[33,34] Unfortunately, the maintenance of these teams is a cost that many hospitals are not willing to bear, even if the cost of treating patients with catheter-related infections exceeds the cost of prevention.

Povidone/iodine-containing ointment is effective at reducing the incidence of catheter-related infection with hemodialysis catheters.[35] A study comparing a triple-antibiotic ointment with iodophor ointment found no significant difference in the incidence of infection, but patients using the triple-antibiotic ointment had an increased incidence of fungemia, with fungal commensals, specially *Candida albicans*.[36] Multiple studies have evaluated the risk of infection with the use of transparent plastic dressing as opposed to gauze bandages for the protection of the catheter entry site; results have been conflicting[37,38] (see Chapter 12).

From a practical standpoint, plastic dressing offers an occlusive barrier that prevents contamination of the exit site during activity and bathing. Plastic dressings also add an element of security against inadvertent catheter removal, especially with peripherally inserted central catheters. Some patients experience irritation that can lead to desquamation and superficial infection as a result of the trauma of tape removal, but these dressings are well tolerated and provide excellent protection for both external devices and during the healing of incisions from implanted device placement.

A large randomized study of gauze dressings versus permeable polyurethane and nonpermeable plastic dressing of nontunneled catheters found an increased incidence of bacterial colonization of the skin under the transparent plastic dressings that had been left in place for 5 days between changes.[38] No statistically significant difference in the incidence of device colonization or catheter-related bacteremia or sepsis was noted, however. Randomized studies of the two dressing types for tunneled, cuffed devices in the renal and bone marrow transplant patients failed to demonstrate an increased risk of catheter-related infection, even when the dressings were left in place up to 7 days.[30,40]

An intriguing scheme to prevent possible bacterial colonization of the catheter tip is the routine use of thrombolytic agents for catheter maintenance. The concept relies on the theory that the biochemistry of the fibrin sheath promotes the adherence of pathogens. By reducing the fibrin sheath, the degree of colonization may be reduced. The thrombolytic agents also have the potential added benefit of reducing catheter malfunction caused by occlusion of the catheter tip by the fibrin sheath. The major drawback is the cost of the thrombolytic agent. In the amounts used for prophylaxis, increased risk of hemorrhage should not be a real clinical concern. The practicality of this approach to prevention of catheter-related bacteremia awaits further clinical study.

PEDIATRIC AND IMMUNOCOMPROMISED PATIENTS

Multiple studies have reported rates of infection for devices in children similar to the rates in adults.[11,12,16,41–43] The inability of children, especially very young children, to care for a device means that special attention in the form of training for device care must be given to the child's parents. Children may be better suited for implanted devices because the absence of external parts that can be damaged by activity and freedom from dressing changes may result in better acceptance of the device.

Patients with acquired immunodeficiency syndrome (AIDS) benefit the same as other chronically ill patients from the placement of long-term venous access devices.

There appears to be a trend toward increased incidence of catheter-related infections in AIDS patients. One study that evaluated Hickman catheters and implanted devices in AIDS patients found a statistically significant difference in the incidence of catheter-related infections favoring implanted devices.[44] The overall rates of infection were acceptable for both types of devices. *S. aureus* was the most common organism involved. Therefore, AIDS should not be a contraindication for the placement of a long-term venous access device unless there is preexisting sepsis. In this situation, the bacteremia should be treated before device placement.

FUTURE DIRECTIONS

The ultimate venous access device has yet to be designed. From the standpoint of catheter-related infection, the implanted devices significantly obstruct microorganisms from the common pathways for colonization and infection; however, these devices still fall prey to contamination during placement, by poor antisepsis during access, and colonization of the fibrin sheath by bacteremia from another source in the body. Active areas of research or areas requiring further research are infection rates for catheters impregnated with antibiotic (cefazolin, rifampin, minocycline), silver, chlorhexidine, benzalkonium, or heparin; use of electric current; and presence of an iodine tincture reservoir in catheter hub.

SUMMARY

Catheter-related infections are well known and many are preventable. Infection prevention requires the commitment of the operator who places the device and of those who will care for the device. Good sterile technique in placement is critical. Operators should accept nothing less than "operating room" standards for patient preparation and in operative technique. Protocols for antibiotic use are quite variable and are based on local practice. Creation of antibiotic resistance is a threat, and there is a need for a randomized study of this problem.

When developing a venous access service, one should consider having a dedicated staff member to teach each patient device care, including instruction on dressing changes and catheter maintenance. Standard written catheter care guidelines to take away also decrease patient confusion and serve as a reference for the patient if problems arise outside the service's offices. Teaching patients device care is essential.

REFERENCES

1. Darouiche RO, Raad II. Prevention of catheter-related infections: the skin. *Nutrition.* 1997;13(suppl):26S–29S.
2. Salzman MB, Rubin LG. Relevance of the catheter hub as a portal for microorganisms causing catheter-related bloodstream infections. *Nutrition.* 1997;13(suppl):15S–17S.
3. Sitges-Serra A, Hernandez R, Maestro S, Pi-Suner T, Garces JM, Segura M. Prevention of catheter sepsis: the hub. *Nutrition.* 1997;13(suppl):30S–33S.
4. Passerini L, Lam K, Costeron JW, et al. Biofilms on indwelling vascular catheters. *Crit Care Med.* 1992;20:665–673.
5. Wadstrom T. Surfaces and infection [abstract]. *J Vasc Surg.* 1998;27:1152.
6. Hoyle BD, Jass J, Costeron JW. The biofilm glycocalyx as a resistance factor. *J Antimicrob Chemother.* 190;26:1–6.
7. Herrmann M, Vaudaux PE, Pittet D, et al. Fibronectin, fibrinogen and laminin act as mediators of adherence of clinical staphylococcal isolates to foreign material. *J Infect Dis.* 1988;158:693–701.
8. Maki DG, Weise CE, Sarafin HW. A semiquantitative culture method for identifying intravenous catheter-related infection. *N Engl J Med.* 1977;296:1305–1309.
9. Mosca R, Curtas S, Forbes B, Meguid MM. The benefit of isolator cultures in the management of suspected catheter sepsis. *Surgery.* 1987;102:718–723.
10. Benezra D, Kien TE, Gold JWM, Brown A, Turnbull ADM, Armstrong D. Prospective study of infections in indwelling central

venous catheters using quantitative blood cultures. *Am J Med.* 1998;85:495–498.

11. Raucher HS, Hyatt AC, Barzilai A, et al. Quantitative blood cultures in the evaluation of septicemia in children with Broviac catheters. *J Pediatr.* 1984;104:29–34.

12. Flynn PM, Shenep JL, Stokes DC, Barrett FF. In-situ management of central venous catheter-related bacteremia. *Pediatr Infect Dis J.* 1987;6:729–734.

13. Maki DG, Mermel LA. Infections due to infusional therapy. In: Bennet JV, Brachman PS, eds. *Hospital Infections.* 4th ed. Philadelphia, PA: Lippincott; 1998:689–724.

14. Cercenado E, Ena J, Rodriguez-Creixems RI, Bouza E. A conservative procedure for the diagnosis of catheter-related infections. *Arch Intern Med.* 1990;150:1417–1420.

15. Kappers-Klunne MC, Degener JE, Stijnen T, Abels J. Complications from long-term indwelling central venous catheters in hematologic patients with special reference to infection. *Cancer.* 1989;64:1747–1752.

16. Kelin JF, Shahrivar F. Use of percutaneous silastic central venous catheters in neonates and the management of infectious complications. *Am J Perinatol.* 1992;9:261–264.

17. May GS, Davis C. Percutaneous catheters and totally implantable access systems: a review of reported infection rates. *J Intrav Nurs.* 1988;11:97–102.

18. Pauley SY, Vallande NC, Riely EN, Jenner NM, Gulbinas DG. Catheter-related colonization associated with percutaneous inserted central catheters. *J Intrav Nurs.* 1993;16: 50–55.

19. Farakas JC, Liu N, Bleriot JP, et al. Single-versus triple-lumen central catheter-related sepsis: a prospective randomized study in a critically ill population. *Am J Med.* 1992;93: 277–282.

20. Flowers RH III, Schwenzer KJ, Kopel RJ, et al. Efficacy of an attachable subcutaneous cuff for the prevention of intravascular catheter-related infection. *JAMA.* 1989;261: 878–883.

21. Maki DG, Cobb L, Garman JK, Shapiro JM, Ringer M, Helgerson RB. An attachable silver-impregnated cuff for prevention of infection with central venous catheters: a prospective randomized multicenter trial. *Am J Med.* 1988;85:307–314.

22. Groeger JS, Lucas AB, Coit D, et al. A prospective, randomized evaluation of the effect of silver-impregnated subcutaneous cuffs for preventing tunneled chronic venous access catheter infections in cancer patients. *Ann Surg.* 1993;218:206–210.

23. Dahlberg PJ, Agger WA, Singer JR, et al. Subclavian hemodialysis catheter infections: a prospective, randomized trial of an attachable silver-impregnated cuff for prevention of catheter-related infection. *Infect Control Hosp Epidemiol.* 1995;16:506–511.

24. Maki DG, Stoz SM, Wheeler S, Mermel LA. Prevention of central venous catheter-related bloodstream infection by use of an antiseptic-impregnated catheter: a randomized controlled trial. *Ann Intern Med.* 1997; 127:257–266.

25. Pemberton LB, Ross V, Cuddy P, Kremer H, Fessler T, McKurck E. No difference in catheter sepsis between standard and antiseptic central venous catheters: a prospective randomized trial. *Arch Surg.* 1996;131: 986–989.

26. Tennenberg S, Lieser M, McCurdy B, et al. A prospective randomized trial of an antibiotic-and-antiseptic–coated central venous catheter in the prevention of catheter-related infection. *Arch Surg.* 1997;132:1348–1351.

27. Darouche RO, Raad II, Wall M, et al. Antimicrobial efficacy, durability and safety of ventral venous catheters coated with minocycline and rifampin [abstract]. *Crit Care Med.* 1996;24(suppl):A121.

28. Maki DG, Alvarado CJ, Ringer M. A prospective randomized trial of povidone-iodine, alcohol, and chlorhexidine for prevention of infection with central venous and arterial catheters. *Lancet.* 1991;338:339–343.

29. Kaiser AB, Clayson KR, Muljerin JR Jr. Antibiotic prophylaxis in vascular surgery. *Ann Surg.* 1978;188:283–289.

30. Zibari GB, Gadallah MF, Landrenea M, et al. Preoperative vancomycin prophylaxis decreases the incidence of postoperative hemodialysis vascular access infections. *Am J Kidney Dis.* 1997;30:343–348.

31. DaCosta A, Kirkorian G, Cucherat M, et al. Antibiotic prophylaxis for permanent pacemaker implantation: a meta-analysis. *Circulation.* 1998;97:1796–1801.

32. Guidelines for the prevention of intravascular catheter-related infections. MMWR recommendations and reports. Vol. 51, No. RR-10. Atlanta, GA: Centers for Disease Control; 2002:1–29.

33. Fridkin SK, Pear SM, Williamson H, et al. The role of understaffing in central venous catheter-associated bloodstream infections. *Infect Control Hosp Epidemiol.* 1996;17:150–158.

34. Tomford JW, Hershey CO. The I.V. therapy team: impact on patient care and the cost of hospitalization. *NITA.* 1985;8:387–389.

35. Levin A, Mason AJ, Jindal KK, et al. Prevention of hemodialysis subclavian vein catheter infections by topical povidone-iodine. *Kidney Int.* 1991;40:934–938.

36. Maki DG, Band JD. A comparative study of polyantibiotic and iodophor ointments in prevention of catheter-related infection. *Am J Med.* 1981;70:739–744.

37. Conloy JM, Grieves K, Peters B. A prospective, randomized study comparing transparent and dry gauze dressings for central venous catheters. *J Infect Dis.* 1989;159:310–319.

38. Maki DG, Stolz SS, Wheller S, et al. A prospective, randomized trial of gauze and two polyurethane dressings for site care of pulmonary artery catheter: implications for catheter management. *Crit Care Med.* 1994;32:1729–1737.

39. Maki DG, Will L. Colonization and infection associated with transparent dressings for central venous, arterial and Hickman cath-eters: a comparative trial [abstract]. In: *Program and Abstracts of the Thirty-fourth Inter-science Conference on Antimicrobial Agents and Chemotherapy.* October 1994, Orlando, Florida. Washington, DC: American Society for Microbiology; 1984:253.

40. Shivnan JC, McGuire D, Freeman S, et al. Comparison of transparent adherent and dry sterile gauze dressings for long-term central catheters in patients undergoing bone marrow transplant. *Oncol Nurs Forum.* 1991;18:1349–1356.

41. Daghistani D, Horn M, Rodriguez S, Shoenike S, Toledano S. Prevention of indwelling catheter sepsis. *Med Pediatr Oncol.* 1996;26:405–408.

42. Duboi J, Garel L, Tapiero B, Dube J, Lafambroise S, David M. Peripherally inserted catheters in infants and children. *Radiology.* 1997;204:622–626.

43. Crowley JJ, Pereira JK, Harris LS, Becker CJ. Radiologic placement of subcutaneous venous access ports for children. *AJR Am J Roentgenol.* 1998;17:257–260.

44. Muscadere G, Bennett JD, Lee TY, Mackie L, Vanderburgh L. Complications of radiologically placed central venous ports for Hickman catheters in patients with AIDS. *Can Assoc Radiol J.* 1998;49:84–89.

Chapter 15

Catheter and Port Removal: Techniques and Follow-Up Care

Janice Newsome
Jaime Tisnado

The use of central venous catheters has increased dramatically over the past 20 years. These devices now are considered essential in providing dependable venous access for both acute and chronically ill patients. Whereas much emphasis is placed on the insertion and management of central catheters, little attention has been given to their removal, and this task is often assigned to junior physicians or nurses who are inexperienced in removal procedures. This chapter discusses the techniques for removal of the various types of venous catheters and ports; briefly mentions the complications of catheter removal; and provides therapeutic measures to deal with infected catheters, tunnels, and pockets.

Once the decision is made to remove a catheter or port either because an infection clearly has occurred, because infection is suspected to be present, or because the vascular access is no longer needed, the patient is counseled about what to expect during the removal procedure and thereafter. Informed consent is not routinely obtained for a simple catheter removal unless another catheter is going to be inserted or an associated procedure will be performed. Some operators may wish to obtain consent, however, particularly if the catheter being removed was placed initially by someone else. Necessary equipment for catheter removal includes a cut-down tray and a small table with basic instruments.

A bed that allows placement of the patient in a head-down position (Trendelenburg) is ideal although not required. This special bed is not routinely available in most radiology departments. Removals are done in any suitable room, not necessarily in the angiographic laboratory; so the laboratory can be used for other purposes.

REMOVAL OF TUNNELED CATHETERS

Tunneled catheters should be removed when they are infected or no longer needed. In general, the longer a catheter has been in place, the more difficult the removal may be; however, this is not necessarily true. In fact, some infected catheters or ports will slide out easily regardless of how long they have been in place. Some patients develop thick scar tissue and cheloid very rapidly. We have seen patients in whom removal of a catheter placed a few weeks earlier was rather difficult.

The skin over the catheter exit site, the tunnel, and the area overlying the entrance site into the vein is prepared using povidone–iodine (7.5–10%) or alcohol. Sterile drapes and towels are placed to establish a sterile field. Adequate local anesthesia is obtained with lidocaine, with or without epinephrine, and infiltrated in the soft tissues, making sure that the entire subcutaneous tunnel and the skin over the site of entry into the vein are well anesthetized.

Special care must be taken not to puncture the catheter during the administration of local anesthetic because bleeding may follow if the catheter is damaged. Initially, the catheter is released from the skin at the exit site by cutting the anchoring sutures, if present. If the catheter was placed recently, that is, less than 2 weeks ago, removal requires little dissection, but this is not always true.

HELPFUL HINTS

If the catheter cuff has not yet scarred in place, administration of local anesthesia, which can be painful, especially in inflamed tissues, may not be necessary. A gentle tug on the catheter may be given before anesthetizing to determine whether the catheter will slide out of the tunnel, thereby eliminating the need for local anesthesia. We routinely mix lidocaine with sodium bicarbonate (1 mL of NaHCO$_3$ for 10 mL of lidocaine) to decrease significantly the pain and burning associated with lidocaine.

The patient should be instructed to suspend respiration temporarily to prevent the serious risk of air embolism, which may occur if the patient takes a deep inspiration as the catheter exits the vein. The catheter is grasped with one hand, at or near the hub, and pulled slowly and steadily to ensure that the force of traction follows the path of the tunnel. Excessive force or tension must be avoided because the catheter may rupture, with resultant bleeding in the tunnel or fragment embolization. The operator must immediately hold pressure at the venous insertion site with the other hand as soon as the catheter exits the vein at the puncture site. In certain cases, such as infection, care

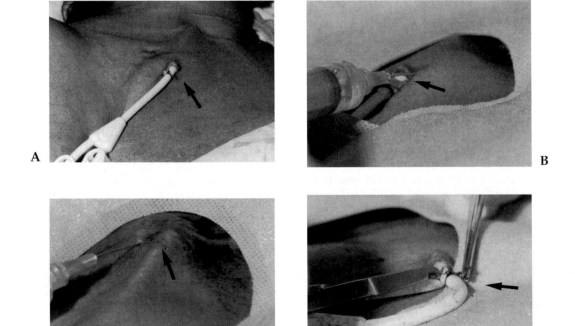

Figure 15–1   Removal of tunneled catheter. **(A)** Catheter exit site prepped and draped. **(B, C)** Exit site and tunnel infiltrated with lidocaine with 1% epinephrine. **(D)** The stitch holding the catheter is removed. (*Continued*) **(E)** Blunt dissection of the tunnel with a Kelly clamp. **(F)** The catheter is withdrawn from the tunnel. **(G)** Hemostasis is obtained. **(H)** Dressing is applied. Patient is sent home.

should be taken to prevent contamination of the catheter if the tip is needed for culture. Hemostasis usually is achieved by holding gentle pressure on the vein for about 10 minutes. Elevation of the head of the bed more than 30 degrees may help with hemostasis.

When the catheter has been in place a long time, scarring and granulation at the cuff site(s) and elsewhere require blunt and sharp dissection along the entire tunnel to free the scar tissue. This is done using a long hemostat or a straight Kelly clamp. The dissection must be done circumferentially around the entire catheter, that is, front, back, medial, and lateral. The aim is to loosen the scar tissue and allow the catheter to become free. Progressively increasing tension may be needed, but special care must be taken to avoid rupturing the catheter. The point of greatest resistance, scarring, and adherence is usually around the Dacron cuff (or cuffs if two or more are present).

HELPFUL HINTS
Applying steady tension to the catheter may result in dimpling of the skin overlying the cuff because this is the point of "attachment." This "dimpling" will give the operator the expected location of the cuff(s). As the closed hemostat is inserted into the subcutaneous tunnel, alongside the catheter, resistance will be encountered at the site of granulation and scar tissue. Continuing to apply tension to the catheter, forcefully advancing the closed hemostat into the scar tissue, and opening the hemostat will bluntly dissect the scar tissue and free the catheter from the tunnel.

HELPFUL HINTS
During pulling the catheter, enough tension must be applied to release the catheter free of the remaining granulation and scar tissue; however, care must be taken not to apply so much tension that the catheter breaks. Some large catheters, such as

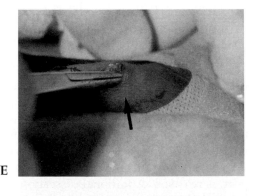
E

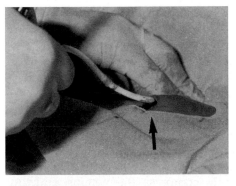
F

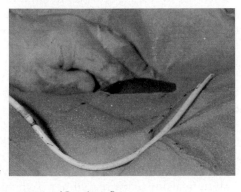
G

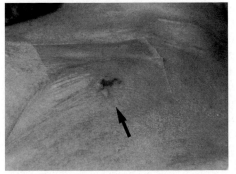
H

Figure 15–1 (*Continued*)

dialysis (12–14 F) catheters, are quite sturdy, and a great deal of tension can be applied during removal, but these catheters can rupture. The smaller 7 to 10 F tunneled catheters, especially Silastic catheters, will break with the application of even a little tension. When the catheters break, they usually tear on the hub side of the Dacron cuff. This is a serious situation that requires prompt action because brisk bleeding into the subcutaneous tract may occur and air embolization into the venous system is likely. The catheter must be compressed immediately. If the procedure was being done unassisted, one must get help immediately because it is impossible to hold pressure over the catheter while dissecting the tract. Once the bleeding has been controlled with compression, another incision should be made at the venous entry site or over the subcutaneous tunnel near this site. Using a hemostat, blunt dissection is done until the underlying catheter is seen and retrieved. The catheter must be clamped to stop bleeding from its torn end. The clamped catheter should then slide easily out of the vein as pressure is applied at the venous puncture site. When hemostasis is obtained, the remaining segment of catheter with the Dacron cuff may be dissected free through the new skin incision.

The patient must stop breathing momentarily while the catheter is being removed to prevent air embolism. The operator must promptly compress the venous puncture site, which is usually apparent on examination of the scar of the healed puncture site. Once hemostasis is achieved, antibiotic ointment may be applied to the exit wound and an airtight occlusive dressing placed over the site and left there for 2 to 3 days. If the exit site is large, a single interrupted stitch must be placed; otherwise, Steri-strips are used to close the skin. Tunneled catheters placed in the femoral vein are removed in a similar fashion (Fig. 15–1).

On occasion, during tension and pulling of the catheter, the Dacron cuff may be separated off the catheter and remain in the subcutaneous tissue. The cuff is left there because it is of no clinical significance and nothing needs to be done. If for cosmetic or other reasons (infected tunnel) cuff removal is desired, a direct cut-down over the region of the retained cuff may be needed for the cuff to be removed.

REMOVAL OF SUBCUTANEOUS PORTS

Ports must be removed by an experienced operator. A surgical cut-down tray is required. The skin over the pocket, the subcutaneous tunnel, and the venous puncture site are prepped with povidone–iodine (7.5–10%) and alcohol. Sterile towels and drapes are placed to create a sterile surgical field. Adequate local anesthesia is obtained using generous amounts of 1% buffered (with sodium bicarbonate) lidocaine. Care must be taken not to puncture the catheter within the tunnel while injecting the local anesthetic. Ideally, if a special table is available, the patient can be placed in a Trendelenburg position with the head turned away from the working site. A no. 10 or 15 scalpel is used to make an adequate skin incision over the previous scar, which will result in only one scar with better cosmetic results. Forceps are used to elevate and separate the tissues directly over the port. Using blunt and sharp dissection with scissors and scalpels, the scar tissue, which usually surrounds and encases the port, is released. Additional dissection may be needed to release scar tissue often found at the port stem/catheter lock as well as at the proximal portion of the tunnel. Dissection along the tunnel is rarely needed to free the catheter because the Silastic catheter is biocompatible and does not promote scar tissue. The catheter is withdrawn from the vein and tunnel easily. Once the port and catheter are free, the patient is instructed to suspend respirations to prevent air embolism. The catheter is grasped distal to the connection with the port and withdrawn in a slow, steady manner. To achieve hemostasis, the venous puncture site must be compressed for 10 minutes as soon as the catheter tip exits the vein. Dry gauze can be placed inside the pocket and pressure applied for hemostasis. The gauze is removed and the pocket examined to ensure that it is "dry" and no hematoma is forming. If bleeding sites are noted, they should be ligated or controlled. Absorbable sutures are placed to approximate the deeper subcutaneous tissues and, depending on the operator's preferences, buried subcutaneous running absorbable sutures or simple interrupted nonabsorbable sutures are used to close the skin. Antibiotic ointment can be applied to the wound, and an airtight dressing is left in place for 2 to 3 days.

REMOVAL OF NONTUNNELED CATHETERS

Nontunneled access catheters are used for a few weeks to 3 months. Because these catheters require minimal tissue disruption, and no tunnel is formed, removal of the catheter is easy and straightforward. Nontunneled catheters are removed in a manner similar to tunneled catheters, although tunnel dissection is not needed. Once the external fixation tape and suture are removed, the patient is instructed to stop breathing, and the catheter is withdrawn in a firm and steady manner along the axis of the central vein. Hemostasis is achieved by holding pressure on the vein for 10 minutes or longer.

Peripherally inserted central catheters (PICCs) are removed easily at the bedside or at home by nursing personnel. Once the anchoring suture and tape are removed, the catheter is withdrawn from the vein and compression is applied for 3 to 5 minutes. On rare occasions, PICCs are difficult to remove. Tourniquet application and warm soaks have been tried with success. Venospasm (as confirmed by ultrasound) may be the cause of difficulty in some cases. Gentle traction usually can overcome a mild vasospasm; however, aggressive pulling may

result in catheter breakage and embolism with serious consequences and embarrassment for the operator. This will require retrieval using conventional techniques. If any resistance is felt during removal by nursing personnel, the procedure should be aborted and an experienced operator or radiologist consulted. If catheter fragments and embolism occur during removal, percutaneous retrieval is done by an experienced operator in the conventional manner.

COMPLICATIONS

The incidence of complications of placement of central venous catheters and ports is low and ranges from 0.4 to 11%, including major and minor complications. There are, however, no accurate statistics for complications associated with catheter or port removal. This topic has received little attention and is not mentioned in most reviews. It is clear from the available information that the risks of central venous catheter removal are low but still may create a problem for some operators. Furthermore, the life-threatening nature of some complications (such as air embolism) may contribute to high morbidity.

Air Embolism

Besides bleeding, one of the most common and feared complications of catheter and port removal is air embolism. The signs and symptoms may be nonspecific, and the diagnosis can be made based on clinical assumption, often after an unsuspected transient cardiopulmonary collapse or neurologic dysfunction has occurred. Few documented cases are reported in the literature of air embolism during placement of central venous catheters,[1-4] and even fewer documented cases are reported of air embolism during catheter removal.[5-8] Breathing during removal by uncooperative patients is the cause. Also, if a fibrin sheath is present along the catheter tract in the tunnel, the sheath can be a pathway for air to enter the venous system if prompt hemostasis is not performed.

After removal of a central venous catheter, regardless of the site, a short tract between the skin and the vein may stay patent momentarily. The tract, if large enough, can allow air to enter the venous system during inspiration. Enough air to cause embolism and cardiorespiratory collapse can enter the venous system in one inspiration. For this reason, it is critical that patients suspend respiration during the withdrawal phase of catheter removal until firm pressure is maintained on the vein to occlude the puncture site. It has been reported that a tract diameter of 4.5 mm needed to insert a 14 F catheter can allow conduction of 200 cc of air in 1 second, according to Poiseuille's law.[7] The documented lethal amount of injected air in humans is 70 to 105 cc per second.[1] If the embolized air is trapped in the right ventricle, it may produce right ventricular obstruction, resulting in acute right heart failure, shock, and death.

Furthermore, it has been reported that in humans the foramen ovale may remain patent in 10 to 24% of the population.[9] Therefore, if a patient has a patent foramen ovale, serious and catastrophic arterial air embolism can occur. Air in the left ventricle can migrate into the carotid arteries, causing cerebral air embolism.

In addition, air can enter the venous system directly through the catheter, especially if it becomes disconnected from the intravenous line or if the hub of the catheter is open or incompletely locked. The sound of sucking air through the catheter or tract is highly suggestive of air embolism. Fluoroscopy and other radiologic examinations, such as chest radiographs, computed tomography, or echocardiogram, may show air embolized in the heart or brain. Prompt recognition of air emboli is critical to allow therapeutic intervention. Patients should be given 100% oxygen immediately. Embolized air can produce right ventricular outflow obstruction, acute right-sided heart failure, and shock. If the embolized air remains in the right side of the heart, immediately place the patient in the left lateral decubitus position with the patient's left side down (Durant) and the head down (Trendelenburg) to allow blood to flow out of the right ventricle into the pulmonary outflow tract and preventing obstruction.[10] Furthermore, the air can be trapped in the right atrium, and a catheter can be inserted into the right side of the heart and the air aggressively aspirated (as much as possible) to prevent the serious sequelae.[11]

Pulmonary Embolism

Pericatheter thrombus is a common complication of long-term indwelling central venous catheters. It is estimated that 42 to 100% of venous catheters become covered by a fibrin sheath.[12] During withdrawal of the catheters, thrombi and fibrin may be stripped from the catheter and embolize into the lungs. These pulmonary emboli are usually small and of no clinical significance in most patients, unless they have a borderline pulmonary reserve. Furthermore, if the patient has a patent foramen ovale, the emboli can gain access to the left ventricle and embolize into the carotid circulation, leading to a stroke. Moreover, it was recently reported that the sleeve surrounding the catheters is not a true fibrin sleeve but, rather, an organized cellular–collagen tissue covered by endothelium.[12]

It is important to know that the cellular–collagen sleeve can be present as early as 24 hours, be complete in 1 week, and last up to 10 months after catheter removal. This process may play an important role in the withdrawal occlusion of veins. Some investigators have suggested the prophylactic use of aspirin, and even oral warfarin, to decrease the incidence of catheter-related venous thrombus formation, as is almost routinely done for arterial thrombus prevention.[13] Other researchers have found no correlation between thrombus formation, duration of catheterization, type of catheter used, or regimen of anticoagulation with heparin, either therapeutic or low-dose.[14]

Catheter Rupture

Catheter breakage during removal is an infrequent complication. Repeated handling of the external portion of the catheter by health care personnel and patients may result in fatigue and fragmentation of the catheter material. During withdrawal, the catheter may break, leaving a segment of catheter inside the vein or in the tunnel. If this occurs, the broken segment may embolize into right heart or pulmonary arteries. The fragment can be removed percutaneously from a femoral approach with conventional retrieval methods. If the segment stays in the tunnel or at the entry site, it can be removed by direct cut-down on the vein. In our experience, the retained fragment remains in position in the tunnel and usually does not embolize.

Arterial Trauma

It is important to remember the relationship of the internal jugular veins to the carotid arteries in the neck. The puncture site in the neck is always close to the carotid artery. Too much pressure or forceful rubbing in this region may cause arteriosclerotic plaque dislodgment and embolization, causing stroke. Furthermore, stimulation of the carotid sinus during hemostasis compression may result in unwanted vasovagal bradycardia, hypotension, and even loss of consciousness. Fortunately, this event is very rare.

Infection

Catheter-related infection is a serious and significant complication of central venous catheter placement. Whether the infection is confined to the skin exit site, involves the pocket or tunnel, or has entered the bloodstream (bacteremia/sepsis), it is imperative that the interventional radiologist be knowledgeable and prepared to provide treatment and make recommendations for appropriate care.

The incidence of infectious complications differs significantly with the different types of catheters. There is a higher infection rate in nontunneled catheters. The incidence of infection of tunneled catheters is as high as 10 to 30%.[15,16] The infection rate for Hickman catheters is 1.9 per 1000 catheter days when a radiologist places the catheter and 4.0 per 1000 catheter days when a surgeon places the catheters.[17]

Subcutaneous ports have lower infection rates, ranging from 0.03 to 0.1 per 1000 catheter days.[18] On the other hand, PICCs have infection rates of 3.1 per 1000 catheter days.[15] The diagnosis of catheter-related infection can be difficult. Subtle clinical signs, such as unexplained leukocytosis, low-grade fever, or an isolated positive blood culture, might be the only feature of a raging infection. Unfortunately, the frequently used parameters for diagnosing a catheter infection are nonspecific. Pain, local erythema, and swelling may be more significant indicators of catheter infection than other clinical and laboratory parameters.[19]

The treatment for a catheter-related infection depends on the extension of the process. Exit-site infections are the easiest to diagnose and usually present with tenderness and erythema about 1 cm around the exit site. Occasionally, a purulent exudate may be present. These infections can be treated successfully with local measures and antibiotics.

Tissue disruption of the port pocket or tunnel and tenderness and cellulitis over the port or along the tunnel indicate a serious infection or abscess. The port or tunneled catheter must be removed. Pus or cloudy fluid should be cultured and intravenous antibiotics started. The pocket must be opened and thoroughly irrigated with saline and packed with iodoform gauze twice daily until the drainage has stopped. The pocket eventually will heal by secondary intention. If the tunnel is infected, the skin over the tunnel can be incised and the tunnel drained. Alternatively, the tunnel can be enlarged, irrigated, and packed from both ends with gauze twice daily until drainage stops and eventually heals by secondary intention as the gauze is progressively withdrawn.

Occasionally, an infection is suspected, but there is no purulent drainage when the port or catheter is removed. The wound can be packed for a few days and then closed primarily, a process called *delayed primary closure* or *tertiary healing*. Because most patients who require ports and tunneled catheters are immunocompromised, the absence of pus does not exclude an infected port pocket or catheter tunnel.

Diagnosing catheter-related infections early and providing aggressive treatment reduce the morbidity and may allow salvage of the access device. Most catheter infections are caused by skin flora; therefore, antibiotic coverage of gram-positive microorganisms with cefazolin or vancomycin is usually sufficient. A 10- to 14-day course of oral or intravenous treatment is given, with modifications depending on the patient's clinical response, or bacterial culture and sensitivity results.

SUMMARY

Catheter and port removal is done when a catheter-related infection is present or suspected or when the device is no longer needed. Care must be taken during catheter removal because complications, some of them serious (e.g., air embolism, catheter rupture, embolization) could occur.

The vascular and interventional radiologist must be prepared to remove catheters and ports and must educate ancillary personnel and home caregivers about the methods and problems associated with catheter or port removal.

REFERENCES

1. Coppa GF, Gouge TH, Hofstetter SR. Air embolism: a lethal but preventable complication of subclavian vein catherization. *Int Surg.* 1972;57:42–45.

2. Feliciano DV, Mattox KL, Graham JM, et al. Major complications of percutaneous subclavian vein catheters. *Am J Surg.* 1979;138:869–874.

3. Kashuk JL, Penn I. Air embolism after central venous catherization. *Surg Gynecol Obstet.* 1984;159:249–252.

4. Grace DM. Air embolism with neurologic complications: a potential hazard of central venous catheters. *Can J Surg.* 1977;20:51–53.

5. Sing RF, Steffe TJ, Branas CC. Fatal venous air embolism after removal of a central venous catheter. *J Am Osteopath Assoc.* 1995; 95:204–205.

6. Mennim P, Coyle CF, Taylor JD. Venous air embolism associated with removal of central venous catheter. *BMJ.* 1992;305:171–172.

7. Phifer TJ, Bridges M, Conrad SA. The residual central venous catheter tract: an occult source of lethal air embolism: case report. *J Trauma.* 1991;31:1558–1560.

8. McCarthy PM, Wang N, Birchfield F, et al. Air embolism in single-lung transplant patients after central venous catheter removal. *Chest.* 1995;107:1178–1179.

9. Papadopoulous G, Kuhly P, Brock M, et al. Venous and paradoxical embolism in the sitting position: a prospective study with transesophageal endocardiology. *Acta Neurol.* 1994;126:140–143.

10. Durant TM, Oppenheimier MJ, Lynch PR, et al. Body position in relation to venous air embolism: a roentgenologic study. *Am J Med Sci.* 1954;227:509–520.

11. Minchenfelder JD, Martin JT, Altenberg BM, et al. Air embolism during neurosurgery: an evaluation of right atrial catheters for diagnosis and treatment. *JAMA.* 1969;208:1353–1358.

12. Xiang DZ, Verbeken EK, Van Lommel AT, et al. Composition and formation of the sleeve enveloping of a central venous catheter. *J Vasc Surg.* 1998;28:260–271.

13. Bern MM, Lokich JJ, Wallach SR, et al. Very low doses of warfarin can prevent thrombosis in central venous catheters: a randomized prospective trial. *Ann Intern Med.* 1990;112:423–428.

14. Randolph AG, Cook DJ, Gonzales CA, et al. Benefit of heparin in peripheral venous and arterial catheters: systematic review and meta-analysis of randomized controlled trials. *BMJ.* 1998;316:969–975.

15. Clarke DE, Raffin TA. Infectious complications of indwelling long-term central venous catheters. *Chest.* 1990;97:966–972.

16. Johnson A, Oppenheim BA. Vascular catheter-related sepsis: diagnosis and prevention. *J Hosp Infect.* 1992;20:67–78.

17. McBride KD, Fisher R, Warnock N, et al. Comparative analysis of radiological and surgical placement of central venous catheters. *Cardiovasc Interv Radiol.* 1997;20:17–22.

18. Hills JR, Cardella JF, Cardella K, et al. Experience with 100 consecutive central venous access arm ports placed by interventional radiologists. *J Vasc Interv Radiol.* 1997;8:983–989.

19. Barnes JR, Lucas N, Broadwater JR, et al. When should the "infected" subcutaneous infusion be removed? *Am Surg.* 1996;62:203–206.

INDEX

Numbers in italics indicate figure references.